Cardioembolic Stroke

Editors

RANJAN K. THAKUR
ZIYAD M. HIJAZI
ANDREA NATALE

CARDIOLOGY CLINICS

www.cardiology.theclinics.com

Consulting Editors
ROSARIO FREEMAN
JORDAN M. PRUTKIN
DAVID M. SHAVELLE
AUDREY H. WU

May 2016 • Volume 34 • Number 2

ELSEVIER

1600 John F. Kennedy Boulevard • Suite 1800 • Philadelphia, Pennsylvania, 19103-2899

http://www.theclinics.com

CARDIOLOGY CLINICS Volume 34, Number 2
May 2016 ISSN 0733-8651, ISBN-13: 978-0-323-44457-6

Editor: Lauren Boyle
Developmental Editor: Alison Swety

Cardiology Clinics (ISSN 0733-8651) is published quarterly by Elsevier Inc., 360 Park Avenue South, New York, NY 10010-1710. Months of issue are February, May, August, and November. Business and Editorial Offices: 1600 John F. Kennedy Blvd., Ste. 1800, Philadelphia, PA 19103-2899. Customer Service Office: 3251 Riverport Lane, Maryland Heights, MO 63043. Periodicals post-age paid at New York, NY and additional mailing offices. Subscription prices are $320.00 per year for US individuals, $581.00 per year for US institutions, $100.00 per year for US students and residents, $390.00 per year for Canadian individuals, $729.00 per year for Canadian institutions, $455.00 per year for international individuals, $729.00 per year for international institutions and $220.00 per year for Canadian and international students/residents. To receive student/resident rate, orders must be accompanied by name of affiliated institution, data of term, and the *signature* of program/residency coordinator on institution letterhead. Orders will be billed at individual rate until proof of status is received. Foreign air speed delivery is included in all *Clinics* subscription prices. All prices are subject to change without notice. **POSTMASTER:** Send address changes to *Cardiology Clinics*, Elsevier Health Sciences Division, Subscription Customer Service, 3251 Riverport Lane, Maryland Heights, MO 63043. **Customer Service: 1-800-654-2452 (U.S. and Canada); 314-447-8871 (outside U.S. and Canada). Fax: 314-447-8029. E-mail: journalscustomerservice-usa@ elsevier.com (for print support); journalsonlinesupport-usa@elsevier.com (for online support).**

Reprints. For copies of 100 or more, of articles in this publication, please contact the Commercial Reprints Department, Elsevier Inc., 360 Park Avenue South, New York, NY 10010-1710. Tel.: 212-633-3874; Fax: 212-633-3820; E-mail: reprints@elsevier.com.

Cardiology Clinics is also published in Spanish by McGraw-Hill Interamericana Editores S. A., P.O. Box 5-237, 06500, Mexico D. F., Mexico; in Portuguese by Reichmann and Alfonso Editores Rio de Janeiro, Brazil; and in Greek by Dimitrios P. Lagos, 8 Pondon Street, GR115-28 Ilissia, Greece.

Cardiology Clinics is covered in *MEDLINE/PubMed (Index Medicus)*, *Excerpta Medica*, *The Cumulative Index to Nursing and Allied Health Literature* (CINAHL).

Contributors

AUTHORS

PHILIP AAGAARD, MD, PhD
Department of Medicine, Albert Einstein
College of Medicine, Montefiore Hospital,
Bronx, New York

CONOR BARRETT, MD
The Al-Sabah Arrhythmia Institute at
Mount Sinai St. Luke, New York,
New York

DAVID BRICENO, MD, PhD
Department of Medicine, Albert Einstein
College of Medicine, Montefiore Hospital,
Bronx, New York

ELCHANAN BRUCKHEIMER, MBBS
Director, Cardiac Catheterization, Section of
Pediatric Cardiology, Schneider Children's
Medical Center Israel, Petach Tikva, Israel

J. DAVID BURKHARDT, MD, PhD, FACC
Department of Cardiology, Texas Cardiac
Arrhythmia Institute, St. David's Medical
Center, Austin, Texas

ANTONIO CAROLEI, MD, FAHA
Department of Biotechnological and Applied
Clinical Sciences, Neurological Institute,
University of L'Aquila, L'Aquila, Italy

JOHN D. CARROLL, MD
Professor of Medicine, University of Colorado
Denver, Aurora, Colorado

TAHMEED CONTRACTOR, MD
Department of Cardiology, Lehigh Valley
Health Network, Allentown, Pennsylvania

ZOLTAN CSANADI, MD, PhD
Department of Cardiology, University of
Debrecen, Debrecen, Hungary

CLIFFORD L. CUA, MD
Associate Professor of Clinical Pediatrics,
The Ohio State University; The Heart Center,
Nationwide Children's Hospital, Columbus,
Ohio

STEPHAN DANIK, MD
The Al-Sabah Arrhythmia Institute at Mount
Sinai St. Luke, New York, New York

DIANA DEGAN, MD
Department of Biotechnological and Applied
Clinical Sciences, Neurological Institute,
University of L'Aquila, L'Aquila, Italy

LUIGI DI BIASE, MD, PhD, FACC, FHRS
Section Head Electrophysiology; Director of
Arrhythmia Services, Montefiore-Einstein
Center for Heart and Vascular Care, Montefiore
Medical Center; Department of Cardiology,
Albert Einstein College of Medicine, Montefiore
Hospital, Bronx, New York; Texas Cardiac
Arrhythmia Institute, St. David's Medical
Center, Austin, Texas; Department of
Cardiology, University of Foggia, Foggia, Italy;
Department of Biomedical Engineering,
University of Texas, Austin, Texas

JENNIFER FRANKE, MD
CardioVascular Center Frankfurt, Frankfurt,
Germany

SAMEER GAFOOR, MD
CardioVascular Center Frankfurt, Frankfurt,
Germany

CAROLA GIANNI, MD
Department of Cardiology, Texas Cardiac
Arrhythmia Institute, St. David's Medical
Center, Austin, Texas

**ZIYAD M. HIJAZI, MD, MPH, FACC,
MSCAI, FAHA**
Sidra Cardiovascular Center of Excellence,
Sidra Medical and Research Center, Weill
Cornell Medicine, Doha, Qatar

RALF J. HOLZER, MD, MSc, FSCAI
Professor of Clinical Pediatrics, Weill Cornell
Medical College, New York, New York; Chief of
Pediatric Cardiology (Acting); Director, Sidra
Medical and Research Center, Doha, Qatar

MARIUS HORNUNG, MD
CardioVascular Center Frankfurt, Frankfurt,
Germany

SANDIA ISKANDAR, MD
Division of Cardiovascular Diseases,
Cardiovascular Research Institute, Mid
America Cardiology, University of Kansas
Medical Center and Hospital, Kansas City,
Kansas

VISHAL JANI, MD
Department of Neurology and Opthalmology,
Clinical Center, Michigan State University,
East Lansing, Michigan

SHADI KALANTARIAN, MD, MPH
Internal Medicine Residency Program,
Yale New Haven Hospital, New Haven,
Connecticut

**DHANUNJAYA LAKKIREDDY, MD, FACC,
FHRS**
Director, Center for Excellence in Atrial
Fibrillation and EP Research; Professor of
Medicine, Division of Cardiovascular Diseases,
Bloch Heart Rhythm Center, Cardiovascular
Research Institute, University of Kansas
Medical Center, Mid America Cardiology,
University of Kansas Hospitals, Kansas City,
Kansas

ROBERTO M. LANG, MD, FASE
Section of Cardiology, Department of Medicine, University of Chicago Medicine, University of Chicago, Chicago, Illinois

MADHAV LAVU, MD
Division of Cardiovascular Diseases, Cardiovascular Research Institute, Mid America Cardiology, University of Kansas Medical Center and Hospital, Kansas City, Kansas

MICHELLE LEPPERT, MD, MBA
Fellow, Department of Neurology, University of Colorado Denver, Aurora, Colorado

GREGORY Y.H. LIP, MD
Institute of Cardiovascular Sciences, University of Birmingham, City Hospital, Birmingham, United Kingdom; Aalborg Thrombosis Research Unit, Department of Clinical Medicine, Aalborg University, Aalborg, Denmark

SANGHAMITRA MOHANTY, MD
Department of Cardiology, Texas Cardiac Arrhythmia Institute, St. David's Medical Center, Austin, Texas

EDINA NAGY-BALÓ, MD, PhD
Department of Cardiology, University of Debrecen, Debrecen, Hungary

AKHIL NARANG, MD
Section of Cardiology, Department of Medicine, University of Chicago Medicine, University of Chicago, Chicago, Illinois

ANDREA NATALE, MD, PhD, FACC, FESC, FHRS
Department of Cardiology, Texas Cardiac Arrhythmia Institute, Center for Atrial Fibrillation at St. David's Medical Center, Austin, Texas; Division of Cardiology, Stanford University, Stanford, California; Case Western Reserve University, Cleveland, Ohio; EP Services, California Pacific Medical Center, San Francisco, California; Interventional Electrophysiology, Scripps Clinic, San Diego, California; Dell Medical School, University of Texas, Austin, Texas

RAFFAELE ORNELLO, MD
Department of Biotechnological and Applied Clinical Sciences, Neurological Institute, University of L'Aquila, L'Aquila, Italy

ROD S. PASSMAN, MD, MSCE
Professor of Medicine and Preventive Medicine, Clinical Cardiac Electrophysiology Section, Division of Cardiology, Departments of Medicine and Preventative Medicine, The Bluhm Cardiovascular Institute, Northwestern Memorial Hospital, Northwestern University Feinberg School of Medicine, Chicago, Illinois

MEHUL B. PATEL, MD
Department of Clinical Cardiac Electrophysiology, The Bay Pines Veterans Affairs Health Care System, University of South Florida, Tampa, Bay Pines, Florida

FRANCESCA PISTOIA, MD, PhD
Department of Biotechnological and Applied Clinical Sciences, Assistant Professor of Neurorehabilitation, Neurological Institute, University of L'Aquila, L'Aquila, Italy

SHARON N. POISSON, MD
Assistant Professor, Department of Neurology, University of Colorado Denver, Aurora, Colorado

MARCO PROIETTI, MD
Institute of Cardiovascular Sciences, University of Birmingham, City Hospital, Birmingham, United Kingdom; Department of Internal Medicine and Medical Specialties, Sapienza-University of Rome, Rome, Italy

ANMAR RAZAK, MD
Department of Neurology and Opthalmology, Clinical Center, Michigan State University, East Lansing, Michigan

SUKIT M. RINGWALA, MD, MPH
Fellow, Clinical Cardiac Electrophysiology Section, Northwestern Memorial Hospital, Chicago, Illinois

JEREMY N. RUSKIN, MD
Professor of Medicine, Harvard Medical School; Director, Cardiac Arrhythmia Service, Massachusetts General Hospital, Boston, Massachusetts

SIMONA SACCO, MD
Department of Biotechnological and Applied
Clinical Sciences, Neurological Institute,
University of L'Aquila, L'Aquila, Italy

GAUTAM SACHDEVA, MD
Department of Neurology and Opthalmology,
Clinical Center, Michigan State University,
East Lansing, Michigan

ALI SAEED, MD
Department of Neurology and Opthalmology,
Clinical Center, Michigan State University,
East Lansing, Michigan

ABDUL SAFADI, MD
Sparrow Thoracic and Cardiovascular Institute,
Michigan State University, Lansing, Michigan

JAVIER SANCHEZ, MD
Department of Cardiology, Texas Cardiac
Arrhythmia Institute, St. David's Medical
Center, Austin, Texas

FRANCESCO SANTORO, MD
Department of Cardiology, University of
Foggia, Foggia, Italy

HORST SIEVERT, MD
CardioVascular Center Frankfurt, Frankfurt,
Germany

HUSSAM S. SURADI, MD, FACC, FSCAI
Assistant Professor of Internal Medicine and
Pediatrics, Interventional Cardiology, Rush
Center for Congenital and Structural Heart
Disease, Rush University Medical Center,

Chicago, Illinois; Department of Cardiology,
St. Mary Medical Center, Community
HealthCare Network, Community Healthcare
System, Hobart, Indiana

PHANI SURAPANENI, MD
Sparrow Thoracic and Cardiovascular Institute,
Michigan State University, Lansing, Michigan

**RANJAN K. THAKUR, MD, MPH, MBA,
FACC, FHRS**
Sparrow Thoracic and Cardiovascular Institute,
Michigan State University, Lansing, Michigan

CINDY TISEO, MD
Department of Biotechnological and Applied
Clinical Sciences, Neurological Institute,
University of L'Aquila, L'Aquila, Italy

TODD T. TOMSON, MD
Fellow, Clinical Cardiac Electrophysiology
Section, Northwestern Memorial Hospital,
Chicago, Illinois

CHINTAN TRIVEDI, MD, MPH
Department of Cardiology, Texas Cardiac
Arrhythmia Institute, St. David's Medical
Center, Austin, Texas

JAMES VACEK, MD, MS
Division of Cardiovascular Diseases,
Cardiovascular Research Institute, Mid
America Cardiology, University of Kansas
Medical Center and Hospital, Kansas City,
Kansas

Contents

Preface: Cardioembolic Stroke   xiii

Ranjan K. Thakur, Ziyad M. Hijazi, and Andrea Natale

Cardioembolic Stroke and Postmyocardial Infarction Stroke   207

Marius Hornung, Jennifer Franke, Sameer Gafoor, and Horst Sievert

Ischemic stroke following acute myocardial infarction (AMI) is a rare but serious complication due to left ventricular thrombus formation and atrial fibrillation. Early revascularization of the culprit coronary lesion is essential. Treatment trends may affect the risk. Conversely, the greater use of antiplatelet agents to reduce the risk of ischemic stroke could increase the risk of hemorrhagic stroke. The risk of stroke after AMI has decreased significantly with more use of percutaneous coronary intervention and antithrombotic therapies in the acute setting, and statins, antihypertensive medications, and dual antiplatelet therapy as secondary prevention strategies.

Embolic Stroke in Cardiomyopathy: Should Patients be Anticoagulated?   215

Akhil Narang and Roberto M. Lang

Despite advances in the treatment of patients with heart failure, mortality is still substantial. Part of this mortality is explained by cardioembolic stroke. Patients with heart failure are predisposed to developing cardioembolic strokes owing to abnormalities in Virchow's triad (endothelial function, relative hypercoagulable state, and static blood flow). Several randomized controlled trials have addressed whether patients with heart failure benefit from anticoagulation. Overall, the results suggest the risk of bleeding with anticoagulation outweighs any small benefit conferred by anticoagulation.

Atrial Septal Defects and Cardioembolic Strokes   225

Michelle Leppert, Sharon N. Poisson, and John D. Carroll

Atrial septal defects (ASDs) can be complicated by cardioembolic strokes, but the exact incidence is unknown. Patients with large and small shunts may present with a cardioembolic stroke. Patients with cryptogenic strokes should have cardiac ultrasound to see if an ASD is present. Cardioembolic strokes associated with ASD principally occur with 2 mechanisms. The first is paradoxic embolism involving a venous-based source of thrombus, which may subsequently pass through the ASD by right-to-left shunting, causing a cardioembolic stroke. The second is atrial fibrillation that can complicate the course of patients with ASDs, especially as they age.

Patent Foramen Ovale: Stroke and Device Closure   231

Hussam S. Suradi and Ziyad M. Hijazi

Patent foramen ovale (PFO) is a common finding in healthy adults and has long been implicated in cryptogenic stroke. The pathogenesis is hypothesized to be caused by microemboli gaining access into the systemic circulation via a PFO. Proposed treatment options include medical therapy and/or PFO closure. Despite numerous studies and several randomized trials, much debate persists regarding the efficacy of this approach in reducing the risk of recurrent stroke in cryptogenic stroke patients. This article reviews the association between PFO and cryptogenic stroke, as well as current evidence for PFO device closure.

Pulmonary Arteriovenous Malformations and Risk of Stroke

241

Ralf J. Holzer and Clifford L. Cua

Pulmonary arteriovenous malformations (PAVMs) are rare, with an estimated incidence of 2 to 3 cases per 100,000, with most PAVMs (50%–80%) occurring in patients with hereditary hemorrhagic telangiectasia. Hypoxemia and orthodeoxia are some of the more common clinical presentations. The estimated risk of stroke secondary to PAVMs is as high as 2.6% to 25.0%. A combination of chest radiograph and contrast echocardiography is a good screening evaluation in patients with suspected PAVMs. Transcatheter therapy is the most suitable therapeutic option in most patients with PAVMs, and a variety of devices can be used to occlude the PAVMs.

Congenital Malformations Leading to Paradoxical Embolism

247

Elchanan Bruckheimer

The absolute separation of the right and left circulations and the filtration of blood by the pulmonary circulation are essential to prevent the passage of thrombotic material from the venous system into the systemic arterial circulation. Any breach of the intracardiac septae or circumvention of the pulmonary capillary network may cause a paradoxical embolus. The most common causes are atrial septal defects and pulmonary arteriovenous malformations. This article discusses unusual connections and pathways related to congenital malformations. Although anticoagulation is necessary to prevent paradoxical emboli, the hematologic disturbances and the most appropriate therapy in these patients warrant further investigation.

The Epidemiology of Atrial Fibrillation and Stroke

255

Francesca Pistoia, Simona Sacco, Cindy Tiseo, Diana Degan, Raffaele Ornello, and Antonio Carolei

The burden of stroke is increasing due to aging population and unhealthy lifestyle habits. The considerable rise in atrial fibrillation (AF) is due to greater diffusion of risk factors and screening programs. The link between AF and ischemic stroke is strong. The subtype most commonly associated with AF is cardioembolic stroke, which is particularly severe and shows the highest rates of mortality and permanent disability. A trend toward a higher prevalence of cardioembolic stroke in high-income countries is probably due to the greater diffusion of AF and the control of atherosclerotic of risk factors.

Radiological Portrait of Embolic Strokes

269

Gautam Sachdeva, Ali Saeed, Vishal Jani, and Anmar Razak

Stroke is the leading cause of adult disability and the fifth leading cause of death in the United States. In 2010, the cost of stroke to the health care system in the United States was estimated to be $71.55 billion, and it is projected to double over the next 20 years. Cardioembolism is a leading pathophysiologic cause of stroke. Along with a careful review of the presenting history and clinical symptomatology, early radiographic studies including computed tomography (CT) and MRI, may demonstrate certain characteristics that may be suggestive of a cardioembolic origin to a stroke of concern.

Atrial Fibrillation and Cognitive Decline: Phenomenon or Epiphenomenon? 279

Shadi Kalantarian and Jeremy N. Ruskin

Atrial fibrillation is associated with cognitive impairment ranging from mild to overt dementia, and this association is independent of clinical stroke and multiple shared risk factors. Whether the use of the novel anticoagulants will offer greater protection than warfarin remains to be determined. Rate control strategies may improve brain perfusion and memory but this has not been studied in a randomized controlled trial. Overall, this is a novel field that requires multiple observational studies with long-term follow-up and large-scale randomized controlled trials with accurate neurocognitive testing and brain imaging to ultimately define effective preventive.

Cardiac Monitoring for Atrial Fibrillation in Cryptogenic Stroke 287

Sukit M. Ringwala, Todd T. Tomson, and Rod S. Passman

Despite an extensive initial evaluation, the cause of up to a third of ischemic strokes remains undetermined. The detection of atrial fibrillation (AF) in these patients with cryptogenic stroke is critical as the diagnosis of AF would warrant anticoagulation to reduce the risk of recurrent stroke. Observational studies and prospective randomized controlled trials have shown that a substantial proportion of patients with cryptogenic stroke have AF detected by post-stroke cardiac monitoring with higher AF detection rates observed with longer monitoring periods.

Device-Detected Atrial Fibrillation—Perils and Pitfalls: An Update 299

Phani Surapaneni, Abdul Safadi, Tahmeed Contractor, Mehul B. Patel, and Ranjan K. Thakur

Stroke and thromboembolism are catastrophic complications of atrial fibrillation (AF). Cardiac implantable electronic devices (CIED) with an atrial lead can reliably detect atrial high-rate events (AHRE). However, this correlation may be imperfect because of oversensing and undersensing of atrial signals and spurious arrhythmias. The critical duration, frequency, or overall burden of AHRE that increases stroke risk is still unknown; thus, the threshold level of AHRE (duration and frequency) that warrants anticoagulation in patients with CIED-detected AHRE is still unclear. This article reviews current literature on the risk of stroke with CIED-detected AHRE and raises questions that need further clarification.

Atrial Fibrillation Ablation and Stroke 307

Philip Aagaard, David Briceno, Zoltan Csanadi, Sanghamitra Mohanty, Carola Gianni, Chintan Trivedi, Edina Nagy-Baló, Stephan Danik, Conor Barrett, Francesco Santoro, J. David Burkhardt, Javier Sanchez, Andrea Natale, and Luigi Di Biase

Catheter ablation has become a widely available and accepted treatment to restore sinus rhythm in atrial fibrillation patients who fail antiarrhythmic drug therapy. Although generally safe, the procedure carries a non-negligible risk of complications, including periprocedural cerebral insults. Uninterrupted anticoagulation, maintenance of an adequate ACT during the procedure, and measures to avoid and detect thrombus build-up on sheaths and atheters during the procedure, appears useful to reduce the risk of embolic events. This is a review of the incidence, mechanisms, impact, and methods to reduce catheter ablation related cerebral insults.

Atrial Fibrillation and Stroke: Making Sense of Recent Observations on Anticoagulation   **317**

Marco Proietti and Gregory Y.H. Lip

Atrial fibrillation (AF) is the most prevalent heart rhythm disorder. AF accounts for a great proportion of deaths because it independently increases all-cause mortality and cardiovascular mortality risks. Ischemic stroke is the most common cardiovascular adverse event in AF patients. Oral anticoagulation (OAC) therapy with vitamin K antagonists (VKA) has been central for stroke prevention. Several drugs with a direct inhibitory effects on thrombin and factor Xa have been developed. These non-vitamin K antagonist oral anticoagulants (NOACs) are as effective and safer than warfarin. This review provides an overview of current guidelines and summarizes current evidence for the prevention of stroke in AF patients according to most relevant patients' subgroups and clinical features.

Left Atrial Appendage Closure for Stroke Prevention: Devices, Techniques, and Efficacy   **329**

Sandia Iskandar, James Vacek, Madhav Lavu, and Dhanunjaya Lakkireddy

Left atrial appendage closure can be performed either surgically or percutaneously. Surgical approaches include direct suture, excision and suture, stapling, and clipping. Percutaneous approaches include endocardial, epicardial, and hybrid endocardial-epicardial techniques. Left atrial appendage anatomy is highly variable and complex; therefore, preprocedural imaging is crucial to determine device selection and sizing, which contribute to procedural success and reduction of complications. Currently, the WATCHMAN is the only device that is approved for left atrial appendage closure in the United States.

Index   **353**

CARDIOLOGY CLINICS

FORTHCOMING ISSUES

August 2016
Pulmonary Hypertension
Ronald J. Oudiz, *Editor*

November 2016
Sports Cardiology
Aaron Baggish and Andre La Gerche,
Editors

February 2017
**Hypertension: Pre-Hypertension to Heart
Failure**
Kenneth Jamerson and James Brian Byrd, *Editors*

RECENT ISSUES

February 2016
Nuclear Cardiology
Sharmila Dorbala and Piotr Slomka, *Editors*

November 2015
Adult Congenital Heart Disease
Karen K. Stout, *Editor*

August 2015
**Clinical and Electrophysiologic Management
of Syncope**
Antonio Raviele and Andrea Natale, *Editors*

ISSUE OF RELATED INTEREST

Cardiac Electrophysiology Clinics, September 2015 (Vol. 7, No. 3)
Controversies in Electrophysiology
Emile G. Daoud and Raul Weiss, *Editors*
Available at: http://www.cardiacep.theclinics.com/

THE CLINICS ARE AVAILABLE ONLINE!
Access your subscription at:
www.theclinics.com

Preface
Cardioembolic Stroke

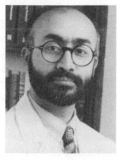

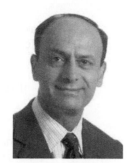

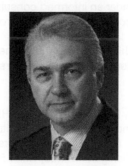

| Ranjan K. Thakur, MD, MPH, MBA, FACC, FHRS | Ziyad M. Hijazi, MD, MPH, FACC, MSCAI, FAHA | Andrea Natale, MD, PhD, FACC, FESC, FHRS |

Editors

Stroke is the leading cause of disability and the second most common cause of death worldwide. While the incidence of stroke is decreasing in advanced economies, the trend is the opposite in low- and middle-income countries (LMIC). In some LMICs, stroke incidence is increasing at an alarming rate, and in the aggregate, the global burden of stroke morbidity and mortality is on the rise.

To facilitate diagnosis and treatment at the time of initial presentation, strokes can be classified as ischemic or hemorrhagic, depending on the presence of intracranial hemorrhage on the initial imaging studies. The classification helps to triage care using the appropriate care pathways.

Roughly 80% to 90% of strokes are ischemic (embolic or thrombotic occlusion), and the remainder are hemorrhagic. Cardioembolism is the mechanism for one-third of ischemic strokes. Cardioembolism may result from one of three mechanisms: (1) blood stasis and thrombus formation in a left cardiac chamber (eg, left atrial appendage, left ventricular aneurysm, or endocardial surface post-myocardial infarction [MI]); (2) release of material from an abnormal valvular surface (eg, prosthetic valve); and (3) abnormal passage of a thrombus from the venous to the arterial circulation (paradoxical embolism).

The relationship between atrial fibrillation (AF) and stroke has been known since the initial description by Gowers in 1875. In fact, among the above mechanisms of cardioembolism, nonvalvular AF is the leading cause for cardioembolism, wherein the thrombus generally originates in the left atrial appendage. Finally, in roughly 30% to 40% of strokes, the cause remains uncertain after extensive evaluation; these are called cryptogenic strokes. Paroxysmal AF, due to its transient and intermittent nature, may elude detection and is the leading cause of cryptogenic stroke. So, AF, manifest or cryptogenic, is inextricably related to stroke.

Since cardioembolism is a leading cause of stroke, and cryptogenic strokes arise predominantly due to paroxysmal AF, cardiologists are increasingly called to participate in the care of stroke patients. Using various diagnostic tools, cardiologists can help identify or confirm the cause of stroke and give advice regarding further treatment and/or prevention. Interventional cardiologists can also deploy intracardiac devices to provide the definitive therapy for prevention of future strokes.

Since cardiologists have an important role in the care of stroke patients, we were pleased to have been invited to edit this issue of the *Cardiology Clinics* on Cardioembolic Stroke. We have called upon thought-leaders in cardiology to contribute articles to elucidate relevant issues in the purview of consulting cardiologists.

The contributors have discussed the various cardiac conditions that may lead to a stroke; these include stroke post-MI, stroke in the setting of a cardiomyopathy, atrial septal defect, and patent foramen ovale. A significant part of this issue of *Cardiology Clinics* is devoted to various aspects of AF and stroke, including the epidemiology of AF and stroke, silent strokes due to AF ablation, management of AF detected in patients with pacemakers and implantable cardioverter defibrillators, cognitive decline in AF patients and whether it may be related to silent embolism, a review of left atrial

Cardiol Clin 34 (2016) xiii–xiv
http://dx.doi.org/10.1016/j.ccl.2016.02.001
0733-8651/16/$ – see front matter © 2016 Published by Elsevier Inc.

cardiology.theclinics.com

appendage closure for stroke prevention in AF, and importantly, reviewing the evidence on anticoagulation in patients with AF. We feel that cardiologists should be thoroughly familiar with these concepts in order to render an informed consultation to their neurology colleagues caring for stroke patients.

We hope the readership will enjoy reading these cutting-edge, well-written reviews from leaders in the field.

Ranjan K. Thakur, MD, MPH, MBA, FACC, FHRS
Sparrow Thoracic and Cardiovascular Institute
Michigan State University
1200 East Michigan Avenue, Suite 585
Lansing, MI 48912, USA

Ziyad M. Hijazi, MD, MPH, FACC, MSCAI, FAHA
Weill Cornell Medicine &
Sidra Medical and Research Center
PO Box 26999
Doha, Qatar

Andrea Natale, MD, PhD, FACC, FESC, FHRS
Texas Cardiac Arrhythmia Institute
Center for Atrial Fibrillation at
St. David's Medical Center
1015 East 32nd Street, Suite 516
Austin, TX 78705, USA

E-mail addresses:
thakur@msu.edu (R.K. Thakur)
zhijazi@sidra.org (Z.M. Hijazi)
andrea.natale@stdavids.com (A. Natale)

Cardioembolic Stroke and Postmyocardial Infarction Stroke

Marius Hornung, MD, Jennifer Franke, MD,
Sameer Gafoor, MD, Horst Sievert, MD*

KEYWORDS

- Stroke • Myocardial infarction • Thrombus • Atrial fibrillation • Inflammation

KEY POINTS

- The stroke risk is highest in the acute phase after myocardial infarction, but persists even thereafter.
- The pathophysiology leading to ischemic stroke following acute coronary syndrome is multifactorial: the leading subtype is the cardioembolic stroke, second is stroke of undetermined pathogenesis.
- The risk of cardiac thromboembolism originating from the left ventricle is mainly caused by akinetic segments of the left ventricle predisposing to mural thrombus formation.
- New onset of atrial fibrillation following acute myocardial infarction not only increases the risk of ischemic stroke but is also accompanied by a significant increase in overall mortality.

INTRODUCTION

Epidemiologic studies have proven that patients who have recently suffered an acute myocardial infarction (AMI), in consequence have an increased risk for the occurrence of ischemic stroke. These patients not only have a higher incidence for strokes when compared with the general population,[1,2] ischemic strokes after AMI remain associated with a worse mortality rate when compared with patients without cerebrovascular complications.[3,4] The odds ratio of in-hospital death is 4.3 in case of a stroke. The in-hospital mortality after ischemic stroke can be up to 10% to 20%, and even higher in patients with hemorrhagic stroke.[2,5] The mortality rates after 30 days and in long-term follow-up have been estimated to be 45% and up to 28%, respectively.[1,6–8]

The stroke risk is highest in the acute phase after myocardial infarction but persists even thereafter. The stroke risk is increased up to 44-fold within the first month but is also increased 3 years after the acute event.[9] The incidence of stroke during a hospital stay after acute coronary syndrome ranges from 0.7% to 2.2%.[10–15] Hachet and colleagues[16] reported the results of 8485 patients admitted to their intensive care unit for AMI between 2001 and 2010. Of those, 168 patients (1.9%) had a stroke within 1 year after AMI. Two-thirds (n = 123) were in-hospital strokes, of which the most occurred within the first 5 days after admission with a 30-day mortality of 34%. One year after the AMI, mortality was significantly increased: 57 patients with an in-hospital stroke died (46%) compared with 1056 patients (12%) without a stroke complicating the AMI (P<.001). Although the stroke risk progressively decreases in the months after AMI, the annual stroke rate (in-hospital and postdischarge) remained stable over the period 2001 to 2010.[16]

These rates could be confirmed by observational studies of American and Swedish patient registries showing the results of representative patient populations.[3,17,18] The evaluation of the

CardioVascular Center Frankfurt, Sankt Katharinen Krankenhaus, Seckbacher Landstrasse 65, 60389 Frankfurt, Germany
* Corresponding author.
E-mail address: info@cvcfrankfurt.de

Cardiol Clin 34 (2016) 207–214
http://dx.doi.org/10.1016/j.ccl.2015.12.003

American Nationwide Inpatient Sample revealed 1,924,413 patients admitted for AMI between 2006 and 2008. The overall rate of in-hospital neurologic complications was 2%: ischemic stroke 1.5%, transient ischemic attack (TIA) 0.3%, and hemorrhagic stroke 0.2%.[17] Female gender, age older than 65 years, and black race were found to be predictive of an increased risk for in-hospital neurologic complications. Independent risk factors were congestive heart failure, peripheral vascular disease, and the presence of atrial fibrillation.[17] Data collected from 173,233 patients from the Swedish Register of Information and Knowledge about Swedish Heart Intensive Care Admission registry for 1998 to 2008 showed an ischemic stroke rate within 1 year of 4.1% (7185 patients). The 1-year mortality rate of these patients was 36.5%, compared with 18.3% for AMI patients without cerebral event.[3] But the mortality decreased over time (1998–2000 vs 2007–2008) in patients with and without a complicating stroke. There is an absolute decrease of 9.4% and 7.5%, and a relative decrease of 24% and 35%, respectively ($P<.001$).[3,18] This is mainly caused by the implementation of early reperfusion strategies in the therapy for myocardial infarction and secondary preventive therapies. A Cox regression of the registry results reveals age, female gender, transmural myocardial infarction, history of previous stroke, diabetes, reduced ejection fraction at admission, and atrial fibrillation as independent predictors of stroke complicating AMI, whereas reperfusion strategies using fibrinolysis or percutaneous coronary intervention (PCI) and medical treatment with aspirin, adenosine diphosphate (ADP)-receptor blockers, and statins reduce the stroke risk.[18]

Van de Graaff and colleagues[19] evaluated the beneficial effect of early reperfusion strategies for diminishing the risk of ischemic stroke following AMI. They used the National Registry of Myocardial Infarction to identify a total of 93,873 patients with an AMI. Of these, 45,997 patients were treated with thrombolytic therapy and 47,876 patients underwent primary PCI. The in-hospital stroke rates were 0.5% and 0.3%. Univariate analysis showed a statistically significant linear correlation between time to revascularization and the in-hospital stroke risk. A multivariate analysis revealed a significantly lower ischemic stroke risk in case of thrombolytic therapy, beginning within 15 minutes (odds ratio 0.58), and a nonsignificant trend toward a lower stroke risk in PCI started within 90 minutes of hospital arrival. However, the mechanism of decreasing the ischemic stroke risk did not seem to be related to an improved left ventricular ejection fraction (LV-EF).[19]

NONCARDIOEMBOLIC STROKES FOLLOWING ACUTE MYOCARDIAL INFARCTION

The pathophysiology leading to ischemic stroke following acute coronary syndrome is multifactorial. An evaluation of in-hospital strokes according to the Trial of Org 10172 in Acute Stroke Treatment (TOAST) classification showed 2 dominant stroke types: the leading subtype was the cardioembolic stroke (60%), the second was stroke of undetermined pathogenesis (36%).[16]

Regarding the group of noncardioembolic strokes, the underlying pathophysiological processes are multifactorial. Ischemia itself induces a systemic procoagulant effect, facilitating thrombus formation and embolization in the cerebral circulation. Although in patients with AMI a hypercoagulable state can be detected by increased prothrombin fragment 1 and 2, and fibrinopeptide A levels, which remain increased for up to 6 months after the index event, the appropriate blood levels in patients with stable coronary artery disease do not increase.[20] Furthermore, ischemia results in the release of inflammatory cytokines, causing the activation of neutrophils and the synthesis of acute phase reactants.[21,22] These might trigger the destabilization and rupture of plaques in the cerebral circulation.[23] The acute mediators of inflammation serve as both propagators and markers of plaque instability. The C-reactive protein (CRP) has a proinflammatory and a procoagulant effect.[20,24] CRP levels are increased in response to myocardial injury.[25,26] The inflammatory effect of the released cytokines is not limited to the coronary vasculature. Therefore, complex and unstable carotid plaques are common in patients with AMI (42% vs 8% in patients with stable angina).[27] This may cause plaque rupture and subsequent thrombus formation in supra-aortic vessels and cerebral circulation. These ischemia and cytokine-mediated processes also explain the beneficial effect of a fast restoration of coronary flow with respect to the risk of ischemic strokes following AMI.

CARDIOEMBOLIC STROKES FOLLOWING MYOCARDIAL INFARCTION

The previously listed cytokine mediated reactions also play a role in the development of cardiac thrombi. However, cardioembolic strokes following an AMI are mainly caused by (1) the formation of left ventricular thrombi and (2) atrial fibrillation.

Left Ventricular Thrombus Formation

The risk of cardiac thromboembolism originating from the left ventricle is mainly caused by an akinetic segment of the left ventricular myocardium, resulting in local blood stasis predisposing to mural thrombus formation. It is a common complication, especially in patients with an anterior ST-segment elevation myocardial infarction (STEMI) with focal dyskinesia leading to an aneurysmatic dilatation of the anterior or apical wall of the left ventricle. The thrombi usually occur within 2 weeks after the AMI, in median 5 days after the acute event.[28] In the prethrombolytic era, the incidence of thrombus formation was reported to range from 20% up to 55% in patients with an anterior STEMI. In the reperfusion era, and despite the routine use of fibrinolytics and acute PCI, the incidence of left ventricular thrombus formation seems to be lower but remains substantial.[29] In addition, the thrombotic risk increases with decreasing of LV-EF. For every 5% decrease of the LV-EF, there is an 18% increase of the relative risk of thrombus formation.[22] Analyzing the results of the GISSI-3 database of 8326 patients at low-to-medium risk for thrombus formation, left ventricular thrombi were seen in 427 patients (5.1%).[30] Thrombi were found in 292 of 2544 patients with an anterior AMI (11.5%) compared with 135 of 5782 patients with an AMI in another location (2,3%; $P<.0001$). Furthermore, the incidence was significantly higher in patients with an LV-EF of less than 40%, both in total (10.5% vs 4%) and in the subgroup with anterior AMI (17.8% vs 9.6%).[30] Along with early revascularization, an adjunctive pharmacologic therapy with antiplatelet and antithrombotic agents is needed for a reduction in left ventricular thrombus formation. Buss and colleagues[31] used an institutional database to identify survivors of an anterior STEMI with an LV-EF of 40% or less. They analyzed the influence of oral anticoagulation with vitamin K antagonists on the incidence of ischemic stroke, death, and clinically relevant bleeding complications within 6 months after the AMI. There was no significant difference in the rate of bleeding or death between the 2 groups. Although 4 of the anticoagulated patients (2.5%) suffered an ischemic stroke, only 1 of the nonanticoagulated patients was affected (0.9%). A population-based cohort analysis by Udell and colleagues[32] could also demonstrate no positive effect in terms of a lower ischemic stroke rate due to oral anticoagulation. They analyzed 10,383 patients who survived an AMI in Ontario, Canada, between 1999 and 2001. The use of warfarin up to 90 days after an anterior AMI was not associated with a reduction in ischemic strokes. In contrast, the use of beta-blockers and angiotensin-converting-enzyme inhibitors was associated with a significantly decreased risk of ischemic stroke.[32]

In the recent years, catheter procedures have been developed to reduce the end-diastolic volume of the left ventricle and thus to improve the LV-EF. An influence of these procedures on the development of ventricular thrombi and ischemic strokes has not been studied in particular yet. The Parachute system (Cardiokinetix, Menlo Park, CA, USA) is a device for the treatment apical aneurysms. A total of 16 nitinol wires are deployed that carry a polytetrafluoroethylene membrane to separate the aneurysm from the vital left ventricular myocardium. As the nitinol wires anchor in healthy myocardium, they transmit the rotary screw movement of the ventricle to the implant and thus lead to an ejection of blood from the apex.[33] However, it must be noted, that each intracardiac implant is also associated with the risk of device-associated thrombus formation. Another system for the restoration of left ventricular aneurysms is the Revivent system (BioVentrix, Inc, San Ramon, CA, USA). It is a hybrid procedure using a venous and a thoracoscopic access to the left ventricle. Titanium anchors gather the scarred heart muscle to restore the natural conical shape of the ventricle. By multiple repetitions along the entire length of the aneurysm, the natural shape of the left ventricle can be reconstructed. First clinical experiences have been favorable. A relevant increase of the LV-EF was achieved by significant reductions of the end systolic and end diastolic left ventricular volumes. Furthermore, improvements in exercise capacity, the heart failure degree, and an increase in the quality of life were reached.[34] Whether these procedures may also cause a reduction in left ventricular thrombi and cerebral embolism needs to be evaluated in future investigations.

Atrial Fibrillation

Another strong predictor of an increased stroke risk following AMI is the presence or new onset of atrial fibrillation. Data from the Framingham Study show that a myocardial infarction, or even ischemia, is a risk factor for new onset of atrial fibrillation.[35] Despite improved reperfusion strategies, the incidence of atrial fibrillation during hospitalization for AMI is still between 8% and 22%.[36] The increased rate of atrial fibrillation results from an increased left atrial pressure. This can either be a direct consequence of atrial ischemia[37] or be indirectly caused by an enhanced left ventricular filling pressure or a restricted left ventricular function.[38,39] To evaluate whether the CHADS$_2$ (congestive heart failure, hypertension, age ≥ 75 years, diabetes mellitus, stroke) and CHA$_2$DS$_2$-VASc (congestive heart failure, hypertension, age

≥75 years, diabetes mellitus, stroke or TIA, vascular disease, age 65–74 years, sex category) scores can be used to predict the risk of new onset of atrial and ischemic stroke in patients with AMI, Lau and colleagues[40] analyzed the data of 617 consecutive patients who survived a STEMI. After a mean follow-up of 63 months, new atrial fibrillation was found in 83 patients (13.7%). Patients at risk for new onset of atrial fibrillation were older, more likely to be female, had a decreased LV-EF, and had significantly higher CHADS$_2$ (1.71 ± 1.04 vs 1.21 ± 0.98, $P<.0001$) and CHA$_2$DS$_2$-VASc scores (3.90 ± 1.34 vs 2.97 ± 1.40, $P<.001$). In addition, Cox proportional hazards regression showed female gender, hypertension, a history of stroke, CHADS$_2$, and CHA$_2$DS$_2$-VASc score were associated with stroke following AMI.[40]

However, the new onset of atrial fibrillation following an acute coronary syndrome increases not only the risk of developing a stroke but is also accompanied by a significant increase in overall mortality. Bang and colleagues[41] identified 89,703 patients from Danish nationwide registries who had a first AMI without prior atrial fibrillation between 1997 and 2009. They found a negative influence of the new-onset of atrial fibrillation following AMI on all-cause mortality, as well as on the incidence of cardiovascular complications at an average follow-up of 5 years. The all-cause mortality in patients with atrial fibrillation (n = 10,708) was 173.9 per 1000 patient years compared with 69.4 deaths per 1000 patient years among the 78,992 patients who stayed in sinus rhythm. During follow-up, there were 610 fatal (5.7%) and 606 nonfatal (5.6%) strokes registered in the atrial fibrillation group, compared with 2414 (3.1%) and 2172 (0.3%) events in the control-group. Therefore, new onset of atrial fibrillation remained predictive of increased all-cause mortality (hazard ratio 1.9), fatal and nonfatal stroke rate (hazard ratio 2.3 and 2.5), and fatal and nonfatal re-infarction rate (hazard ratio 1.7 and 1.8; all $P<.001$).[41] Furthermore, myocardial ischemia represents an independent risk factor for the occurrence of atrial fibrillation. The rate of patients admitted for atrial fibrillation was significantly higher after AMI discharge (23.9 per 1000 patient years) than in the Danish population of the same age without prior myocardial infarction (about 6 per 1000 patient years).[42]

There is evidence that atrial fibrillation is associated with impairment of endothelial function even in the absence of hypertension or heart failure. This could explain the increased incidence of atrial fibrillation caused by ischemia-reperfusion injury after AMI.[43] In addition, inflammatory responses are a common pathophysiological mechanism in atrial fibrillation and AMI.[44] CRP reduces the endothelial production of nitric oxide but it also causes an increased expression of adhesion molecules. It also influences the chemotaxis of monocytes and the foam cell formation in atherosclerotic plaques and aggravates the vasoreactivity of unstable plaques.[44] This may explain the association among acute myocardial ischemia, new onset of atrial fibrillation, and the risk of reinfarction (cerebral and coronary).

Not only previous or new-onset atrial fibrillation (paroxysmal or persistent) is associated with worse short-term and long-term prognosis. The same applies for silent atrial fibrillation, which may occur in the setting of an acute coronary syndrome. Because atrial fibrillation is often asymptomatic, it is important to improve the detection rate by systematic screening in AMI. Continuous ECG monitoring demonstrated a 3 times higher rate of silent atrial fibrillation when compared with symptomatic atrial fibrillation, with an incidence of 16%.[45] In 2015, Stamboul and colleagues[46] published the results on 737 patients with an AMI. Among them, in 106 cases (14.3%) silent atrial fibrillation was detected and 32 patients (4.3%) had symptomatic atrial fibrillation. At 1-year follow-up, 24 patients (3.2%) had died from cardiovascular complications, with an increased risk of death among patients with silent or symptomatic atrial fibrillation compared with patients in sinus rhythm (5.7% vs 18.8% vs 2%; $P<.001$). The same was seen with regard to rehospitalization for acute heart failure: this was significantly higher in patients with silent and symptomatic atrial fibrillation (6.6% and 6.3%). Patients in sinus rhythm suffered acute heart failure in only 1.3%; $P<.001$. Compared with patients without atrial fibrillation, those with silent atrial fibrillation were markedly older, more frequently hypertensive, less likely to be smokers, and were more likely to have an impaired LV-EF. Therefore, risk factors for silent and symptomatic atrial fibrillation are similar. However, a history of stroke or atrial fibrillation was less frequent in patients with silent than in patients with symptomatic atrial fibrillation.[46]

Because even silent atrial fibrillation is associated with a dramatic up to 3 times higher rate of cardiovascular death at 1 year after AMI, it may severely impair the prognosis. It is, therefore, necessary to optimize the patients' drug therapy. Acute revascularization by implantation of drug-eluting stents requires dual antiplatelet therapy but also only anticoagulation can achieve effective protection against cerebral ischemia by cardiac thrombi. The European Heart Rhythm Association survey reported a strong consensus (78.1%) for a triple therapy (dual antiplatelet plus anticoagulation) after the first, even single, episode of silent atrial fibrillation in patients with an AMI and CHA_2DS_2-VASc-Score of 1 point or more.[47]

For patients with AMI, current guidelines favor periprocedural dual antiplatelet therapy with prasugrel or ticagrelor due to their faster onset, greater potency, and proven superiority compared with clopidogrel, although these agents have not yet been evaluated properly in combination with any oral anticoagulant.[48,49] Following stent implantation, patients with atrial fibrillation are at risk for both stroke and stent thrombosis and, therefore, have an indication for triple therapy. The benefits of triple therapy are outweighed by a substantial increase in the risk of bleeding complications.[50] Until more data are available, especially on the use of the new oral anticoagulants, the current guidelines recommend triple therapy with aspirin plus clopidogrel and warfarin (with an international normalized ratio of 2–2.5) with duration of triple therapy for 1 month after implantation of a bare metal stent, and 3 to 6 months after implantation of a drug-eluting stent.[48,49]

In patients at high risk for bleeding complications under triple therapy, interventional occlusion of the left atrial appendage (LAA) may be a reasonable alternative. Because nearly 90% of all thrombi in patients with atrial fibrillation arise in the LAA,[51] various surgical and catheter-based techniques have been developed to exclude the LAA as a source for thromboembolic complications. Following successful LAA occlusion, an oral anticoagulant to protect against cardiac embolism can be waived to decrease the risk of bleeding complications. The current commercially available systems include endocardial implants with the ACP/Amulet (St. Jude Medical, Inc, St. Paul, MN, USA), the Watchman (Boston Scientific Corporation, Marlborough, MA, USA), and the WaveCrest (Coherex Medical, Salt Lake City, UT) devices, as well as the Lariat technique (SentreHEART, Redwood City, CA, USA) for combined endocardial-epicardial closed-chest ligation of the LAA. The Watchman device demonstrated noninferiority and, later, even superiority when compared with warfarin in a controlled randomized trial (PROTECT AF [WATCHMAN Left Atrial Appendage System for Embolic PROTECTion in Patients with Atrial Fibrillation]).[52,53] This resulted in approval by the Food and Drug Administration in March 2015 for the use of the Watchman device in the United States as an alternative to warfarin. The Amplatzer Cardiac Plug (St. Jude Medical, Inc., St. Paul, MN, USA) was presented as a device designed specifically for percutaneous occlusion of the LAA in 2008. In December of the same year,

the system received the Conformité Européene (CE) mark. In August 2013, and subsequent to the results of the WAVECREST I trial, CE mark approval was granted to the Coherex WaveCrest occluder, which is, since then, the third commercially available device for percutaneous occlusion of the LAA. The main indication for percutaneous sealing of the LAA is a relative or absolute contraindication to oral anticoagulation in patients with atrial fibrillation and an increased stroke-risk ($CHADS_2$-score ≥ 1 or CHA_2DS_2-VASc-score ≥ 2). Following the results of the PROTECT AF trial, however, LAA occlusion may be discussed as an alternative in all patients with an indication to oral anticoagulation because the procedural complication rates are low and, as of this writing, at least the Watchman device has proven its superiority in long-term follow-up.[52,53]

SUMMARY

Ischemic stroke following AMI is a rare but serious complication, both in terms of individual as well as socioeconomic consequences. In the acute phase after acute coronary syndrome, the risk of ischemic stroke is the highest due to left ventricular thrombus formation and occurrence of atrial fibrillation. The most important method in relation to the acute treatment of myocardial infarction and in the secondary prevention of stroke is early revascularization of the culprit coronary lesion. Improved secondary prevention with statins and antiplatelet therapy to avoid adverse events after AMI could also contribute to risk reduction. Moreover, the trends in revascularization treatments may affect the risk of stroke. Conversely, the greater use of antiplatelet agents recommended by recent guidelines intended to reduce the risk of ischemic stroke, such as clopidogrel and aspirin, could increase the risk of hemorrhagic stroke. Thus, the risk of stroke after AMI has significantly reduced over the last decade. During this period, patients have been increasingly treated with PCIs and antithrombotic therapies in the acute setting and have received improved secondary prevention strategies, such as statins and antihypertensive medications, and more patients were recommended to receive dual antiplatelet therapy.

REFERENCES

1. Spencer FA, Gore JM, Yarzebski J, et al. Trends (1986 to 1999) in the incidence and outcomes of in-hospital stroke complicating acute myocardial infarction (The Worcester heart attack study). Am J Cardiol 2003;92(4):383–8.

2. Tanne D, Gottlieb S, Hod H, et al. Incidence and mortality from early stroke associated with acute myocardial infarction in the prethrombolytic and thrombolytic eras. Secondary Prevention Reinfarction Israeli Nifedipine Trial (SPRINT) and Israeli Thrombolytic Survey Groups. J Am Coll Cardiol 1997;30(6):1484–90.

3. Brammas A, Jakobsson S, Ulvenstam A, et al. Mortality after ischemic stroke in patients with acute myocardial infarction: predictors and trends over time in Sweden. Stroke 2013;44(11):3050–5.

4. Mooe T, Olofsson BO, Stegmayr B, et al. Ischemic stroke. Impact of a recent myocardial infarction. Stroke 1999;30(5):997–1001.

5. Cronin L, Mehta SR, Zhao F, et al. Stroke in relation to cardiac procedures in patients with non-ST-elevation acute coronary syndrome: a study involving >18 000 patients. Circulation 2001; 104(3):269–74.

6. Budaj A, Flasinska K, Gore JM, et al. Magnitude of and risk factors for in-hospital and postdischarge stroke in patients with acute coronary syndromes: findings from a Global registry of acute coronary events. Circulation 2005;111(24):3242–7.

7. Mahaffey KW, Harrington RA, Simoons ML, et al. Stroke in patients with acute coronary syndromes: incidence and outcomes in the platelet glycoprotein IIb/IIIa in unstable angina. Receptor suppression using integrilin therapy (PURSUIT) trial. The PURSUIT Investigators. Circulation 1999;99(18): 2371–7.

8. Saczynski JS, Spencer FA, Gore JM, et al. Twenty-year trends in the incidence of stroke complicating acute myocardial infarction: Worcester Heart Attack Study. Arch Intern Med 2008;168(19):2104–10.

9. Witt BJ, Brown RD Jr, Jacobsen SJ, et al. A community-based study of stroke incidence after myocardial infarction. Ann Intern Med 2005; 143(11):785–92.

10. Al Suwaidi J, Al Habib K, Asaad N, et al. Immediate and one-year outcome of patients presenting with acute coronary syndrome complicated by stroke: findings from the 2nd Gulf Registry of Acute Coronary Events (Gulf RACE-2). BMC Cardiovasc Disord 2012;12:64.

11. Kajermo U, Ulvenstam A, Modica A, et al. Incidence, trends, and predictors of ischemic stroke 30 days after an acute myocardial infarction. Stroke 2014; 45(5):1324–30.

12. Longstreth WT Jr, Litwin PE, Weaver WD. Myocardial infarction, thrombolytic therapy, and stroke. A community-based study. The MITI Project Group. Stroke 1993;24(4):587–90.

13. Indications for fibrinolytic therapy in suspected acute myocardial infarction: collaborative overview of early mortality and major morbidity results from all randomised trials of more than 1000 patients. Fibrinolytic Therapy Trialists' (FTT) Collaborative Group. Lancet 1994;343(8893):311–22.

14. Becker RC, Burns M, Gore JM, et al. Early assessment and in-hospital management of patients with acute myocardial infarction at increased risk for adverse outcomes: a nationwide perspective of current clinical practice. The National Registry of Myocardial Infarction (NRMI-2) Participants. Am Heart J 1998;135(5 Pt 1):786–96.

15. Wienbergen H, Schiele R, Gitt AK, et al. Incidence, risk factors, and clinical outcome of stroke after acute myocardial infarction in clinical practice. MIR and MITRA study groups. Myocardial Infarction Registry. Maximal Individual Therapy in Acute Myocardial Infarction. Am J Cardiol 2001;87(6): 782–5. A788.

16. Hachet O, Guenancia C, Stamboul K, et al. Frequency and predictors of stroke after acute myocardial infarction: specific aspects of in-hospital and postdischarge events. Stroke 2014;45(12):3514–20.

17. Naderi N, Masoomi H, Mozaffar T, et al. Patient characteristics and comorbidities associated with cerebrovascular accident following acute myocardial infarction in the United States. Int J Cardiol 2014; 175(2):323–7.

18. Ulvenstam A, Kajermo U, Modica A, et al. Incidence, trends, and predictors of ischemic stroke 1 year after an acute myocardial infarction. Stroke 2014; 45(11):3263–8.

19. Van de Graaff E, Dutta M, Das P, et al. Early coronary revascularization diminishes the risk of ischemic stroke with acute myocardial infarction. Stroke 2006;37(10):2546–51.

20. Merlini PA, Bauer KA, Oltrona L, et al. Persistent activation of coagulation mechanism in unstable angina and myocardial infarction. Circulation 1994;90(1): 61–8.

21. Kassem-Moussa H, Mahaffey KW, Graffagnino C, et al. Incidence and characteristics of stroke during 90-day follow-up in patients stabilized after an acute coronary syndrome. Am Heart J 2004;148(3):439–46.

22. Loh E, Sutton MS, Wun CC, et al. Ventricular dysfunction and the risk of stroke after myocardial infarction. N Engl J Med 1997;336(4):251–7.

23. Neumann FJ, Ott I, Gawaz M, et al. Cardiac release of cytokines and inflammatory responses in acute myocardial infarction. Circulation 1995; 92(4):748–55.

24. Motro M, Barbash GI, Hod H, et al. Incidence of left ventricular thrombi formation after thrombolytic therapy with recombinant tissue plasminogen activator, heparin, and aspirin in patients with acute myocardial infarction. Am Heart J 1991;122(1 Pt 1):23–6.

25. Buffon A, Biasucci LM, Liuzzo G, et al. Widespread coronary inflammation in unstable angina. N Engl J Med 2002;347(1):5–12.

26. Mauriello A, Sangiorgi G, Fratoni S, et al. Diffuse and active inflammation occurs in both vulnerable and stable plaques of the entire coronary tree: a histopathologic study of patients dying of acute myocardial infarction. J Am Coll Cardiol 2005; 45(10):1585–93.

27. Lombardo A, Biasucci LM, Lanza GA, et al. Inflammation as a possible link between coronary and carotid plaque instability. Circulation 2004;109(25): 3158–63.

28. Nihoyannopoulos P, Smith GC, Maseri A, et al. The natural history of left ventricular thrombus in myocardial infarction: a rationale in support of masterly inactivity. J Am Coll Cardiol 1989;14(4):903–11.

29. Shacham Y, Leshem-Rubinow E, Ben Assa E, et al. Frequency and correlates of early left ventricular thrombus formation following anterior wall acute myocardial infarction treated with primary percutaneous coronary intervention. Am J Cardiol 2013; 111(5):667–70.

30. Chiarella F, Santoro E, Domenicucci S, et al. Predischarge two-dimensional echocardiographic evaluation of left ventricular thrombosis after acute myocardial infarction in the GISSI-3 study. Am J Cardiol 1998;81(7):822–7.

31. Buss NI, Friedman SE, Andrus BW, et al. Warfarin for stroke prevention following anterior ST-elevation myocardial infarction. Coron Artery Dis 2013;24(8): 636–41.

32. Udell JA, Wang JT, Gladstone DJ, et al. Anticoagulation after anterior myocardial infarction and the risk of stroke. PLoS One 2010;5(8):e12150.

33. Costa MA, Mazzaferri EL Jr, Sievert H, et al. Percutaneous ventricular restoration using the parachute device in patients with ischemic heart failure: three-year outcomes of the PARACHUTE first-in-human study. Circ Heart Fail 2014;7(5): 752–8.

34. Faria R, Melica B, Pires-Morais G, et al. New less invasive ventricular reconstruction technique in the treatment of ischemic heart failure. Rev Port Cardiol 2014;33(7–8):469.e1–5.

35. Benjamin EJ, Levy D, Vaziri SM, et al. Independent risk factors for atrial fibrillation in a population-based cohort. The Framingham Heart Study. JAMA 1994;271(11):840–4.

36. Bhatia GS, Lip GY. Atrial fibrillation post-myocardial infarction: frequency, consequences, and management. Curr Heart Fail Rep 2004;1(4):149–55.

37. Hod H, Lew AS, Keltai M, et al. Early atrial fibrillation during evolving myocardial infarction: a consequence of impaired left atrial perfusion. Circulation 1987;75(1):146–50.

38. Aronson D, Mutlak D, Bahouth F, et al. Restrictive left ventricular filling pattern and risk of new-onset atrial fibrillation after acute myocardial infarction. Am J Cardiol 2011;107(12):1738–43.

39. Lopes RD, Elliott LE, White HD, et al. Antithrombotic therapy and outcomes of patients with atrial fibrillation following primary percutaneous coronary intervention: results from the APEX-AMI trial. Eur Heart J 2009;30(16):2019–28.

40. Lau KK, Chan PH, Yiu KH, et al. Roles of the CHADS2 and CHA2DS2-VASc scores in post-myocardial infarction patients: risk of new occurrence of atrial fibrillation and ischemic stroke. Cardiol J 2014;21(5):474–83.

41. Bang CN, Gislason GH, Greve AM, et al. New-onset atrial fibrillation is associated with cardiovascular events leading to death in a first time myocardial infarction population of 89,703 patients with long-term follow-up: a nationwide study. J Am Heart Assoc 2014;3(1):e000382.

42. Frost L, Andersen LV, Vestergaard P, et al. Trend in mortality after stroke with atrial fibrillation. Am J Med 2007;120(1):47–53.

43. Adam O, Neuberger HR, Bohm M, et al. Prevention of atrial fibrillation with 3-hydroxy-3-methylglutaryl coenzyme A reductase inhibitors. Circulation 2008; 118(12):1285–93.

44. Chan AW, Bhatt DL, Chew DP, et al. Relation of inflammation and benefit of statins after percutaneous coronary interventions. Circulation 2003; 107(13):1750–6.

45. Stamboul K, Zeller M, Fauchier L, et al. Incidence and prognostic significance of silent atrial fibrillation in acute myocardial infarction. Int J Cardiol 2014; 174(3):611–7.

46. Stamboul K, Zeller M, Fauchier L, et al. Prognosis of silent atrial fibrillation after acute myocardial infarction at 1-year follow-up. Heart 2015;101(11): 864–9.

47. Potpara TS, Lip GY, Dagres N, et al. Management of acute coronary syndrome in patients with non-valvular atrial fibrillation: results of the European Heart Rhythm Association Survey. Europace 2014; 16(2):293–8.

48. O'Gara PT, Kushner FG, Ascheim DD, et al. 2013 ACCF/AHA guideline for the management of ST-elevation myocardial infarction: a report of the American College of Cardiology Foundation/American Heart Association Task Force on Practice Guidelines. Circulation 2013;127(4): e362–425.

49. Task Force on the management of ST-segment elevation acute myocardial infarction of the European Society of Cardiology (ESC), Steg PG, James SK, et al. ESC guidelines for the management of acute myocardial infarction in patients presenting with ST-segment elevation. Eur Heart J 2012;33(20):2569–619.

50. Lamberts M, Olesen JB, Ruwald MH, et al. Bleeding after initiation of multiple antithrombotic drugs, including triple therapy, in atrial fibrillation patients

following myocardial infarction and coronary intervention: a nationwide cohort study. Circulation 2012;126(10):1185–93.

51. Blackshear JL, Odell JA. Appendage obliteration to reduce stroke in cardiac surgical patients with atrial fibrillation. Ann Thorac Surg 1996; 61(2):755–9.

52. Holmes DR Jr, Kar S, Price MJ, et al. Prospective randomized evaluation of the Watchman Left Atrial Appendage Closure device in patients with atrial fibrillation versus long-term warfarin therapy: the PREVAIL trial. J Am Coll Cardiol 2014;64(1):1–12.

53. Holmes DR, Reddy VY, Turi ZG, et al. Percutaneous closure of the left atrial appendage versus warfarin therapy for prevention of stroke in patients with atrial fibrillation: a randomised non-inferiority trial. Lancet 2009;374(9689):534–42.

Embolic Stroke in Cardiomyopathy
Should Patients be Anticoagulated?

Akhil Narang, MD, Roberto M. Lang, MD*

KEYWORDS

- Heart failure • Stroke • Anticoagulation • Warfarin • Prevention

KEY POINTS

- A number of studies have shown that patients with heart failure have greater incidence of stroke when compared with patients without heart failure.
- The combination of endothelial dysfunction, a relative hypercoagulable state, and static blood flow (from cardiac remodeling) predisposes patients with heart failure to develop thrombus that leads to cardioembolic stroke. This is mediated by the release of prothrombotic factors.
- To date, 4 major randomized trials have investigated the role of anticoagulation in patients with heart failure (in sinus rhythm). Data pooled from these studies suggested the risk for bleeding with anticoagulation counterbalanced the small benefit observed in preventing strokes with anticoagulation.
- The decision to anticoagulate patients with heart failure with atrial fibrillation should be based on the $CHADS_2$-VASC score. The choice of anticoagulation (warfarin or a novel oral anticoagulant) should be individualized for each patient.

INTRODUCTION

Heart failure (HF) is a growing public health concern. The aging population and advancements in medical therapies have led to the increased prevalence of HF. Recent survey data from the American Heart Association estimated that at least 5.1 million American adults have HF.[1] Worldwide, approximately 23 million people are thought to have HF.[2] Additionally, the economic burden of HF is significant. By 2030, the total direct medical costs of HF in the United States are projected to exceed $50 billion,[3] with an average lifetime expenditure of more than $100,000 per patient.[4]

Despite the use of interventions that improve outcomes in HF (resynchronization therapy and neurohormonal modulation with β-blockers, renin-angiotensin inhibitors, and aldosterone antagonism),

mortality is still substantial. Nearly half of the patients with HF will die within 5 years of diagnosis.[5] A significant contribution to the overall mortality in HF is the predisposition of these patients to experience stroke and thromboembolic disease.

This review focuses on the role of anticoagulation in patients with HF. The epidemiology and pathogenesis of embolic stroke in HF will be discussed. In addition, we review the outcomes data available for anticoagulation in patients with HF.

EPIDEMIOLOGY OF STROKE IN HEART FAILURE

Patients with HF have higher rates of thromboembolic events compared with the general population

Disclosure: Advisory Board for Philips Medical Imaging (R.M. Lang).
Section of Cardiology, Department of Medicine, University of Chicago Medicine, University of Chicago, 5841 South Maryland Avenue, MC5084, Chicago, IL 60637, USA
* Corresponding author.
E-mail address: rlang@medicine.bsd.uchicago.edu

Cardiol Clin 34 (2016) 215–224
http://dx.doi.org/10.1016/j.ccl.2015.11.001
0733-8651/16/$ – see front matter © 2016 Elsevier Inc. All rights reserved.

(**Fig. 1**). Several studies lend insight into the risk HF poses for stroke.

In a large Danish prospective study of 51,553 adults between the ages of 50 and 64 years who were followed for 14 years, 1239 patients with incident HF (and no concomitant atrial fibrillation) were identified. In the initial 30 days following the diagnosis of HF, patients experienced a greater risk for death (Hazard Ratio [HR] 42.8) or the composite of death and stroke (HR 38.4) compared with patients without HF. At more than 6 months after the diagnosis of HF, the risk for death or death and stroke remained elevated (HR 4.9 and 4.0, respectively). When adjusted for previous use of vitamin K antagonists, gender, and systolic blood pressure, HF continued to pose a greater risk for death (HR 2.9), death and stroke (HR 2.3), and ischemic stroke (HR 3.2) compared with patients without HF.[6]

In the Rotterdam study, 7546 patients aged 55 years or older without a history of stroke were followed for an average of 9.7 years. A total of 1014 patients developed HF, whereas strokes occurred in 827 patients (470 ischemic, 75 hemorrhagic, and 282 unclassified). In the first 30 days after the diagnosis of HF, an increased risk for ischemic stroke was observed (HR 4.6) even after adjusting for a number of risk factors, including age, gender, smoking, diabetes, ankle-brachial index, hypertension, use of antithrombotics, presence of atrial fibrillation, or history of myocardial infarction (MI). After 6 months, unlike what was observed in the Danish study, HF did not confer additional risk for stroke compared with patients without HF.[7]

Older community-based studies also have demonstrated the impact of HF on stroke. In the initial cohort from the Framingham Heart Study, composed of 5184 adults aged 30 to 62 years for which 24-year follow-up data are available, the relative risk (adjusted for age, systolic blood pressure, cholesterol, and smoking) for having an ischemic stroke in patients with HF was 2.7 for men and 2.1 for women.[8] In the Olmsted County Study of 630 patients with incident HF, a significant relative risk (17.4) for ischemic stroke was noted when compared with the general population in the first 30 days after the diagnosis of HF. The risk for ischemic stroke between patients with and without HF did not equalize at 5 years.[9]

Population and community-based studies often rely on diagnosis coding and lack complete information on left ventricular ejection fraction (LVEF) as it pertains to stroke. Analyses of several trials have shed light on the impact of LVEF and stroke incidence in patients with HF.

In a retrospective analysis of the SOLVD trial (6378 patients), the overall incidence of thromboembolic events (stroke, pulmonary embolism, and peripheral embolism) in patients with LV dysfunction (mean LVEF 27%) in sinus rhythm was 1.8% in men and 2.4% in women. In a multivariate analysis, a decrease in LVEF (per 10% intervals) remained an independent predictor of thromboembolic events in women but not in men.[10]

The SCD-HeFT trial also demonstrated a similar incidence of thromboembolism in patients with HF. When 2114 patients with New York Heart Association (NYHA) functional class II or III (mean LVEF 25%) and in sinus rhythm were examined for a median follow-up of 46 months, the annual risk of thromboembolism was approximately 1% per year.[11]

Similarly, when the V-HeFT I and II cohorts (1446 men with a mean LVEF or 29%) were examined retrospectively after a follow-up period of approximately 2.5 years, the incidence of all

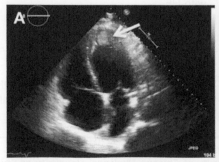
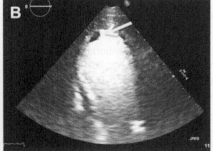

Fig. 1. (*A*) A 70-year-old man with a history nonischemic cardiomyopathy presented with acute decompensated HF. Transthoracic echocardiography demonstrated apical thrombus (*arrow*). (*B*) A 61-year-old man with a history of ischemic cardiomyopathy and acute lymphocytic leukemia presented in septic shock. Hospital course was complicated by left frontal ischemic stroke. Contrast transthoracic echocardiography demonstrated apical thrombus (*arrow*).

thromboembolic events was estimated at 2.4 per 100 patient-years. Atrial fibrillation was not associated with increased rates of thromboembolic events in this study.[12]

A well-recognized complication after acute MI is left ventricular dysfunction. After a mean follow-up of 42 months in 2231 patients with MI who developed LV dysfunction (mean LVEF 31%), 103 patients experienced a stroke. Of these patients with stroke, most experienced an ischemic (96%) as opposed to a hemorrhagic event. The 5-year rate of stroke in this study was 8.1% (which corresponded to 1.5% per patient-year). Moreover, for each 5% reduction in LVEF, there was an 18% increase in the risk of stroke.[13]

Less is known about the risk for stroke in patients with HF with preserved ejection fraction (HFpEF). Two studies suggest that the risk for stroke in patients with HFpEF is not diminished. In the I-PRESERVE study, which compared the effects of irbesartan versus placebo in patients with HFpEF (defined as NYHA functional class II-IV and LVEF >45%), the annual risk of stroke was 0.93% per year (79 strokes in 2061 patients during a mean follow-up period of 49.5 months).[14] The CHARM investigators analyzed outcomes for 7599 patients who ranged from NYHA functional class II-IV with severely reduced to normal LVEF.

This study showed that although there was greater all-cause mortality in patients with LVEF of 22% or less compared with patients with LVEF greater than 52%, this was not due to the combined endpoint of fatal or nonfatal strokes. After adjusting for a variety of risk factors including age, gender, NYHA class, diabetes, smoking, atrial fibrillation, and blood pressure, the HR per 10% reduction in LVEF was 0.95 (confidence interval [CI] 0.83–1.09).[15]

PATHOGENESIS OF STROKE IN HEART FAILURE

The pathogenesis of stroke in HF is multifactorial, with changes occurring at the molecular level in addition to abnormalities in blood flow dynamics. Many studies have investigated the pathophysiology in hopes of better understanding the mechanisms of cardioembolic stroke[16] (**Fig. 2**).

Named after the prominent German physician, Rudolph Virchow, the triad of endothelial (and endocardial) dysfunction, hypercoagulable state, and stasis of blood flow has been implicated in cardioembolic stroke. Endothelial dysfunction, although often associated with arterial and venous thrombus, has been shown to play an important role in HF. Normal endothelial function allows for

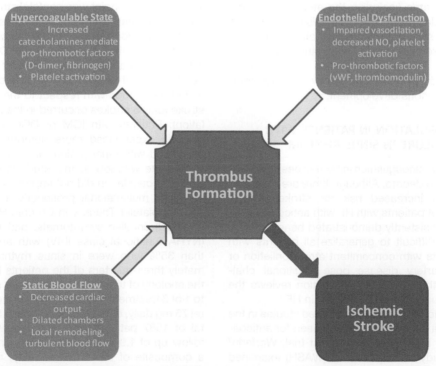

Fig. 2. Pathogenesis of stroke in HF. Hypercoagulable state, endothelial dysfunction, and static blood flow can lead to thrombus formation and subsequently ischemic stroke. vWF, von Willebrand Factor.

release of nitric oxide, thus mitigating static blood flow by promoting vasodilation and platelet inhibition. Decreased endothelium-mediated vasodilation has been observed in patients with HF and shown to be an independent predictor of death and hospitalization.[17] Additionally, several pro-thrombotic biomarkers released in response to endothelial damage are elevated in patients with HF. Most notably, compared with healthy controls, higher levels of von Willebrand factor (vWF) and thrombomodulin have been demonstrated in both acute and chronic HF.[18]

Beyond endothelial dysfunction leading to a milieu favorable for thrombus development, HF leads to an inherent hypercoagulable state. Although there is overlap in the molecular cascade resultant from endothelial dysfunction, other pro-thrombotic factors mediated by neuroendocrine activation are present in patients with HF. Notably, elevated concentrations of D-dimer (a fibrin degradation product) and fibrinogen are seen in patients with HF.[19,20] Elevated levels of catecholamines (particularly norepinephrine) are thought to mediate the cross-talk between these prothrombotic factors (and others) and the coagulation cascade in HF.[16]

HF resulting in poor contractility and low cardiac output leads to static blood flow. This in turn leads to endothelial dysfunction and facilitates a hyper-coagulable state. In addition, compensatory dilation of the atria (including the atrial appendage) and ventricles results in local stasis that increases the propensity of thrombus formation.[21] In addition, local remodeling, including aneurysmal segments or regional wall-motion abnormalities, further leads to static blood flow and increased risk for thrombus development.[22]

ANTICOAGULATION IN PATIENTS WITH HEART FAILURE IN SINUS RHYTHM

The role of anticoagulation in HF has been the subject of much debate. Although there are data linking HF to increased risk for stroke, routine treatment of patients with HF with anticoagulation has not consistently demonstrated benefit. Moreover, it is difficult to generalize all patients with HF. Patients with concomitant atrial fibrillation or coronary artery disease pose additional challenges to the clinician. This section reviews the data surrounding anticoagulation in HF.

Four major randomized controlled studies in the modern era have addressed the need for anticoagulation in HF (Table 1). The first trial, Warfarin/Aspirin Study in Heart Failure (WASH) examined 279 patients (mostly in the United Kingdom) who were randomized to no antithrombotic therapy,

aspirin (300 mg/d), or warfarin (international normalized ratio [INR] goal 2.0–3.0). All patients had an LVEF less than 35%. Most patients in the study were in sinus rhythm with only 6% in atrial fibrillation. The primary outcome was death, nonfatal MI, and nonfatal stroke, and the mean follow-up time was 27 months. There was no significant difference in the primary outcome among the 3 groups; this was also true when analysis was performed in patients in sinus rhythm. There were a total of 4 strokes (2 each in the patient arms who received no antithrombotic therapy or aspirin); the absence of strokes in the warfarin group was not statistically significant. Notably, the aspirin group had a higher rate of all-cause hospitalization ($P < .05$) compared with other groups; an exploratory analysis suggested this was due to worsening HF.[23]

A similar European study examining antithrombotic therapy in patients with HF in sinus rhythm also concluded there was no benefit with anticoagulation. The Heart Failure Long-term Antithrombotic Study (HELAS) enrolled 197 patients with an LVEF less than 35%, all in sinus rhythm. Patients were stratified according to etiology of HF, with 115 patients diagnosed with ischemic cardiomyopathy (ICM) and 82 patients with dilated cardiomyopathy (DCM). The ICM group received either aspirin 325 mg daily or warfarin, whereas the DCM group received warfarin or placebo. The primary endpoint was nonfatal stroke, peripheral or pulmonary embolism, MI, rehospitalization, HF exacerbation, or death; the follow-up period was 2 years. Although patients with DCM treated with warfarin had the lowest endpoint occurrence per 100 patient-years, there was no difference in any of the groups with respect to the endpoint of stroke (only 5 strokes occurred in the study population). Patients with ICM or DCM treated with warfarin experienced more hemorrhagic events compared with other patient groups. Overall, the stroke rate was low in this study and treatment with anticoagulation did not improve outcomes.[24]

A large, multinational, prospective trial, Warfarin and Antiplatelet Therapy in Chronic Heart Failure (WATCH) enrolled symptomatic patients with HF (NYHA functional class II-IV) with an LVEF less than 35% who were in sinus rhythm. Approximately three-quarters of the patients had ICM as the etiology of their HF. Patients were randomized to 1 of 3 treatment arms: aspirin 162 mg, clopidogrel 75 mg daily, or warfarin (INR goal 2.5–3.0). A total of 1587 patients were enrolled with a mean follow-up of 1.9 years. The primary endpoint was a composite of all-cause mortality, nonfatal MI, and nonfatal stroke. Comparisons between warfarin and aspirin and clopidogrel and aspirin

Table 1
Summary of 4 major randomized trials of treating patients with heart failure (in sinus rhythm) with anticoagulation

Trial	No. of Patients	Randomization	Primary Outcome	Follow-up Period	Results	Comments
WASH (2004)	279 (LVEF<35%)	1. No therapy 2. ASA (300 mg/d) 3. Warfarin	Death, nonfatal MI, nonfatal stroke	27 mo	No difference in outcomes	More hospitalization in ASA group, more bleeding in Warfarin group
HELAS (2006)	197 (LVEF<35%)	ICM: ASA (325 mg/d) or Warfarin DCM: Warfarin or Placebo	Nonfatal stroke, peripheral or pulmonary embolism, MI, rehospitalization, HF exacerbation, death	2 y	No difference in stroke outcomes	More bleeding in Warfarin group
WATCH (2009)	1587 (LVEF<35%)	1. ASA (162 mg/d) 2. Clopidogrel (75 mg/d) 3. Warfarin	All-cause mortality, nonfatal MI, and nonfatal stroke	1.9 y	Lower stroke rate in Warfarin vs ASA and Warfarin vs Clopidogrel	More bleeding in Warfarin vs Clopidogrel but not Warfarin vs ASA
WARCEF (2012)	2305 (LVEF<35%)	1. ASA (325 mg/d) 2. Warfarin	Ischemic stroke, intracerebral hemorrhage, or all-cause death	3.5 y	Lower stroke rate in Warfarin vs ASA	More bleeding in Warfarin group

Abbreviations: ASA, aspirin; DCM, dilated cardiomyopathy; HF, heart failure; ICM, ischemic cardiomyopathy; LVEF, left ventricular ejection fraction; MI, myocardial infarction.

showed no difference in occurrence of the primary endpoint. There was a combined total of 21 strokes (9, 11, and 1 in the aspirin, clopidogrel, and warfarin arms, respectively). The reduced incidence of stroke between warfarin and aspirin and warfarin and clopidogrel was statistically significant ($P < .01$). Major bleeding episodes were more common in patients treated with warfarin compared with clopidogrel ($P < .01$) but not when warfarin was compared with aspirin ($P = .22$). Taken together, although warfarin was superior to aspirin for the prevention of stroke, the increased rates of bleeding suggest that widespread use of warfarin is not without risk.[25]

The most comprehensive study to date, Warfarin and Aspirin in Patients with Heart Failure and Sinus Rhythm (WARCEF), followed 2305 patients with HF for a mean of 3.5 years. Notably, patients in this trial were treated with modern HF therapies. All patients had an LVEF less than 35% and fewer than 4% of the patients were in atrial fibrillation. Ischemic cardiomyopathy comprised approximately 40% of patients. Patients were randomized to receive aspirin 325 mg daily or warfarin (INR goal 2.0–3.5). The primary outcome was ischemic stroke, intracerebral hemorrhage, or all-cause death. More than one-quarter of the patients developed the composite primary endpoint (no difference between the treatment arms). There were 29 ischemic strokes in the warfarin group (0.72 events/100 patient-years) and 55 ischemic strokes in the aspirin group (1.36 events/100 patient-years); this difference between stroke rates in the 2 arms was significant ($P < .01$). Similar to the WATCH study, patients treated with warfarin experienced more bleeding in the WARCEF trial; there were 1.78 events of major hemorrhage per 100 patient-years with warfarin versus 0.87 events per 100 patient-years with aspirin ($P < .001$).[26] Subgroup analysis showed improvement in the primary endpoint (and less bleeding) in patients younger than 60 years.[27] In addition, in a post hoc analysis, it was found that risk stratification with bleeding scores, such as HAS-BLED or OBRI, can help identify patients who are at lower risk for bleeding (and may benefit from anticoagulation).[28]

A recent meta-analysis pooled data from the WASH, HELAS, WATCH, and WARCEF studies. Of the 2644 studies screened, only the 4 aforementioned trials met the inclusion criteria for this meta-analysis. When aspirin was compared with warfarin, there was no difference in the endpoint of all-cause mortality (n = 3701, Relative Risk (RR) = 1.00, $P = .94$). When aspirin or warfarin was compared with no anticoagulation, there was a nonsignificant increase in all-cause mortality (n = 295,

RR = 1.33, $P = .22$ and n = 324, RR = 1.21, $P = .41$, respectively).[29]

Overall, the meta-analysis found a 41% relative risk reduction (RRR) for all strokes and a 52% RRR for ischemic strokes (n = 3368, $P < .01$) with the use of warfarin over aspirin. Compared with aspirin, treatment with warfarin resulted in a number needed to treat (NNT) of 58 to prevent any stroke, and the NNT to prevent an ischemic stroke was 49.[29] However, the risk for major hemorrhage resulted in a number needed to harm of 34,[30] again suggesting the widespread use of anticoagulation with warfarin in patients with HF in sinus rhythm carries significant risk.

ANTICOAGULATION IN PATIENTS WITH HEART FAILURE IN ATRIAL FIBRILLATION

It is well known that patients with atrial fibrillation are at higher risk for systemic embolism, with ischemic stroke as the most common manifestation of embolization. Similarly, anticoagulation with aspirin, warfarin, or a novel oral anticoagulant (direct thrombin inhibitor or factor Xa inhibitor) has been shown in multiple meta-analyses to decrease the risk for stroke.[31–33]

HF and atrial fibrillation are intimately intertwined. In a study of 65,807 patients with newly diagnosed ischemic stroke without a prior history of atrial fibrillation, it was shown that a baseline history of HF (after age $\geq$75 years) was the strongest predictor, in a multivariate analysis, for the development of atrial fibrillation.[34] Similarly, the prevalence of atrial fibrillation increases from approximately 10% to nearly 50% with worsening NYHA functional class I to IV.[35]

Patients with HF and atrial fibrillation are thought to have rates of ischemic stroke predominantly determined by the presence of other risk factors, as determined by the CHADS$_2$-VASC score. In a recent analysis of 3487 patients with HF and atrial fibrillation, the degree of LV dysfunction or NYHA functional class were not independently associated with embolic events. Additionally, the risk for embolic events was similar in patients with LV dysfunction and those with HFpEF. Overall, the biggest risk factors remained those identified by the CHADS$_2$-VASC score.[36] Accordingly, the decision to anticoagulate patients with both HF and atrial fibrillation is typically based on the CHADS$_2$-VASC score.

Increasingly common are patients with HF, atrial fibrillation, and vascular disease (either coronary artery disease or peripheral arterial disease). In a large study of 37,464 patients with HF and vascular disease who were followed for a mean of 3 years, 20.8% had prevalent atrial fibrillation and 17.1% developed incident atrial fibrillation. When aspirin or clopidogrel was added to warfarin therapy in these patients, there was no reduction in the risk for thromboembolism, but bleeding rates were significantly higher (HR 1.31).[37]

NOVEL ORAL ANTICOAGULATION IN HEART FAILURE

There is much excitement surrounding the development of novel oral anticoagulants (NOAC) for the treatment of atrial fibrillation and veno-thromboembolic disease. These direct thrombin and factor Xa inhibitors allow for effective anticoagulation without the routine monitoring required with warfarin administration. There are compelling data demonstrating the efficacy and safety of NOACs when compared with warfarin for the prevention of stroke in patients with atrial fibrillation.[38] Similarly, the treatment of veno-thromboembolic disease with NOACs compared with warfarin has been shown to be efficacious and safe.[39,40]

Although novel oral anticoagulants have not been studied for the prevention of stroke in patients with HF in sinus rhythm, data are available demonstrating the efficacy of NOACs in patients with HF in atrial fibrillation.[41]

Dabigatran, a direct thrombin inhibitor, was approved for stroke prophylaxis in patients with atrial fibrillation based on the RE-LY trial. More than 25% of patients in this study had symptomatic HF. The patients with HF treated with dabigatran had rates of stroke noninferior to those treated with warfarin.[42]

The factor Xa inhibitor, apixaban, was also shown to be noninferior compared with warfarin in the prevention of stroke in atrial fibrillation in the ARISTOTLE study. More than one-third of the patients in this study had HF (symptomatic or LVEF $\leq$40%) and the risk for stroke was not different for patients treated with apixaban or warfarin.[43] In the AVERROES study, patients deemed unsuitable to receive warfarin for atrial fibrillation received apixaban or aspirin; apixaban was shown to be superior for the prevention of stroke. Subgroup analysis in patients with LVEF less than 35% also confirmed these findings.[44]

Moreover, the ROCKET-AF study showed that rivaroxaban, another factor Xa inhibitor, was non-inferior compared with warfarin in the prevention of stroke in atrial fibrillation. Most patients (63%) in the study had HF (either LVEF $\leq$40% or by symptoms), and outcomes in this subgroup did not differ from the overall study findings.[45]

Overall, in patients with HF with atrial fibrillation, treatment with a novel oral anticoagulant is effective and safe for the prevention of stroke.

The advent of reversal agents for NOACs will make these medications more attractive for greater use.

GUIDELINES FOR ANTICOAGULATION IN HEART FAILURE

Guidelines from a variety of societies reflect the body of evidence that exits on the topic of anticoagulation in HF (**Table 2**).

The most recent HF guidelines published in 2013 from American College of Cardiology (ACC)/American Heart Association (AHA) argue against anticoagulation (class III recommendation) for patients with chronic HF with LV systolic dysfunction without atrial fibrillation, a prior thromboembolic event, or a cardioembolic source (such as LV thrombus). These guidelines reference the aforementioned randomized controlled trials as the predominant source for this recommendation.

Furthermore, the ACC/AHA guidelines offer a class I indication for anticoagulation in patients with HF with atrial fibrillation and an additional risk factor for cardioembolic stroke as defined by the CHADS$_2$-VASC score. The choice of anticoagulation (warfarin vs novel oral anticoagulants) should be individualized to each patient. In patients with HF and atrial fibrillation but without an additional risk factor, these guidelines issue a class IIa indication for anticoagulation.[46]

Similarly, the European Society for Cardiology (ESC) published guidelines for HF in 2012. For patients with HF and atrial fibrillation, the CHADS$_2$-VASC determines recommendations for anticoagulation. For patients with a CHADS$_2$-VASC score of 0, no anticoagulation is recommended. For a CHADS$_2$-VASC score of $\geq$1, guidelines recommend anticoagulation (class I indication). There is no recommendation for anticoagulation in patients with HF not in atrial fibrillation.[47]

The ESC Heart Failure Association Working Group on Thrombosis published a consensus document in 2012 that reiterates the ESC recommendations on anticoagulation. The document recommends proactive monitoring for AF and other comorbidities in patients with HF. If AF is documented, the benefits for anticoagulation should be weighed against the risk for bleeding through assessment of CHADS$_2$-VASC and HAS-BLED scores. Additionally, if concomitant coronary disease is present with HF, the combination of antiplatelet therapy and anticoagulation should not continue past 12 months from the acute coronary event. For patients in sinus rhythm with HF, the authors recommend against routine anticoagulation; however, certain patient populations (previous stroke, intracardiac thrombus, right HF

Table 2
Society-based guidelines of treating patients with heart failure with anticoagulation

Guideline	Recommendations
ACC/AHA (2013)	• Do not recommend anticoagulation in patients with HF in sinus rhythm • Recommend anticoagulation in patients with HF with atrial fibrillation and additional risk factors for a cardioembolic event (defined by $CHADS_2$-VASC score) • Reasonable to consider anticoagulation in patients with HF with atrial fibrillation without additional risk factors for a cardioembolic event
ESC (2012)	• For patients with HF with atrial fibrillation, calculate $CHADS_2$-VASC score; for score of 0, do not recommend anticoagulation; for score ≥ 1, recommend anticoagulation
ESC Heart Failure Working Group on Thrombosis (2012)	• Recommend proactive monitoring for presence of atrial fibrillation in patients with HF • When atrial fibrillation present in patients with HF, weigh benefits of anticoagulation vs risks of bleeding • Routine anticoagulation of patients with HF in sinus rhythm not recommended but consider in certain patient groups (previous stroke, intracardiac thrombus, right heart failure with pulmonary hypertension)
HFSA (2010)	• Recommend anticoagulation in patients with HF with atrial fibrillation • Recommend anticoagulation in patients with HF with ischemic cardiomyopathy and large recent anterior MI • Recommend anticoagulation in patients with HF with LV thrombus

Abbreviations: ACC, American College of Cardiology; AHA, American Heart Association; ESC, European Society of Cardiology; HF, heart failure; HFSA, Heart Failure Society of America; LV, left ventricle; MI, myocardial infarction.

with pulmonary hypertension) may benefit, and an individualized approach should be taken.[22]

The Heart Failure Society of America (HFSA) issued guidelines in 2010. Similar to others, these guidelines recommend anticoagulation for patients with HF and atrial fibrillation. Additionally, anticoagulation is recommended in patients with ischemic cardiomyopathy and recent large anterior MI or recent MI with documented LV thrombus. Patients with nonischemic cardiomyopathy and LV thrombus also should receive anticoagulation.[48]

SUMMARY

Although patients with HF and sinus rhythm are at risk for stroke, randomized controlled trials largely have failed to demonstrate consistent benefit with anticoagulation. The risk for bleeding, hospitalization, and other adverse cardiac events often negates any incremental benefit derived from anticoagulation. As such, recent guidelines avoid recommending anticoagulation for patients with HF in sinus rhythm. When patients with HF develop AF, however, there is little doubt that anticoagulation is important. Similarly, those with previous cardioembolic stroke or LV thrombus benefit from anticoagulation. As the HF population continues to grow, it is imperative we identify additional populations at greater risk for stroke and

investigate therapies that will ultimately improve outcomes and survival.

REFERENCES

1. Go AS, Mozaffarian D, Roger VL, et al. Heart disease and stroke statistics–2014 update: a report from the American Heart Association. Circulation 2014;129:e28–292.
2. McMurray JJ, Petrie MC, Murdoch DR, et al. Clinical epidemiology of heart failure: public and private health burden. Eur Heart J 1998;19(Suppl P):P9–16.
3. Heidenreich PA, Albert NM, Allen LA, et al. Forecasting the impact of heart failure in the United States: a policy statement from the American Heart Association. Circ Heart Fail 2013;6:606–19.
4. Dunlay SM, Shah ND, Shi Q, et al. Lifetime costs of medical care after heart failure diagnosis. Circ Cardiovasc Qual Outcomes 2011;4:68–75.
5. Roger VL, Weston SA, Redfield MM, et al. Trends in heart failure incidence and survival in a community-based population. JAMA 2004;292:344–50.
6. Lip GY, Rasmussen LH, Skjøth F, et al. Stroke and mortality in patients with incident heart failure: the Diet, Cancer and Health (DCH) cohort study. BMJ Open 2012;2(4).
7. Alberts VP, Bos MJ, Koudstaal P, et al. Heart failure and the risk of stroke: the Rotterdam Study. Eur J Epidemiol 2010;25:807–12.

8. Kannel WB, Wolf PA, Verter J. Manifestations of coronary disease predisposing to stroke. The Framingham study. JAMA 1983;250:2942–6.

9. Witt BJ, Brown RD, Jacobsen SJ, et al. Ischemic stroke after heart failure: a community-based study. Am Heart J 2006;152:102–9.

10. Dries DL, Rosenberg YD, Waclawiw MA, et al. Ejection fraction and risk of thromboembolic events in patients with systolic dysfunction and sinus rhythm: evidence for gender differences in the studies of left ventricular dysfunction trials. J Am Coll Cardiol 1997;29:1074–80.

11. Freudenberger RS, Hellkamp AS, Halperin JL, et al. Risk of thromboembolism in heart failure: an analysis from the Sudden Cardiac Death in Heart Failure Trial (SCD-HeFT). Circulation 2007;115:2637–41.

12. Dunkman WB, Johnson GR, Carson PE, et al. Incidence of thromboembolic events in congestive heart failure. The V-HeFT VA Cooperative Studies Group. Circulation 1993;87:VI94–101.

13. Loh E, Sutton MS, Wun CC, et al. Ventricular dysfunction and the risk of stroke after myocardial infarction. N Engl J Med 1997;336:251–7.

14. Massie BM, Carson PE, McMurray JJ, et al. Irbesartan in patients with heart failure and preserved ejection fraction. N Engl J Med 2008;359:2456–67.

15. Solomon SD, Anavekar N, Skali H, et al. Influence of ejection fraction on cardiovascular outcomes in a broad spectrum of heart failure patients. Circulation 2005;112:3738–44.

16. Zannad F, Stough WG, Regnault V, et al. Is thrombosis a contributor to heart failure pathophysiology? Possible mechanisms, therapeutic opportunities, and clinical investigation challenges. Int J Cardiol 2013;167:1772–82.

17. Fischer D, Rossa S, Landmesser U, et al. Endothelial dysfunction in patients with chronic heart failure is independently associated with increased incidence of hospitalization, cardiac transplantation, or death. Eur Heart J 2005;26:65–9.

18. Chong AY, Freestone B, Patel J, et al. Endothelial activation, dysfunction, and damage in congestive heart failure and the relation to brain natriuretic peptide and outcomes. Am J Cardiol 2006;97:671–5.

19. Sbarouni E, Bradshaw A, Andreotti F, et al. Relationship between hemostatic abnormalities and neuroendocrine activity in heart failure. Am Heart J 1994;127:607–12.

20. Yamamoto K, Ikeda U, Furuhashi K, et al. The coagulation system is activated in idiopathic cardiomyopathy. J Am Coll Cardiol 1995;25:1634–40.

21. Freudenberger RS, Schumaecker MM, Homma S. What is the appropriate approach to prevention of thromboembolism in heart failure? Thromb Haemost 2010;103:489–95.

22. Lip GY, Piotrponikowski P, Andreotti F, et al. Thromboembolism and antithrombotic therapy for heart failure in sinus rhythm: an executive summary of a joint consensus document from the ESC Heart Failure Association and the ESC Working Group on Thrombosis. Thromb Haemost 2012;108:1009–22.

23. Cleland JG, Findlay I, Jafri S, et al. The Warfarin/Aspirin Study in Heart failure (WASH): a randomized trial comparing antithrombotic strategies for patients with heart failure. Am Heart J 2004;148:157–64.

24. Cokkinos DV, Haralabopoulos GC, Kostis JB, et al. Efficacy of antithrombotic therapy in chronic heart failure: the HELAS study. Eur J Heart Fail 2006;8: 428–32.

25. Massie BM, Collins JF, Ammon SE, et al. Randomized trial of warfarin, aspirin, and clopidogrel in patients with chronic heart failure: the Warfarin and Antiplatelet Therapy in Chronic Heart Failure (WATCH) trial. Circulation 2009;119:1616–24.

26. Homma S, Thompson JL, Pullicino PM, et al. Warfarin and aspirin in patients with heart failure and sinus rhythm. N Engl J Med 2012;366:1859–69.

27. Homma S, Thompson JL, Sanford AR, et al. Benefit of warfarin compared with aspirin in patients with heart failure in sinus rhythm: a subgroup analysis of WARCEF, a randomized controlled trial. Circ Heart Fail 2013;6:988–97.

28. Ye S, Cheng B, Lip GY, et al. Bleeding risk and antithrombotic strategy in patients with sinus rhythm and heart failure with reduced ejection fraction treated with warfarin or aspirin. Am J Cardiol 2015; 116(6):904–12.

29. Hopper I, Skiba M, Krum H. Updated meta-analysis on antithrombotic therapy in patients with heart failure and sinus rhythm. Eur J Heart Fail 2013;15:69–78.

30. Kumar G, Goyal MK. Warfarin versus aspirin for prevention of stroke in heart failure: a meta-analysis of randomized controlled clinical trials. J Stroke Cerebrovasc Dis 2013;22:1279–87.

31. Friberg L, Rosenqvist M, Lip GY. Net clinical benefit of warfarin in patients with atrial fibrillation: a report from the Swedish atrial fibrillation cohort study. Circulation 2012;125:2298–307.

32. Agarwal S, Hachamovitch R, Menon V. Current trial-associated outcomes with warfarin in prevention of stroke in patients with nonvalvular atrial fibrillation: a meta-analysis. Arch Intern Med 2012;172:623–31 [discussion: 631–3].

33. Dentali F, Riva N, Crowther M, et al. Efficacy and safety of the novel oral anticoagulants in atrial fibrillation: a systematic review and meta-analysis of the literature. Circulation 2012;126:2381–91.

34. Fauchier L, Clementy N, Pelade C, et al. Patients with ischemic stroke and incident atrial fibrillation: a nationwide cohort study. Stroke 2015;46(9): 2432–7.

35. Maisel WH, Stevenson LW. Atrial fibrillation in heart failure: epidemiology, pathophysiology, and rationale for therapy. Am J Cardiol 2003;91:2D–8D.

36. Sandhu RK, Hohnloser SH, Pfeffer MA, et al. Relationship between degree of left ventricular dysfunction, symptom status, and risk of embolic events in patients with atrial fibrillation and heart failure. Stroke 2015;46:667–72.

37. Lamberts M, Lip GY, Ruwald MH, et al. Antithrombotic treatment in patients with heart failure and associated atrial fibrillation and vascular disease: a nationwide cohort study. J Am Coll Cardiol 2014; 63:2689–98.

38. Ruff CT, Giugliano RP, Braunwald E, et al. Comparison of the efficacy and safety of new oral anticoagulants with warfarin in patients with atrial fibrillation: a meta-analysis of randomised trials. Lancet 2014; 383:955–62.

39. van der Hulle T, Kooiman J, den Exter PL, et al. Effectiveness and safety of novel oral anticoagulants as compared with vitamin K antagonists in the treatment of acute symptomatic venous thromboembolism: a systematic review and meta-analysis. J Thromb Haemost 2014;12:320–8.

40. Gómez-Outes A, Terleira-Fernández AI, Lecumberri R, et al. Direct oral anticoagulants in the treatment of acute venous thromboembolism: a systematic review and meta-analysis. Thromb Res 2014;134:774–82.

41. Shantsila E, Lip GY. Use of novel oral anticoagulants in patients with heart failure. Curr Treat Options Cardiovasc Med 2014;16:285.

42. Connolly SJ, Ezekowitz MD, Yusuf S, et al. Dabigatran versus warfarin in patients with atrial fibrillation. N Engl J Med 2009;361:1139–51.

43. Granger CB, Alexander JH, McMurray JJ, et al. Apixaban versus warfarin in patients with atrial fibrillation. N Engl J Med 2011;365:981–92.

44. Connolly SJ, Eikelboom J, Joyner C, et al. Apixaban in patients with atrial fibrillation. N Engl J Med 2011; 364:806–17.

45. Patel MR, Mahaffey KW, Garg J, et al. Rivaroxaban versus warfarin in nonvalvular atrial fibrillation. N Engl J Med 2011;365:883–91.

46. Yancy CW, Jessup M, Bozkurt B, et al. 2013 ACCF/AHA guideline for the management of heart failure: a report of the American College of Cardiology Foundation/American Heart Association Task Force on Practice Guidelines. J Am Coll Cardiol 2013;62: e147–239.

47. McMurray JJ, Adamopoulos S, Anker SD, et al. ESC guidelines for the diagnosis and treatment of acute and chronic heart failure 2012: the task force for the diagnosis and treatment of acute and chronic heart failure 2012 of the European Society of Cardiology. Developed in collaboration with the Heart Failure Association (HFA) of the ESC. Eur Heart J 2012; 33:1787–847.

48. Lindenfeld J, Albert NM, Boehmer JP, et al. HFSA 2010 comprehensive heart failure practice guideline. J Card Fail 2010;16:e1–194.

Atrial Septal Defects and Cardioembolic Strokes

Michelle Leppert, MD, MBA[a], Sharon N. Poisson, MD[a], John D. Carroll, MD[b],*

KEYWORDS

- Stroke • Paradoxic embolism • Atrial septal defect • Atrial fibrillation • Shunt

KEY POINTS

- Cardioembolic strokes associated with ASDs principally occur with 2 mechanisms. The first is paradoxic embolism involving a venous-based source of thrombus that then becomes an embolism, which may subsequently pass through the ASD by right-to-left shunting, finally causing a cardioembolic stroke. The second is atrial fibrillation that can complicate the course of patients with ASDs, especially as they age. Atrial fibrillation may lead to cardioembolic strokes primarily with the embolism arising from a left atrial appendage thrombus.
- Surgical and transcatheter closure of ASDs will prevent paradoxic embolism but not cardioembolic strokes from atrial fibrillation.
- Surgical and transcatheter closure is recommended if a patient has a stroke from a presumed paradoxic embolism even if the defect is anatomically small with no signs of cardiac volume overload. Early closure in children or adolescents mitigates the risk of developing tachyarrhythmias later in life, whereas patients after ASD closure as an adult continue to carry a high risk of developing tachyarrhythmias.
- Patients with ASDs, both before and after closure, need to have cardiac rhythm monitoring to detect occult paroxysmal atrial fibrillation that would necessitate anticoagulation to prevent cardioembolic stroke. Prolonged, continuous heart rhythm monitoring is more effective at detecting occult atrial fibrillation than short-term monitors.
- Routine full anticoagulation is not recommended as primary prevention of ischemic stroke for all patients with ASDs. An individualized approach is recommended and is principally influenced by the presence or absence of any degree of atrial fibrillation; any indication of venous thromboembolism, such as deep venous thrombophlebitis and pulmonary embolism; and a history of prior systemic embolism, including that causing ischemic stroke.

BACKGROUND AND PRESENTATION

Atrial septal defects (ASDs) are the third most common type of congenital heart disease with an estimated incidence of 56 per 100,000 live births (**Fig. 1**).[1] There are 3 major types of ASDs: ostium secundum, ostium primum, and sinus venosus defect, accounting for 65% to 75%, 20%, and 5% to 10% of all ASDs, respectively. Females compose 65% to 75% of patients with secundum ASDs, but the sex distribution is equal for ostium primum and sinus venosus ASDs.[2] Ostium secundum defect, the most common of the 3, is located in the region of the fossa ovalis and considered a true defect of the atrial septum. It is not confluent with other structures and is most associated with paradoxic embolus leading to stroke.

Dr J.D. Carroll is a member of the RESPECT steering committee, a clinical trial of the Amplatzer PFO Occluder (NCT00465270), and receives compensation for his work from the sponsor, St. Jude Medical, USA.

[a] Department of Neurology, University of Colorado Denver, 12631 East 17th Avenue, Aurora, CO 80045, USA;
[b] Department of Medicine University of Colorado Denver, Leprino Office Building on Anschutz Medical Campus, 12401 East 17th Avenue, Room 524, Mail Stop B132, Aurora, CO 80045, USA
* Corresponding author.
E-mail address: John.carroll@ucdenver.edu

Cardiol Clin 34 (2016) 225–230
http://dx.doi.org/10.1016/j.ccl.2015.12.004
0733-8651/16/$ – see front matter © 2016 Elsevier Inc. All rights reserved.

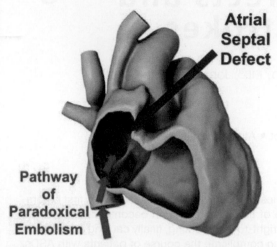

Atrial Septal Defect

Pathway of Paradoxical Embolism

Fig. 1. This graphic shows a cutaway revealing the right atrial side of an ostium secundum ASD. The black arrow identifies the defect. The red arrows show a portion of the pathway of a paradoxic embolism. The embolism travels up the inferior vena cava and in the right atrium can cross the defect during transient right-to-left blood flow that may occur with all ASDs.

Many patients remain asymptomatic throughout most of childhood, although most will become symptomatic at some point in their lives. ASDs account for 25% to 30% of congenital heart disease cases diagnosed in adulthood.[3] Patients most commonly become symptomatic in the second decade of life with exercise intolerance in the form of exertional dyspnea or fatigue as the most common presenting symptom.[4] Atrial fibrillation or flutter is a common complication of ASD and reflects age-related atrial dilation but is uncommon before 40 years of age.[5] Occasionally, a paradoxic embolus or transient ischemic attack may be the first presentation of an ASD. Less commonly, decompensated right heart failure will occur, typically in older patients in association with substantial tricuspid regurgitation.

EPIDEMIOLOGY OF STROKE IN ATRIAL SEPTAL DEFECTS

The overall incidence of strokes due to ASD remains unknown. There has been strong evidence that patent foramen ovale (PFO) and atrial septal aneurysm is strongly associated with strokes in patients younger than 55 years.[6] This finding is consistent with ASDs whereby the average age of stroke onset was 55 years compared with 68 years in risk-matched controls without ASDs.[6]

The risk of stroke seems to be elevated in all patients with ASDs, regardless of closure status. However, there is evidence that patients

with unclosed defects have an increased risk compared with closed defects. Hoffman and colleagues[7] analyzed aggregated European and Canadian databases with a total of 23,253 patients with congenital heart disease excluding patients who had an isolated patent foramen ovale. With a mean follow-up of 36.4 years, they found that the prevalence of stroke was 4.0% in an open ASD and 1.4% in a closed atrial or ventricular defect, compared with 2.0% in all patients with congenital heart disease. Another cohort of Danish patients with ASDs similarly found that the risk of stroke was higher both before and after closure compared with a control population without ASD.[8] The hazard ratio for stroke with an open ASD was 2.6 compared with 1.8 five years after ASD closure, while adjusting for cardiovascular risk factors.

CAUSES OF STROKE

There are 2 major mechanisms of embolic strokes in patients with ASDs, either due to paradoxic emboli or related to atrial fibrillation. Given the high incidence of atrial fibrillation in ASD, as well as the limitations in proving paradoxic emboli, it is difficult to separate the mechanism of strokes in studies and to quantify the number of strokes related to each.

The most obvious cause of stroke in ASD is a paradoxic embolism. Although most patients with ASDs have left-to-right shunts, intermittent right-to-left shunting may occur during transient increases in right heart pressure allowing for the introduction of paradoxic embolus to the brain. Regardless of the size of ASD, paradoxic embolism from any source, including peripheral venous thromboses, atrial arrhythmias, unfiltered intravenous infusions, or indwelling venous catheters, is a risk.[9–11] In fact, one study found that of patients with ASDs undergoing repair, those with a paradoxic embolism had significantly smaller left-to-right shunt (mean ratio of pulmonary blood flow to systemic blood flow Qp:Qs of 1.4) compared with patients with ASD without a paradoxic emboli (mean Qp:Qs of 1.95).[12] These results are likely confounded by the fact that larger defects likely present with symptoms requiring repair. However, it does draw attention to the fact that even small defects are likely at risk of paradoxic emboli.

Another major risk factor for ischemic stroke in patients with ASDs is the development of atrial fibrillation, which can lead to embolism arising most often from a thrombus in the left atrial appendage. The prevalence of atrial tachyarrhythmia was found to be approximately 19% in a large cohort of adult patients with ASDs, which is 4-fold higher than the general population.[13] The development of atrial fibrillation or flutter is an age-related reflection of atrial dilation, which in patients with ASDs older than 60 years can be as high as 50%.[14] Indeed, although paradoxic embolus in the absence of atrial fibrillation was the culprit of strokes in younger patients with ASDs, atrial fibrillation is the major risk factor for stroke in older patients with ASDs regardless of closure status. In patients with stroke after ASD closure, 77% had atrial fibrillation, compared with only 28% of those with stroke before ASD closure, suggesting that other mechanisms were more likely, such as possible paradoxic embolus.

MANAGEMENT
Closure

ASDs can be closed for multiple reasons, including for symptomatic relief, treatment of cardiac volume overload, and prevention of paradoxic embolism, including stroke. Importantly, closure does not prevent cardioembolic strokes due to atrial fibrillation. In general, guidelines for medical versus interventional/surgical management of ASD are based on the size of the defect and current or predicted complications of it (**Table 1**). There is strong evidence that closure of larger defects with findings of right ventricular volume overload can help to prevent long-term complications, such as atrial fibrillation, congestive heart failure, and pulmonary hypertension (class I, level B evidence). Conversely, the indication for closure of a small ASD (<5 mm) with no evidence of right ventricular volume overload is somewhat controversial. In general, these small defects are not thought to change clinical course or outcome, and closure is not recommended. If, however, paradoxic embolism is suspected, such as that leading to stroke, consensus opinion is that closure is reasonable,[15] despite little evidence to support this. Because of the multiple possible causes of stroke in patients with ASDs, it is difficult to distinguish the effect of ASD closure on prevention of paradoxic embolism.

Closure of ASD in older adults does not seem to greatly impact the development of atrial tachyarrhythmias. In a Danish cohort study, 1168 patients with ASD were followed for a median of 9.6 years.[8] They found that the prevalence of atrial fibrillation was no different between the group of patients with ASD closure versus those with unclosed ASDs. Of the patients who did have their ASD closed, 14% had stroke, which was not significantly different from the 15% of those with unclosed ASD, although many of the strokes

occurred before closure, with a rate of only 5% after closure occurred. As discussed earlier, about two-thirds of patients with stroke after ASD closure had concurrent atrial fibrillation, as compared with less than one-third of those with stroke before closure, which suggests that paradoxic embolus was likely responsible for more strokes before closure. Interestingly, half of the strokes in the group with unclosed ASDs had atrial fibrillation, a significantly higher proportion compared with those with stroke before their ASD closure. This finding likely reflects the increased incidence of atrial fibrillation with increasing age, as median age at closure was 45 years. Overall, this study found that patients with ASDs, with or without closure, had a two-fold higher risk of stroke as compared with an age- and sex-matched comparison cohort. Those patients who did not have atrial fibrillation at the time of closure had an 11% incidence of atrial fibrillation in the 10 years after closure, which was 5-fold higher than the age- and sex-matched cohort without ASDs, suggesting that the risk of stroke after ASD closure is mediated by atrial fibrillation. This finding was reproduced in a Canadian cohort of patients with ASD closure, with mean age of 41 years; they found that most patients with prevalent atrial tachyarrhythmias at the time of closure did not revert back to sinus rhythm, but in addition 8% of those aged at least 40 years at the time of closure developed new-onset atrial tachyarrhythmias over a 3.8-year follow-up period.[5]

In contrast with closure in older cohorts, when ASD closure is performed early in life, the risk of developing atrial tachyarrhythmias is low. A study of long-term outcomes after surgical repair of secundum ASDs found that those with repair before 25 years of age had normal long-term survival, as compared with increased mortality in those who had closure after the age of 25.[16] Another single-center study with a follow-up of more than 20 years similarly demonstrated a low incidence of atrial tachyarrhythmias after ASD closure; stroke, right heart failure, and pulmonary hypertension did not occur.[17] One complicating factor is that spontaneous closure does occur in very young patients with small defects. A study of 200 consecutive patients younger than 14 years with isolated secundum ASDs found a 56% rate of spontaneous closure in patients with an initial defect size of 4 to 5 mm, 30% in 6 to 7 mm, and 12% in 8 to 10 mm. It is notable that age at diagnosis was clearly associated with ASD closure, with 39% of patients diagnosed at less than 1 year of age with spontaneous closure, compared with 19% diagnosed at age greater than 1 year.[18]

Table 1
ACC/AHA's 2008 guidelines for adults with CHD: management strategies for ASD

Recommendations for medical therapy	Class I
	1. Cardioversion after appropriate anticoagulation is recommended to attempt restoration of the sinus rhythm if atrial fibrillation occurs (level of evidence: A).
	2. Rate control and anticoagulation are recommended if sinus rhythm cannot be maintained by medical or interventional means (level of evidence: A).
Recommendations for interventional and surgical therapy	Class I
	1. Closure of an ASD either percutaneously or surgically is indicated for right atrial and RV enlargement with or without symptoms (level of evidence: B).
	2. A sinus venosus, coronary sinus, or primum ASD should be repaired surgically rather than by percutaneous closure (level of evidence: B).
	3. Surgeons with training and expertise in CHD should perform operations for various ASD closures (level of evidence: C).
	Class IIa
	1. Surgical closure of secundum ASD is reasonable when concomitant surgical repair/replacement of a tricuspid valve is considered or when the anatomy of the defect precludes the use of percutaneous device (level of evidence: C).
	2. Closure of an ASD, either percutaneously or surgically, is reasonable in the presence of
	a. Paradoxic embolism (level of evidence: C)
	b. Documented orthodeoxia-platypnea (level of evidence: B)
	Class IIb
	1. Closure of an ASD, either percutaneously or surgically, may be considered in the presence of net left-to-right shunting, pulmonary artery pressure less than two-thirds systemic levels, PVR less than two-thirds systemic vascular resistance, or when responsive to either pulmonary vasodilator therapy or test occlusion of the defect (patients should be treated in conjunction with providers who have expertise in the management of pulmonary hypertensive syndromes) (level of evidence: C).
	2. Concomitant maze procedure may be considered for intermittent or chronic atrial tachyarrhythmias in adults with ASDs (level of evidence: C).
	Class III
	1. Patients with severe irreversible PAH and no evidence of a left-to-right shunt should not undergo ASD closure (level of evidence: B).

Abbreviations: ACC, American College of Cardiology; AHA, American Heart Association; CHD, congenital heart disease; PAH, pulmonary artery hypertension; PVR, pulmonary vascular resistance; RV right ventricle.

As described earlier, the current guidelines from the American College of Cardiology/American Heart Association suggest that closure of an ASD either percutaneously or surgically is reasonable in the presence of paradoxic embolism. Early closure in children or adolescents may be beneficial as primary prevention of stroke, both related to paradoxic embolism as well as to tachyarrhythmias. Closure in adults may not completely mitigate stroke risk, as the risk is still high of developing atrial tachyarrhythmias. In general, closure of small ASDs (<5 mm) in asymptomatic older adults without evidence of right ventricular volume overload for the primary prevention of strokes should be avoided. Cardiac rhythm monitoring to detect paroxysmal atrial fibrillation should be performed both before and after closure, and anticoagulation treatment should be considered when atrial fibrillation is found. In general, prolonged continuous heart rhythm monitoring is more effective at detecting silent atrial fibrillation than short-term monitoring. For patients with pre-existing atrial fibrillation undergoing surgery, ablation before closure should be considered, given that access to the left atrium is restricted following closure.[19]

Medical Management

Similarly to the surgical/percutaneous management of ASDs, medical management should be based on symptoms and predicted complications. Patients with asymptomatic small shunts may not require any medical therapy, but patients should be followed closely for symptoms or for evidence of complications. Guidelines recommend annual follow-up to look for signs of pulmonary arterial hypertension, atrial arrhythmias, right or left ventricular dysfunction, or coexisting valvular or other cardiac lesions (level C).[15]

Monitoring for atrial tachyarrhythmias is the most important study for determining the need for medical therapy, regardless of closure status. Patients with atrial fibrillation should be treated in accordance with guidelines for atrial fibrillation, including rate control and anticoagulation.[15]

Patients with ASD and ischemic stroke should be closely evaluated for other risk factors for stroke and treated aggressively with secondary stroke prophylaxis according to guidelines.[20] In those with cryptogenic stroke and ASDs, closure may be reasonable (see earlier section); but the best medical therapy remains unclear. There are currently no trials of medical management of ASDs and stroke, but some information can be extrapolated from the experience in research of PFO and cryptogenic stroke. A meta-analysis of 5 retrospective studies evaluating management in patients with PFO and cryptogenic stroke found that over an average follow-up of 36 months, patients treated with warfarin had a 2.5% estimated annual recurrent cerebral ischemic event rate, compared with 5.1% in those treated with antiplatelet therapy.[21] However, in the PFO in Cryptogenic Stoke Study, there was a trend toward improvements in 2-year rates of recurrent stroke or death in the group with PFO and cryptogenic stroke treated with warfarin (9.5%) versus those treated with aspirin (17.9%), although this difference was not statistically significant, and there was not adequate statistical power to test the superiority of warfarin over aspirin.[22] Current secondary stroke prevention guidelines are that there are insufficient data to establish whether anticoagulation is equivalent or superior to aspirin for secondary stroke prevention in patients with PFO.[20]

Hence, routine full anticoagulation is not currently recommended as the primary prevention of stroke in all patients with ASDs. Instead, an individualized approach is recommended taking into account the presence or absence of atrial fibrillation; any indication of venous thromboembolism, such as deep venous thrombophlebitis and pulmonary embolism; and a history of prior systemic embolism, including that causing ischemic stroke.

REFERENCES

1. Hoffman JL, Kaplan S. The incidence of congenital heart disease. J Am Coll Cardiol 2002;39:1890–900.
2. Webb G, Gatzoulis MA. Atrial septal defects in the adult. Circulation 2006;114:1645–53.
3. Lindsey JB, Hillis LD. Clinical update: atrial septal defects in adults. Lancet 2007;369:1244–6.
4. Geva T, Martins JD, Wald RM. Atrial septal defects. Lancet 2014;383:1921–32.
5. Gatzoulis MA, Freeman MA, Siu SC, et al. Atrial arrhythmia after surgical closure of atrial septal defects in adults. N Engl J Med 1999;340:839–46.
6. Overell JR, Bone I, Lees KR. Interatrial septal abnormalities and stroke. Neurology 2000;888:1172–9.
7. Hoffman A, Chockalingam P, Balint OH, et al. Cerebrovascular accidents in adult patients with congenital heart disease. Heart 2010;96:1223–6.
8. Nyboe C, Olsen MS, Nielsen-Kudsk JE, et al. Atrial fibrillation and stroke in adult patients with atrial septal defect and long-term effect of closure. Heart 2015;101:706–11.
9. Loscalzo J. Paradoxical embolism: clinical presentation, diagnostic strategies, and therapeutic options. Am Heart J 1986;112:141–5.
10. Silka MJ, Rice MJ. Paradoxic embolism due to altered hemodynamic sequencing following transvenous pacing. Pacing Clin Electrophysiol 1991;14:499–503.
11. Ward R, Jones D, Haponik EF. Paradoxical embolism. An underrecognized problem. Chest 1995;108:549–58.
12. Bannan A, Shen R, Silvestry FE, et al. Characteristics of adult patients with atrial septal defects presenting with paradoxical embolism. Catheterization and Card Inter 2009;74:1066–9.
13. Bouchardy J, Therrien J, Pilote L, et al. Atrial arrhythmias in adults with congenital heart disease. Circulation 2009;120:1679–86.
14. John Sutton MG, Tajik AJ, McGoon DC. ASD in patients ages 60 years or older: operative results and long-term postoperative follow up. Circulation 1981;64:402–9.
15. Warnes CA, Williams RG, Bashore TM, et al. ACC/AHA 2008 guidelines for the management of adults with congenital heart disease: a report of the American College of Cardiology/American Heart

Association task force on practice guidelines. J Am Coll Cardiol 2008;52:e143–263.

16. Murphy JG, Gersh BJ, McGoon MD, et al. Long-term outcome after surgical repair of isolated atrial septal defect: follow-up at 27 to 32 years. N Engl J Med 1990;323:1645–50.

17. Roos-Hesselink JW, Meiboom FJ, Spitaels SE, et al. Excellent survival and low incidence of arrhythmias, stroke and heart failure long-term after surgical ASD closure at young age: a prospective follow-up study of 21-33 years. Eur Heart J 2003;24:190–7.

18. Hanslik A, Prospisil U, Salzer-Muhar U, et al. Predictors of spontaneous closure of isolated secundum atrial septal defect in children: a longitudinal study. Pediatrics 2006;11:1560–5.

19. Yap SC. Atrial fibrillation and stroke after atrial septal defect closure. Is earlier closure warranted? Heart 2015;101:661–2.

20. Kernan WN, Ovbiagele B, Black HR, et al. Guidelines for the prevention of stroke in patients with stroke and transient ischemic attack: a guideline for healthcare professionals from the American Heart Association/American Stroke Association. Stroke 2014;45:2160–236.

21. Orgera MA, O'Malley PG, Taylor AJ. Secondary prevention of cerebral ischemia in patent foramen ovale: systematic review and meta-analysis. South Med J 2001;94:699–703.

22. Homma S, Sacco RL, Di Tullio MR, et al. Effect of medical treatment in stroke patients with patent foramen ovale. Circulation 2002;105:2625–31.

Patent Foramen Ovale
Stroke and Device Closure

Hussam S. Suradi, MD, FACC, FSCAI[a,b,*], Ziyad M. Hijazi, MD, MPH, FACC, MSCAI, FAHA[c]

KEYWORDS

- Patent foramen ovale • Cryptogenic stroke • Closure devices • Shunt closure
- Transient ischemic attack

KEY POINTS

- This article reviews the association between patent foramen ovale (PFO) and cryptogenic stroke, as well as the evidence for PFO device closure in the current era.
- PFO is a common finding in healthy adults and has long been implicated in cryptogenic stroke. The pathogenesis is hypothesized to be caused by microemboli gaining access to the systemic circulation via a PFO.
- Treatment options proposed include medical therapy and PFO closure.
- Despite numerous studies and several randomized trials, much debate persists regarding the efficacy of PFO closure in reducing the risk of recurrent stroke in cryptogenic stroke patients.

INTRODUCTION

Stroke is among the leading causes of mortality and serious long-term disability.[1] Approximately 795,000 strokes occur annually in the United States, with around 185,000 being recurrent attacks.[2] Around 25% of all strokes are cryptogenic and this reaches approximately 50% in the younger age group.[3] A stroke is considered cryptogenic when no apparent cause is detected. Patent foramen ovale (PFO) is a common finding in healthy adults (10%–26%) and has been long implicated in cryptogenic stroke. Its prevalence in patients with cryptogenic stroke has been found to be higher (up to 66%) when compared with patients with stroke from known causes. Paradoxic embolism was first identified as a stroke mechanism by Connheim in 1877.[4] The pathogenesis is hypothesized to be caused by microemboli or neurohormones that would otherwise be filtered by the lungs, escaping into the systemic circulation via the atrial communication, especially during Valsalva maneuver. Despite medical therapy, the rate of stroke recurrence in patients with PFO is estimated to be up to 25% within a 4-year period.[5]

Treatment options that have been proposed are, among others, medical therapy, PFO closure, or both. Currently, controversy exists regarding the optimal treatment approach with some investigators advocating device closure, whereas others recommend a less invasive approach until more supportive data are available. This article reviews the association between PFO and cryptogenic stroke, the risk of recurrence of stroke in patients with PFO, and the current evidence for PFO device closure.

ASSOCIATION BETWEEN PATENT FORAMEN OVALE AND CRYPTOGENIC STROKE

The most common indication for PFO closure in practice today is for prevention of recurrent stroke

---

Disclosure: Dr Z.M. Hijazi is a consultant to Occlutech, a device manufacturing company.
[a] Interventional Cardiology, Rush Center for Congenital & Structural Heart Disease, Rush University Medical Center, 1653 W Congress Pkwy, Chicago, IL 60612, USA; [b] Department of Cardiology, St Mary Medical Center, Community HealthCare Network, Community Healthcare System, 1500 South Lake Park Avenue, Suite 110, Hobart, IN 46342, USA; [c] Sidra Cardiovascular Center of Excellence, Sidra Medical & Research Center, Al Corniche street, P.O. Box 26999, Doha, Qatar
* Corresponding author. Interventional Cardiology, Rush University Medical Center, Chicago, IL 60612.
E-mail address: Hussam_suradi@rush.edu

Cardiol Clin 34 (2016) 231–240
http://dx.doi.org/10.1016/j.ccl.2015.12.001
0733-8651/16/$

or transient ischemic attack (TIA) in patients with a first or second neurologic event. This practice is built on a large database demonstrating an association between PFO and cryptogenic stroke both in the younger and older patient populations. This association began with observational studies that demonstrated a significantly higher prevalence of PFO in patients with cryptogenic stroke compared to non-stroke patients or patients who have stroke with known cause.[6,7] This relationship becomes even more apparent when evaluating patients younger than 55 years. Despite the findings, these observational studies had small sample sizes and hence were not powered to draw concrete conclusions. Subsequent meta-analysis of these case-control studies showed that cryptogenic stroke in patients younger than 55 years are 6 times more likely to have a PFO compared with patients with a known cause of stroke.[8] Similarly, a more recent meta-analysis reproduced the association between PFO and cryptogenic stroke.[9] Bearing in mind the limitations of meta-analysis studies, prospective studies were subsequently conducted.

Among these prospective studies, 2 major studies looked into the association of PFO and first cryptogenic stroke: (1) the Stroke Prevention: Assessment of Risk in a Community (SPARC)[10] study and (2) the Northern Manhattan Study (NOMAS).[11] These studies surveyed a total cohort of 1685 participants with mean age of 68 years. In both studies, PFO was not found to be an independent risk for stroke. These studies failed to achieve statistical significance and they were considered flawed because they focused on older populations in which secondary stroke risk factors would be expected to be present. Furthermore, the modest number of PFO and strokes encountered limited the power of the studies to make any meaningful association between PFO and cryptogenic stroke.

The main hypothesis of the potential mechanism of stroke caused by a PFO is paradoxical embolism of venous emboli to the arterial circulation. Physicians are frequently challenged to confidently identify the stroke mechanism in a patient with cryptogenic stroke in whom a PFO is detected. Given the high prevalence of PFO in the general population, the possibility of having an incidental PFO that has no relationship to the index stroke should be taken into consideration. Other stroke mechanisms may be present in patients with cryptogenic stroke, even in the presence of a PFO. These mechanisms include lacunar disease, undetected atrial fibrillation, hypercoagulable states, and aortic atheroma. Both clinical evidence and Bayes theorem can be used to assist in determining the probability of having detected a PFO as an innocent bystander in patients with cryptogenic stroke.

This methodology was used in a systematic analysis of several case-control studies in which the probability of PFO in cryptogenic stroke being incidental was found to be 20% (16%–25%) in patients younger than 55 years but 48% (34%–66%) in patients older than 55 years, reflecting the importance of conventional vascular risk factors in causing stroke in the older population.[12] Combining clinical and statistical analysis of this type maybe helpful in guiding treatment decisions. Box 1 lists clinical features that suggest causal relationship between PFO and cryptogenic stroke.

PATENT FORAMEN OVALE AND RECURRENT STROKE

Following a first cryptogenic stroke, the risk of stroke recurrence in subjects with PFO is modestly increased, with an average annualized risk across studies of approximately 2%.[13,14] This estimated risk, however, has varied across different studies. For example, in a small study, 33 subjects with apparent PFO-related paradoxical embolism were followed for 18 months without any therapy. The annualized 1-year recurrent event rate was found to be 16%.[15] Despite this, subsequent prospective follow-up studies in subjects with stroke have failed to demonstrate a significant increase in risk of recurrent stroke in subjects with PFO compared with non-PFO controls. In the Patent Foramen Ovale in Cryptogenic Stroke Study (PICSS), the 2-year incidence of recurrent stroke or death in 603 subjects with recent stroke was 14.8% in PFO subjects and 15.4% in those without a PFO.[5] In the Risk of Paradoxic Embolism (RoPE) study, subjects who were the most likely to have stroke-related PFOs were those with the lower recurrence risk compared with non-PFO related events (2% vs 20%), this finding suggested a

---

Box 1
Clinical features suggesting causal relationship of patent foramen ovale and cryptogenic stroke

Sedentary period before onset

Valsalva before onset

Absence of stroke risk factors (eg, hypertension, diabetes, hyperlipidemia)

Atrial septal aneurysm

Large PFO size

Shunt at rest

Hypercoagulable state

Embolic stroke topography

more benign natural history of the former with respect to recurrence.[16]

Certain high-risk PFO features have been implicated in stroke recurrence. The strongest predictor is the coexistence of an interatrial septal aneurysm (ASA).[17] ASA is a hypermobile atrial septum extending at least 10 mm into the right or left atrium; it occurs in 2.2% of the general population and is associated with a PFO in 56% of cases.[18] In a study of 581 subjects with cryptogenic stroke treated with medical therapy, the risk of recurrent stroke in a 4-year period was 15.2% in subjects with concurrent PFO and ASA compared with 4.2% in subjects with neither of these abnormalities.[14] The exact mechanism by which ASA potentiates the risk of stroke remains unclear. Hypotheses include alteration of flow through the PFO by the hypermobile septum or serving as a nidus for thrombus formation.

An additional potential predictor is the anatomic size of the PFO. Several studies have found that stroke subjects with PFOs have a greater frequency of right-to-left shunting at rest compared with controls. Larger PFOs may be associated with greater volumes of paradoxical blood flow, allowing the passage of larger clots into the systemic circulation. This hypothesis was studied by Schuchlenz and colleagues,[19] who looked into 121 stroke subjects and 123 control subjects with the conclusion that the diameter of the PFO was an independent risk factor for recurrent strokes. More specifically, they found that a PFO diameter larger than 4 mm was associated with an odds ratio of 3.4 for TIA, 12 for stroke, and 27 for 2 or more strokes. In contrast, a PFO diameter less than 4 mm was associated only with TIA having an odds ratio of 1.5. Stone and colleagues[20] further examined the PFO characteristics in regard to the degree of shunting. They followed 34 subjects for 21 months and divided the population into large and small shunts based on the agitated saline injections in a peripheral intravenous line. In the large shunt group (≥20 microbubbles), 31% of the subjects had a recurrent adverse neurologic event compared with none in the small shunt group (≥3 but <20 microbubbles). Nevertheless, not all studies have replicated the finding that size of PFO and degree of shunting correlate with degree of stroke risk.

The presence of hypercoagulable state may also potentially increase the risk of stroke by favoring the formation of venous thromboemboli. In a small study, 72 subjects with PFO-associated systemic thrombotic events who were referred for transcatheter device closure were tested for thrombophilia, which was present in 28% of this population. Before device closure, 80% of subjects with thrombophilia had more than 1 thromboembolic event compared with 10% of subjects without thrombophilia. After device closure of PFO, recurrent cerebrovascular events after 20 months of follow-up were 4%, with no significant difference between the groups.[21] This finding further supports the paradoxical embolism hypothesis.

MANAGEMENT OPTIONS FOR PATENT FORAMEN OVALE IN STROKE
Medical Therapy

The optimal medical therapy for patients with a PFO who have had a cryptogenic stroke or TIA is not established. Traditional medical therapy has been either antithrombotic with warfarin or antiplatelet with aspirin, dipyridamole, or clopidogrel. Thus far, novel oral anticoagulants have not been studied in this patient population. In general, studies to date do not favor a specific medical therapy compared with another in subjects with cryptogenic stroke. The PICSS trial was the only study to compare aspirin and warfarin for the treatment of subjects with cryptogenic stroke and PFO (a substudy of the Warfarin vs Aspirin in Recurrent Stroke Study).[5] There was no statistically significant difference between the effects of aspirin and warfarin on the risk of subsequent stroke or death among this subject population. However, PICSS was designed primarily as a prognostic study and was underpowered to demonstrate a treatment effect.

In practice, most patients are treated initially with antiplatelet therapy rather than anticoagulation. The rationale for antiplatelet therapy comes from clinical data showing that the risk of recurrent stroke among patients with PFO and cryptogenic stroke is so low that the risk of hemorrhage from anticoagulation likely outweighs the potential benefits. A clear exception is patients with evidence of deep venous thrombosis in which anticoagulation is indicated. The challenges and problems associated with warfarin therapy are well known. Contemporary warfarin therapy is associated with a 5% to 15% incidence of intracranial hemorrhage[22] and, at any given time, less than one-fourth of patients on warfarin are actually in the desired therapeutic range.[23]

Surgical Therapy

Surgical closure of PFO was once viewed as the gold standard therapy for PFO closure before the advent of percutaneous closure devices. The major disadvantage of surgical closure is that it involves thoracotomy and cardiopulmonary bypass. There have been no randomized trials comparing surgical closure versus medical therapy or percutaneous closure; however, there have been several observational studies with variable reported results.[24,25] The annual event rate for recurrent cerebral ischemia has ranged in different series from 7% to 14% at 1 to 2 years. One report showed that the overall freedom from an ischemic episode of 91 subjects (mean age 44 years) with 1 or more cerebrovascular ischemic events who underwent surgical PFO closure was 93% and 83% at 1 and 4 years, respectively.[25] These events were driven mainly by TIAs with no strokes reported. Transesophageal echocardiography (TEE) showed that the closure was intact in all subjects, suggesting that paradoxical embolization was not the cause for the recurrent events. In another series of 28 subjects with cryptogenic stroke who underwent surgical closure of PFO, there were 4 recurrent neurologic events at a mean follow-up of 19 months that occurred only in subjects older than 45 years of age, underlining the importance of age for subject selection.[24]

Although perioperative mortality is small, significant morbidity maybe encountered, including atrial arrhythmias, pericardial effusion, repeat surgery for bleeding source exploration, and wound infection. Incomplete closure of the PFO had been observed as well. One study, using postoperative TEE, showed that 73% of subjects had residual shunting after surgical closure.[26] This might have occurred due to suboptimal apposition of the septum primum and secundum or inadvertent puncture of the septum primum during surgery. For all these reasons, and the availability of less invasive closure modalities, surgical closure of PFO for the prevention of recurrent neurologic events is currently rarely performed.

Percutaneous Therapy

During the past 4 decades, there has been great technological advancement and refinement of percutaneous techniques for PFO closure.[27,28] The relative ease and efficacy of the currently used transcatheter approaches for PFO closure have caused a rapid adoption of these procedures. Numerous observational studies have shown reduction in the recurrence of neurologic events in subjects with a history of cerebral events who subsequently underwent PFO closure.[29–32] Windecker and colleagues[29] compared the risk of recurrence in 308 subjects with cryptogenic stroke and PFO who were treated medically or underwent PFO closure. After 4-year follow-up, subjects with more than 1 cerebrovascular event at baseline and those with no residual right-to-left shunt were at lower risk for a recurrent stroke or TIA after PFO closure compared with medically

treated subjects (7.3% vs 33.2%; $P = .01$ and 6.5% vs 22.2%; $P = .04$, respectively). In a recent meta-analysis of comparative and single-arm observational studies evaluating closure with various devices or medical therapy, closure was associated with an 86% reduction in the risk of recurrent stroke and 76% reduction in the risk of recurrent TIA.[33] Despite the results noted in this analysis, several limitations of observational data were concerning because these studies enrolled different subject populations with different indications, used a variety of closure devices and medical therapies, and used different methods for endpoint adjudication.

In the United States, the Food and Drug Administration (FDA) granted Humanitarian Device Exemption (HDE) status to the CardioSeal device (NMT Medical, Boston, MA) in 2000 and the Amplatzer PFO occluder (St. Jude Medical, Inc, St. Paul, MN, USA) in 2002 for PFO closure. The subsequent excess number of implanted devices led to the withdrawal of HDE status for both devices in 2006. Currently, FDA approval for transcatheter PFO closure procedures does not exist.

Randomized Trials Evidence

One of the many shortcomings of comparative observational studies examining PFO closure versus medical management included in meta-analysis is failure to adjust for potential confounders; therefore, there was obvious need for randomized studies because they provide the best scientific evidence. The recent availability of randomized trial data refuting the efficacy of PFO closure in reducing the risk of recurrent stroke refueled the debate challenging the large quantity of observational evidence supporting its benefits. To date, 3 randomized clinical trials have evaluated whether PFO closure is superior to antithrombotic therapy alone in preventing recurrent stroke in subjects who have had a cryptogenic stroke or TIA. These trials are (1) the Evaluation of the STARFlex Septal Closure System in Patients with a Stroke or TIA due to the Possible Passage of a Clot of Unknown Origin Through a Patent Foramen Ovale (CLOSURE I) study (device made by the former NMT Medical, Boston, MA, USA), (2) the Randomized Evaluation of Recurrent Stroke Comparing Patent Foramen Ovale Closure to Established Current Standard of Care Treatment (RESPECT) trial, and (3) the Patent Foramen Ovale and Cryptogenic Embolism (PC) trial. **Table 1** summarizes the main characteristics and results of these trials.

First trial

The first trial to test the hypothesis that closure of PFO reduces the risk of recurrent stroke in a

Table 1
Main results of randomized clinical trials

	CLOSURE I	RESPECT	PC
Enrollment Period	Jun 2003–Oct 2008	Aug 2003–Dec 2011	Feb 2000–Feb 2009
Closure Device	STARFlex (NMT)	Amplatzer PFO occluder (St Jude)	Amplatzer PFO occluder (St Jude)
Number of Enrolled Subjects (Closure/Medical)	447/462	499/481	204/210
Mean follow-up period (Year)	2.0	2.6	4.0
Primary endpoint (Closure vs Medical)	5.5% vs 6.8%	1.85% vs 3.3%	3.45% vs 5.2%
Hazard ratio for closure vs medical treatment (95% CI)	0.78 (0.45–1.35)	0.49 (0.22–1.11)	0.63 (0.24–1.62)
Stroke (Closure vs Medical)	2.9 vs 3.1%	1.85 vs 3.3%	0.5% vs 2.4%
Closure Rate	86%	96%	94%
Atrial Fibrillation (Closure vs Medical)	5.75 vs 0.7%	3.05 vs 1.5%	2.95 vs 1.0%
Major Bleeding (Closure vs Medical)	2.65 vs 1.1%	0.4% vs 0.4%	3.9 vs 5.7%
Outcome	No difference in stroke & TIA rate	Reduced recurrent stroke in per-protocol & as- treated analyses in favor of closure	No difference in mortality, stroke, & TIA rate

prospective, randomized setting was the CLOSURE I study.[34] This study randomized 909 subjects between the ages of 18 to 60 with history of TIA or ischemic stroke to either percutaneous PFO closure with the STARFlex device plus antiplatelet therapy with aspirin and clopidogrel, or to medical therapy alone with aspirin, warfarin, or a combination of both. After 2-year follow-up, there was no statistically significant difference between the groups for primary endpoints of stroke or TIA; 5.5% in closure arm versus 6.8% in medical arm (hazard ratio [HR] 0.78, 95% CI 0.45–1.35, $P = .37$). Further, no differences were found comparing the per-protocol with intention-to-treat treatment modalities. Prespecified subgroup analysis did not demonstrate any increased benefit from closure in subgroups such as subjects with atrial septal aneurysm or substantial right-to-left shunt. Unexpectedly, potential alternative explanations for recurrent neurologic events, as opposed to PFO-mediated, were found in 80% of subjects. Procedural success was achieved in 89.4% of subjects with effective closure demonstrated in 86% of subjects at 6 months by TEE. The incidence of both vascular complications (3.2% vs 0%; $P<.001$) and atrial fibrillation (5.7% vs 0.7%; $P<.001$) were significantly higher in the PFO closure group.

CLOSURE I implied that PFO closure offered no significant benefit compared with medical therapy,

while carrying the potential to induce harm. However, the study was criticized for several reasons. First, the closure group demonstrated a suboptimal closure rate with 14% of subjects having significant residual right-to-left shunt at 6-months along with higher thrombotic and arrhythmogenic complications. These findings question the overall efficacy and safety of the STARFlex device (**Fig. 1**A) compared with contemporary devices.[35] In addition, the enrolled subjects may not have represented the true population with cryptogenic stroke because the rate of recurrent stroke among those randomized to receive device closure was nearly 4 times higher than that predicted by non-randomized studies, raising the suspicion that non-PFO related strokes were included in the study. Furthermore, significant number of subjects had other risk factors for stroke and less than two-thirds of the subjects had neuroimaging evidence of acute stroke. The inclusion of subjects with TIAs may have also undermined the study from the onset because it is difficult to distinguish a TIA from a complex migraine with a transient neurologic deficit. Another criticism of the study was the slow enrollment rate and the small number of cases performed by each site, potentially indicating that some of the vascular and other complications encountered were due to inexperienced operators in some of the centers. Finally, given the relatively short follow-up time, there remains

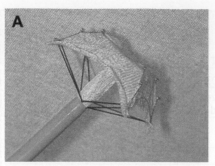 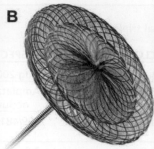 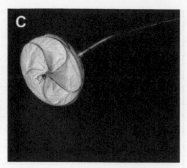

Fig. 1. PFO closure devices (A) STARFlex. (B) Amplatzer PFO occluder. (C) Gore septal occluder. ([A, C] *Courtesy of* W.L. Gore & Associates, Inc, Flagstaff, AZ; with permission; and [B] St. Jude Medical, Inc, St. Paul, MN; with permission. AMPLATZER and St. Jude Medical are trademarks of St. Jude Medical, Inc or its related companies.)

the possibility that the trial was not able to detect a benefit provided by device closure.

Second trial

The RESPECT trial was a randomized clinical trial investigating the safety and efficacy of transcatheter PFO closure using the Amplatzer PFO occluder (**Fig. 1**B) in the secondary prevention of recurrent cryptogenic stroke versus medical management, which could be either therapy with antiplatelets or anticoagulants.[36] RESPECT capitalized on several of the criticized trial design decisions that plagued CLOSURE I.

The trial enrolled 980 subjects with prior cryptogenic stroke and a PFO between the ages of 18 and 60 years. Primary endpoints were recurrence of stroke or death; lacunar strokes or TIAs were not included. Device implantation was attempted in 464 subjects. Atrial septal aneurysms were present in one-third of subjects. Procedural success was 96.1% and effective closure was achieved in 93.5% of subjects. One important distinction from CLOSURE I is the very low incidence of procedural complications, with no device-related thrombus formation or device embolization. Median follow-up time was 2.2 years (range, 0–8.1 years). There were fewer subject dropouts in the device group (n = 48) compared with the medical treatment group (n = 90). During follow-up, recurrent strokes occurred in 9 subjects in the PFO closure group compared with 16 events in the medical treatment group. Of the 9 subjects in the PFO closure group, 3 subjects suffered a recurrent stroke following randomization but before PFO device closure. As a consequence, the primary endpoint was not reached in the intention-to-treat analysis (relative risk reduction, 46.6%; P = .157), whereas the as-treated analysis (classifying subjects into treatment groups according to the treatment they actually received) was statistically significant (relative risk reduction, 72.7%; P = .007). Overall, the recurrent event rate was low; at 5 years, recurrent strokes

occurred in 2.21% of subjects compared with 6.4% in the medically treated subjects. Important findings of the study included 2 groups of subjects with PFO who benefited the most from PFO closure: subjects with substantial shunt size (recurrent event rate 0.8% for PFO closure vs 4.3% for medical management; HR 0.178, 95% CI 0.039–0.813), as well as subjects with atrial septal aneurysm (recurrent event rate 1.1% for PFO closure vs 5.3% for medical management; HR 0.187, 95% CI 0.04–0.867).

Third Trial

The PC trial is a European trial in which 414 subjects were randomized to either undergo closure of PFO using Amplatzer PFO occluder or to medical therapy.[37] Subjects had to be younger than 60 years of age, and strokes and TIAs were allowed as index events. The primary endpoints were a composite of death, stroke, TIA, or peripheral embolism. During a mean follow-up period of approximately 4 years, there was no significant difference in the composite outcome between the 2 treatment strategies (HR 0.63, 95% CI 0.24–1.62, P = .34). Similarly, there was no significant difference in the rates of individual endpoints, including stroke. These results were also consistent across various subgroups, with no evidence of interaction according to age, presence of atrial septal aneurysm, or prior cardiovascular event. Atrial fibrillation was noted in 2.9% of participants in the closure group compared with 1.0% in the medically treated arm (HR 3.15, 95% CI 0.64–15.6, P = .16).

Limitations of the Randomized Trials

Taken together, the results from the 3 randomized trials published to date have failed to demonstrate benefit of percutaneous closure over antithrombotic therapy. However, caution must be exercised in interpreting these trials. As previously discussed, several shortcomings of CLOSURE I are noteworthy and may have contributed to a null finding. All 3 trials were hampered considerably by slow enrollment and a protracted trial length, with the likelihood that the trials did not meet their expected outcome because of low numbers of enrolled subjects and lower than expected event rates. This lack of statistical power may have played a role in the observed null findings because large treatment effects were assumed and observed event rates were lower than anticipated, rendering trials more sensitive to potential bias. Moreover, follow-up of study subjects was likely too short to assess a significant difference in efficacy between the 2 treatment groups. Data from RESPECT showed that event rates in medical therapy versus device closure seemed to separate more after 2 years and continued to diverge at 5 years, suggesting that the postulated benefit may need more time to become apparent. Furthermore, the benefit of device closure noted in the as-treated analysis of RESPECT leaves open the possibility that this approach could be superior to medical therapy, particularly in patients with higher-risk PFO.

As previously discussed, a big concern with all the 3 trials was the lack of statistical power for the primary outcome; an ideal scenario in which a meta-analysis would provide more insight.

A recent meta-analysis of the 3 randomized trials that included 2303 subjects showed beneficial effects of device closure across all cohorts (intention-to-treat, per-protocol, and as-treated cohorts) with 33% to 39% reduction in the HR for a recurrent neurologic event, depending on the population analyzed.[38] The benefits became even more apparent with the pooled results from the RESPECT and PC trials in which only the Amplatzer device was used (46% to 58% reduction).[38] Therefore, it is very likely that the trials failed to meet their expected outcome because of the low numbers of enrolled subjects and low event rates encountered.

Management Approach for Cryptogenic Stroke and Patent Foramen Ovale

Because PFO is common in the general population, it may incidentally coexist in patients with cryptogenic stroke. This consideration should be borne in mind in the approach used to manage patients with cryptogenic ischemia who are found to have a PFO. The relative importance of paradoxical embolism as a potential mechanism for stroke in older patients is likely to be reduced given the higher prevalence of arterial atherosclerosis and atrial fibrillation in this population. Therefore, thorough assessment and exclusion of secondary

causes for stroke are keys to the decision-making regarding PFO closure. Similarly, thrombophilia as a cause of thromboembolism should be evaluated in the young patient when the cause of stroke remains unknown.

The RoPE study was designed with the goal to identify patient-specific factors that would predict the likelihood that a discovered PFO is related to an index stroke or affect the risk of recurrence.[16] Based on this meta-analysis of observational cohorts of cryptogenic stroke subjects, several factors associated with the detection of a PFO were identified, including younger age; the presence of a cortical stroke on neuroimaging; and the absence of diabetes, hypertension, smoking, and prior stroke or TIA (**Table 2**). These factors were incorporated into a 10-point RoPE score that estimates the probability of finding a PFO in cryptogenic stroke patients based on clinical characteristics. High RoPE scores identify younger patients without conventional vascular risk factors and with infarcts located superficially in the brain, features that are more likely to be embolic in nature. On the other hand, lower RoPE scores identify older patients with deep infarcts and multiple conventional risk factors. The probability of finding a PFO increases from 23% in cryptogenic stroke patients with RoPE scores of 0 to 3, to 73% in those with 9 or 10 points, corresponding to PFO-attributable fraction estimates of 0% to 88%, respectively. An interesting finding in this study is that the subjects who were the most likely to have stroke-related PFOs were also those with the lower recurrence risk, with an estimated 2-year risk of stroke or TIA

Table 2 Risk of paradoxical embolism score calculator	
Characteristics	**Points**
No history of hypertension	1
No history of diabetes	1
No history of stroke or TIA	1
Nonsmoker	1
Cortical infarct on imaging	1
Age (years)	
18–29	5
30–39	4
40–49	3
50–59	2
60–69	1
≥70	0

Maximum score (a patient <30 years with cortical infarct, no risk factors, or prior neurologic events).

Minimum score (a patient >70 years with deep infarct, presence of risk factors, and prior neurologic events).

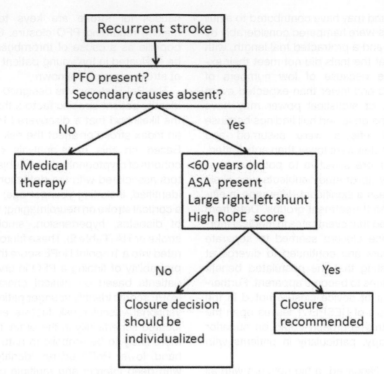

Fig. 2. Proposed approach of PFO closure in cryptogenic stroke.

recurrence of only 2% in subjects with a RoPE score of 9 or 10, suggesting that the natural history of PFO-related events is more benign than the other non-PFO–related stroke mechanisms with respect to recurrence. Although the RoPE score is not yet validated, it can be useful in risk stratification to identify the patients who are likely to benefit from PFO closure.

In addition to clinical findings, certain anatomic features associated with the PFO itself can potentially strengthen the presumption of paradoxic embolism, such as the presence of large magnitude of shunting or the presence of an atrial septal aneurysm, further supporting the decision to proceed with PFO closure (**Fig. 2** demonstrates proposed approach for PFO closure).

Ongoing Studies

Given the uncertainty and shortcomings of the randomized trials to date, further studies are needed regarding percutaneous PFO closure to prevent recurrent cryptogenic stroke. The GORE HELEX Septal Occluder for Patent Foramen Ovale Closure in Stroke Patients (Gore REDUCE) trial aims to demonstrate the reduction of recurrent stroke or imaging-confirmed TIA in subjects with a PFO and history of cryptogenic stroke or imaging-confirmed TIA. Participants were randomized to percutaneous device closure using Gore HELEX

or Gore Septal occluder device (W.L. Gore & Associates, Inc, Flagstaff, AZ, USA) versus medical therapy with antiplatelets alone using a 2:1 randomization scheme (**Fig. 1**C). Enrollment is complete and the scientific community is eagerly waiting for the results.

The Patent Foramen Ovale Closure or Anticoagulants versus Antiplatelet Therapy to Prevent Stroke Recurrence (CLOSE) trial aims to determine whether PFO closure or anticoagulant therapy is superior to antiplatelet therapy for the secondary prevention of stroke. Enrollment is complete; however, results are not available yet. The Device Closure versus Medical Therapy for Cryptogenic Stroke Patients with High-Risk Patent Foramen Ovale (DEFENSE-PFO) trial is an ongoing study that plans to randomize subjects with cryptogenic stroke and high-risk PFO features, defined as PFO size of greater than 2 mm, or presence of atrial septal aneurysm to receive Amplatzer device closure or standard medical therapy.

SUMMARY

The PFO-stroke field has dramatically evolved during the last decade; however, despite 3 trials, the debate of whether clinicians should close a PFO for recurrent stroke prevention is still going strong. It is a common perception among clinicians that there are no data to support PFO closure for secondary stroke prevention; however, as presented in this article, there are several findings that leave open the possibility that this approach could be superior to medical therapy in carefully selected patients. Currently, no device has been granted an indication for PFO closure in the United States. Nevertheless, in carefully selected patients, off-label PFO closure should be considered and expertly performed. The decision to proceed with device closure should only occur after a comprehensive and competent evaluation, shared decision-making with the patient, and a commitment to long-term secondary stroke prevention.

REFERENCES

1. Roger VL, Go AS, Lloyd-Jones DM, et al. Heart disease and stroke statistics–2012 update: a report from the American Heart Association. Circulation 2012;125(1):e2–220.
2. Minino AM, Murphy SL, Xu J, et al. Deaths: final data for 2008. Natl Vital Stat Rep 2011;59(10):1–126.
3. Sacco RL, Ellenberg JH, Mohr JP, et al. Infarcts of undetermined cause: the NINCDS Stroke Data Bank. Ann Neurol 1989;25(4):382–90.
4. Kim JH, Kim YJ. Thrombus in Transit within a Patent Foramen Ovale: Gone with the Cough! Journal of cardiovascular ultrasound. 2011;19(4):196–8.
5. Homma S, Sacco RL, Di Tullio MR, et al. Effect of medical treatment in stroke patients with patent foramen ovale: patent foramen ovale in cryptogenic stroke study. Circulation 2002;105(22):2625–31.
6. Lechat P, Mas JL, Lascault G, et al. Prevalence of patent foramen ovale in patients with stroke. N Engl J Med 1988;318(18):1148–52.
7. Webster MW, Chancellor AM, Smith HJ, et al. Patent foramen ovale in young stroke patients. Lancet 1988;2(8601):11–2.
8. Overell JR, Bone I, Lees KR. Interatrial septal abnormalities and stroke: a meta-analysis of case-control studies. Neurology 2000;55(8):1172–9.
9. Davis D, Gregson J, Willeit P, et al. Patent foramen ovale, ischemic stroke and migraine: systematic review and stratified meta-analysis of association studies. Neuroepidemiology 2013;40(1):56–67.
10. Meissner I, Khandheria BK, Heit JA, et al. Patent foramen ovale: innocent or guilty? Evidence from a prospective population-based study. J Am Coll Cardiol 2006;47(2):440–5.
11. Di Tullio MR, Sacco RL, Sciacca RR, et al. Patent foramen ovale and the risk of ischemic stroke in a multiethnic population. J Am Coll Cardiol 2007; 49(7):797–802.
12. Alsheikh-Ali AA, Thaler DE, Kent DM. Patent foramen ovale in cryptogenic stroke: incidental or pathogenic? Stroke 2009;40(7):2349–55.
13. Homma S, Sacco RL. Patent foramen ovale and stroke. Circulation 2005;112(7):1063–72.
14. Mas JL, Arquizan C, Lamy C, et al. Recurrent cerebrovascular events associated with patent foramen ovale, atrial septal aneurysm, or both. N Engl J Med 2001;345(24):1740–6.
15. Comess KA, DeRook FA, Beach KW, et al. Transesophageal echocardiography and carotid ultrasound in patients with cerebral ischemia: prevalence of findings and recurrent stroke risk. J Am Coll Cardiol 1994;23(7):1598–603.
16. Kent DM, Thaler DE. The Risk of Paradoxical Embolism (RoPE) Study: developing risk models for application to ongoing randomized trials of percutaneous patent foramen ovale closure for cryptogenic stroke. Trials 2011;12:185.
17. Cabanes L, Mas JL, Cohen A, et al. Atrial septal aneurysm and patent foramen ovale as risk factors for cryptogenic stroke in patients less than 55 years of age. A study using transesophageal echocardiography. Stroke 1993;24(12):1865–73.
18. Agmon Y, Khandheria BK, Meissner I, et al. Frequency of atrial septal aneurysms in patients with cerebral ischemic events. Circulation 1999;99(15):1942–4.
19. Schuchlenz HW, Weihs W, Horner S, et al. The association between the diameter of a patent foramen ovale and the risk of embolic cerebrovascular events. Am J Med 2000;109(6):456–62.
20. Stone DA, Godard J, Corretti MC, et al. Patent foramen ovale: association between the degree of shunt by contrast transesophageal echocardiography and the risk of future ischemic neurologic events. Am Heart J 1996;131(1):158–61.
21. Giardini A, Donti A, Formigari R, et al. Comparison of results of percutaneous closure of patent foramen ovale for paradoxical embolism in patients with versus without thrombophilia. Am J Cardiol 2004; 94(8):1012–6.
22. Flaherty ML, Kissela B, Woo D, et al. The increasing incidence of anticoagulant-associated intracerebral hemorrhage. Neurology 2007;68(2):116–21.
23. Bungard TJ, Ackman ML, Ho G, et al. Adequacy of anticoagulation in patients with atrial fibrillation coming to a hospital. Pharmacotherapy 2000;20(9): 1060–5.
24. Homma S, Di Tullio MR, Sacco RL, et al. Surgical closure of patent foramen ovale in cryptogenic stroke patients. Stroke 1997;28(12):2376–81.
25. Dearani JA, Ugurlu BS, Danielson GK, et al. Surgical patent foramen ovale closure for prevention of paradoxical embolism-related cerebrovascular ischemic events. Circulation 1999;100(19 Suppl): II171–5.
26. Schneider B, Bauer R. Is surgical closure of patent foramen ovale the gold standard for treating interatrial shunts? An echocardiographic follow-up study. J Am Soc Echocardiogr 2005;18(12):1385–91.

27. King TD, Thompson SL, Steiner C, et al. Secundum atrial septal defect. Nonoperative closure during cardiac catheterization. JAMA 1976;235(23):2506–9.

28. Bridges ND, Hellenbrand W, Latson L, et al. Transcatheter closure of patent foramen ovale after presumed paradoxical embolism. Circulation 1992;86(6):1902–8.

29. Windecker S, Wahl A, Nedeltchev K, et al. Comparison of medical treatment with percutaneous closure of patent foramen ovale in patients with cryptogenic stroke. J Am Coll Cardiol 2004;44(4):750–8.

30. Thanopoulos BV, Dardas PD, Karanasios E, et al. Transcatheter closure versus medical therapy of patent foramen ovale and cryptogenic stroke. Catheter Cardiovasc Interv 2006;68(5):741–6.

31. Cerrato P, Priano L, Imperiale D, et al. Recurrent cerebrovascular ischaemic events in patients with interatrial septal abnormalities: a follow-up study. Neurol Sci 2006;26(6):411–8.

32. Casaubon L, McLaughlin P, Webb G, et al. Recurrent stroke/TIA in cryptogenic stroke patients with patent foramen ovale. Can J Neurol Sci 2007;34(1):74–80.

33. Kitsios GD, Dahabreh IJ, Abu Dabrh AM, et al. Patent foramen ovale closure and medical treatments for secondary stroke prevention: a systematic review of observational and randomized evidence. Stroke 2012;43(2):422–31.

34. Furlan AJ, Reisman M, Massaro J, et al. Closure or medical therapy for cryptogenic stroke with patent foramen ovale. N Engl J Med 2012;366(11):991–9.

35. Thaler DE, Wahl A. Critique of closure or medical therapy for cryptogenic stroke with patent foramen ovale: the hole truth? Stroke 2012;43(11):3147–9.

36. Carroll JD, Saver JL, Thaler DE, et al. Closure of patent foramen ovale versus medical therapy after cryptogenic stroke. N Engl J Med 2013;368(12):1092–100.

37. Meier B, Kalesan B, Mattle HP, et al. Percutaneous closure of patent foramen ovale in cryptogenic embolism. N Engl J Med 2013;368(12):1083–91.

38. Khan AR, Bin Abdulhak AA, Sheikh MA, et al. Device closure of patent foramen ovale versus medical therapy in cryptogenic stroke: a systematic review and meta-analysis. JACC Cardiovasc Interv 2013;6(12):1316–23.

Pulmonary Arteriovenous Malformations and Risk of Stroke

Ralf J. Holzer, MD, MSc, FSCAI[a,b,*], Clifford L. Cua, MD[c,d]

KEYWORDS

- Pulmonary arteriovenous malformations • Stroke • Risk • Hereditary hemorrhagic telangiectasia
- PAVMs

KEY POINTS

- The incidence of pulmonary arteriovenous malformations (PAVMs) is about 2 to 3 cases per 100,000.
- Most PAVMs (50%–80%) occur in patients with hereditary hemorrhagic telangiectasia.
- Hypoxemia and orthodeoxia are some of the more common clinical presentations.
- Complications include polycythemia, paradoxic systemic (septic) emboli, rupture, migraine, and seizures.
- The estimated risk of stroke secondary to PAVMs is as high as 2.6% to 25.0%.
- A combination of chest radiograph and contrast echocardiography is a good screening evaluation in patients with suspected PAVMs, followed by a high-resolution computed tomography scan.
- Transcatheter therapy is the most suitable therapeutic option in most patients with PAVMs, and a variety of devices can be used to occlude the PAVMs.

INTRODUCTION

Pulmonary arteriovenous malformations (PAVMs) are an abnormal communication between pulmonary arteries and pulmonary veins. They are rare, with an incidence of about 3.2 to 4.5 cases per year[1] or about 2 to 3 per 100,000.[2] Most PAVMs are hereditary; about 50% to 80% occur in patients with hereditary hemorrhagic telangiectasia (HHT), whereas about 10% to 30% of patients with HHT develop PAVMs.[3,4] PAVMs can also present as a congenital malformation or be acquired secondary to liver disease or associated with lack of hepatic flow to the pulmonary circulation, such as in patients with congenital heart disease who have undergone a Glenn procedure. It has been suggested that the absence of a liver-derived inhibitor of vascular proliferation is responsible for some of the acquired PAVMs.[5] Pathologically, PAVMs often appear as dilated vascular channels with abnormalities in the makeup of the vessel wall and may occur either as an isolated malformation (**Fig. 1**) or as multiple (**Fig. 2**) or diffuse (**Fig. 3**) anomalies; about 50% to 70% are located in the lower lobes.[5,6] They may be recurrent, in particular in patients with HHT.

CLINICAL FINDINGS AND DIAGNOSIS

The spectrum of clinical presentations is wide. Hypoxemia and orthodeoxia are some of the more common clinical presentations, and it is not unusual for a PAVM being diagnosed as part of a workup for a suspected patent foramen ovale (PFO) with right-left shunting. Depending

[a] Weill Cornell Medical College, New York, NY, USA; [b] Sidra Medical and Research Center, PO Box 26999, Doha, Qatar; [c] The Ohio State University, Columbus, Ohio, USA; [d] The Heart Center, Nationwide Children's Hospital, The Ohio State University, 700 Children's Drive, Columbus, OH 43205, USA
* Corresponding author. Sidra Medical and Research Center, PO Box 26999, Doha, Qatar.
E-mail address: rholzer@sidra.org

Cardiol Clin 34 (2016) 241–246
http://dx.doi.org/10.1016/j.ccl.2016.01.001
0733-8651/16/$ – see front matter © 2016 Elsevier Inc. All rights reserved.

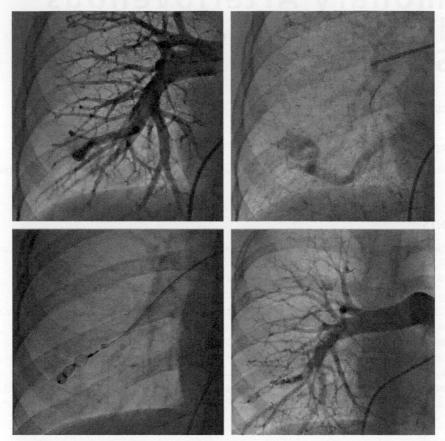

Fig. 1. Isolated PAVM. Isolated PAVM in the right lower lobe draining to the right lower pulmonary vein. The feeder vessel was occluded by placing initially an Amplatzer vascular plug II distally, followed by placement of several nondetachable coils. (*Top left*) Feeder vessel of the PAVM in the right lower lobe. (*Top right*) Draining vessel to the right lower pulmonary vein. (*Bottom left*) Vascular plug II deployed in the feeder vessel. (*Bottom right*) Right pulmonary artery angiography after release of the plug and placement of several additional nondetachable coils. (*Courtesy of* John Cheatham, MD, Columbus, OH.)

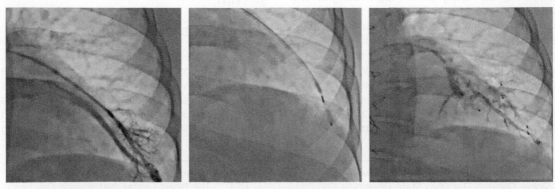

Fig. 2. Multiple PAVMs. Multiple PAVMs in a patient with cyanotic congenital heart disease. (*Top*) One of the PAVMs shown on angiography to the left lower lobe and draining to the left lower pulmonary vein. (*Middle*) Deployment of an Amplatzer vascular plug type IV. (*Bottom*) Angiography after occlusion of multiple AVMs, documenting the various vascular plugs (type II and IV) in different segments of the left lower lobe. (*Courtesy of* John Cheatham, MD, Columbus, OH.)

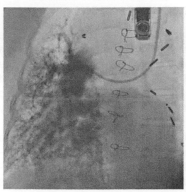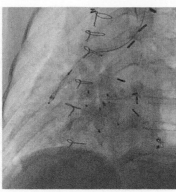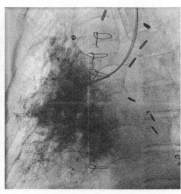

Fig. 3. Diffuse PAVM. A 10-year-old girl with cyanotic congenital heart disease and multiple diffusely small PAVMs throughout the entire right lung. (*Top*) Right pulmonary artery angiography documenting the entire right vasculature with diffuse pulmonary AVMs. (*Middle*) Highlighting multiple vascular plugs (type I) placed inside the right lung. (*Bottom*) Final angiography after occlusion of the entire distal right lung with multiple vascular plugs. This patient had a significant improvement in oxygen saturations and a reduction in symptoms after the procedure.

on the degree of shunting, patients may also present with exercise intolerance. PAVMs can also first present through complications, such as polycythemia, paradoxic systemic emboli (transient ischemic attack, stroke, abscess), or rupture of PAVMs into the pleural space or bronchus (hemoptysis, hemothorax). Other less common forms of presentation include migraine and seizures.

The diagnosis of PAVMs is made through a combination of clinical presentation as well as diagnostic imaging. Patients with clinical features of HHT require a thorough diagnostic workup to evaluate for PAVMs, given the high incidence in that patient population. Desaturations at baseline or with exercise, without being able to normalize the saturations/Po_2 with added oxygen, is very suggestive of a cardiac or extracardiac source of right-to-left shunting.

Echocardiography is the gold standard to evaluate for the presence of cardiac defects that may be associated with right-to-left shunting. Beyond the classic cardiac abnormalities that are associated with right-to-left shunting (and which usually present very early in life), a PFO can occasionally be a source of cyanosis and constant or intermittent right-to-left shunting, especially in patients with a somewhat restrictive right ventricle.[7] The difference on contrast echocardiography between a PFO and PAVMs is the time it takes for the microbubbles to appear within the left atrium. Although a PFO usually results in microbubbles appearing in the left atrium within 1 to 2 cardiac cycles, it can take 3 to 8 or more cardiac cycles for those to appear in the left atrium in patients with PAVMs because the microbubbles have to traverse the

right ventricle and pulmonary circulation before appearing in the left atrium.

Barzilai and colleagues[8] from St Louis, Missouri evaluated contrast echocardiography in 14 patients with PAVMs and used 10 patients with atrial-level right-to-left shunting as control subjects.[6] They injected agitated saline solution in a peripheral vein during echocardiographic imaging and measured the delay in the appearance of microcavitations in the left atrium in number of frames after right atrial appearance. The degree of left ventricular opacification was graded 1 to 4+. Patients with arteriovenous malformation had a significant delay in left atrial appearance of microcavitations compared with those with atrial right-to-left shunt. In patients with 3 to 4+ left ventricular opacification, large or multiple malformations were present, whereas patients with small or isolated malformation had 1 to 2+ left ventricular opacification.[8] The importance here is that in the case of PAVM, there is usually a delay of 3 to 8 cardiac cycles before contrast is visualized in the left atrium because of the time required for the contrast to traverse the pulmonary vasculature.[6] In patients without PAVMs, those microbubbles are usually filtered in the pulmonary circulation and do not appear in the left atrium. Furthermore, being able to visualize the microbubbles directly in the pulmonary veins is virtually diagnostic for PAVMs.

Other imaging modalities to consider include a chest radiograph (CXR), high-resolution computed tomography (CT) scan, MRI, and magnetic resonance angiography (MRA), as well as radionuclide scan. A chest CT scan with a typical round or oval and well-defined mass of equal density is a useful screening test in combination with contrast echocardiography,[4] and the presence of PAVMs is highly unlikely with both tests being negative. A high-resolution CT (HRCT) scan provides excellent anatomic information on PAVMs, whereas an MRI and MRA are less useful tools, with in particular small PAVMs often being indistinguishable from adjacent air-filled lung.

Cottin and colleagues[9,10] looked at the sensitivity, specificity, and positive predictive value of various diagnostic imaging modalities used for the detection and diagnosis of PAVMs. Clinical symptoms, such as dyspnea, had a fairly low sensitivity and specificity, whereas the combination of CXR and contrast echocardiography had a very high sensitivity of 100%. Evaluating the alveolar-arterial Po_2 gradient in 100% oxygen has a high specificity and a high positive predictive value but is less useful as a screening test because of the fairly low sensitivity. However, placing patients in 100% oxygen is fairly simple; transcutaneous saturation in excess of 97% in essence rules out a significant right-to-left shunting.[3] The researchers, therefore, suggested a diagnostic pathway that uses contrast echocardiography and an anteroposterior CXR as a basic screening tool.[6,9] In case of either test being positive, they suggest a HRCT scan. A negative CT scan virtually rules out PAVMs. In case of a positive CT scan, the researchers suggested therapy for those PAVMs that are larger than 2 to 3 mm. The gold standard for diagnosis of PAVMs though is angiography, which not only provides a definitive diagnosis but also at the same time serves as a therapeutic vehicle to be used for transcatheter embolotherapy.

PAVMs have significant associated potential complications, such as stroke, abscess, endocarditis, and rupture. Although the estimated risk of stroke secondary to PAVMs has been reported to be as high as 2.6% to 25.0%,[6] PAVMs are clearly not the most common cause of stroke and only limited case reports have been published.[11–16] Further complicating is the fact that PAVMs can cause a multitude of other neurologic complications, such as brain abscess, seizure, or migraine.[6] However, with a reported incidence of cerebrovascular accidents and brain abscesses of up to 10% to 15%, any cryptogenic stroke in a young adult requires evaluation for the possibility of PAVMSs.[3,14,17]

Although many congenital PAVMs are asymptomatic during infancy, beyond infancy incidence of complications is high, with up to 25% mortality.[6] Gossage and Kanj[6] summarized a variety of articles looking at the incidence of complications in patients with PAVMs, with total mortality and morbidity ranging between 1% and 14%.

THERAPEUTIC CONSIDERATIONS

In general, therapy is indicated in patients who are symptomatic, present with complications, or have larger PAVMs. Transcatheter therapy is the preferred treatment modality for isolated and selected multiple PAVMs. Surgical therapy is rarely indicated or necessary but can occasionally be considered in patients with very diffuse/micro-PVAMs. Surgical therapeutic options include segmental resection, lobectomy, and pneumonectomy.[18–20] Beyond surgical and transcatheter therapy, anticoagulation as a palliative measure as well as estrogen therapy to stabilize the vessel wall of the malformation are therapeutic options. In addition, because of the right-to-left shunting and potential risk for cerebral embolic abscesses, for paradoxic embolic abscess, antibiotic prophylaxis before dental and other surgical procedures is required.[3]

TRANSCATHETER THERAPY

The current recommendations from the American Heart Association for occlusion of pulmonary arteriovenous fistulas list as class I indication patients with discrete PAVMs who have evidence of significant cyanosis or patients who are at risk for or who have a documented history of a systemic embolic event.[21] Before establishment of those guidelines, articles have suggested to consider PAVMs with a diameter of 2 to 3 mm or more for embolotherapy or any PAVM in symptomatic patients or patients presenting with complications.[4,6] Technically, even smaller PAVMs with a diameter of just 1 to 2 mm may be suitable for transcatheter therapy, even though there is no clinical evidence that therapy is indicated in asymptomatic patients with an incidental finding of PAVMs.

Although a HRCT scan can provide detailed information on the size of PAVMs and suitability for transcatheter therapy, some conclusions can already be drawn from the results of contrast echocardiography.[22,23] Van Gent and colleagues[22,23] from the Netherlands tried to evaluate for a correlation between the results of transthoracic contrast echocardiography and the suitability for endovascular therapy/occlusion.[6] They reported on 282 patients who were prospectively enrolled and underwent transthoracic echocardiography (TTCE) and HRCT scan. Opacification of the left ventricle was graded as 1 (maximum of 30 microbubbles in left ventricle), 2 (30–100 microbubbles in left ventricle), or 3 (100 microbubbles in left ventricle), based on the maximum number of microbubbles counted in one still frame. There was a significantly higher positive predictive value for the presence of PAVMs in patients with grade 3 opacification. PAVMs seen on chest CT scans with a feeding tube diameter of 3 mm were considered suitable for endovascular occlusion. All patients with grade 3 positive TTCE eventually underwent transcatheter embolotherapy after the CT scan, in contrast to none of the patients with grade 1 or grade 2 opacifications.

Once patients are selected for transcatheter occlusion of the PAVMs, the procedure itself is technically usually fairly straightforward. Procedures can be performed under sedation or general anesthesia, depending on the age and cooperation of patients, and require full heparinization per activated clotting time during the procedure. Although not mandatory, a basic left and right heart catheterization are helpful, in particular to identify lower systemic arterial saturations and evaluate the alveolar-arterial Po_2 gradient of less than 100% oxygen. In the absence of a confirmatory CT scan, a main pulmonary angiography should be performed at baseline, which will provide an overview of the location of the PAVMs. This angiography should then be followed by selective angiographies.

It can be very helpful to have a long sheath positioned close to the segment in which the PAVM is located. This position allows using a catheter to occlude the vessel while being able to perform an angiography through the sheath to confirm the appropriate device position. Alternatively, a second venous catheter may be helpful in some patients.

Occasionally it can be tricky to enter the PAVM, in which case a venovenous loop can be created by snaring a wire within the left atrium that is advanced through the PAVM, which requires either the presence of a PFO or a transseptal puncture. This procedure, however, is rarely necessary; in most cases, a catheter suitable of delivering the appropriate device can be advance into the feeder vessel of the PAVM. In some cases, a PAVM has more than one feeder vessel, which requires that each of them be closed individually.

One of the most important aspects of occluding PAVM is to spare perfusion to healthy lung tissue. This approach can occasionally be difficult, as the runoff through the fistula may hide side branches of the feeder vessel that perfuse pulmonary tissue. In those cases, it can help occluding the more distal or draining AVM and then inject proximally, which because of the reduced runoff will more readily display the location of side branches that contribute to pulmonary perfusion. An approach such as this may also allow to occlude both the afferent as well as the efferent arm of the PAVM (starting with positioning a device distally at the exit), which is the most efficient way to achieve a secure occlusion and avoids embolization of thrombus that forms distal TO a device solely placed in the feeder vessel.

In general, a wide variety of devices are available that can be used to occlude the PAVMs, usually being used on an off-label basis. Embolization coils, such as the Gianturco coils (Cook, Bloomington, IN), have been used for almost 3 decades; many other devices are suitable for therapeutic occlusion of PAVMs provided they fit the morphology and size.[24] These devices includes a variety of Amplatzer devices, such as vascular plugs (in particular type I, II, and IV, St. Jude Medical, St Paul, MN) and duct occluders (St. Jude Medical, St Paul, MN), Nit-Occlud (pfm AG, Cologne, Germany), or even covered stents.[25,26] In essence, any device that may fit can be successfully used. If the sack of a larger aneurysm that can be associated with the PAVM is being filled, even larger devices, such as septal occluders, may be used. The exact device that should be used depends on the morphology and size of the feeding vessel; in many cases, there is more than one device option available.

It can help placing first a larger device more distally and then stacking up the more proximal feeding vessel with smaller devices or coils to achieve a solid occlusion (see **Fig. 1**). When nitinol plugs are being used, one has to bear in mind that it may take 10 to 20 minutes for occlusion to occur, especially in heparinized patients. Angiographies should be taken through the long delivery sheath or a second catheter after every device placement to confirm accurate positioning.

Very occasionally, in patients with multiple and diffuse PAVMs, occluding each individual communication may not be feasible. In those selected and severely symptomatic and cyanotic patients, it may be possible to occlude even an entire lung (see **Fig. 3**). However, this is generally a last resort; usually other treatment alternatives are available to remedy the situation.

SUMMARY

As a summary, although PAVMs are rare, they have a significant associated incidence of stroke. It is important to be vigilant to their presence in particular in patients with HHT. Transcatheter occlusion is usually straight forward and the preferred therapeutic modality in patients with significant cyanosis or patients who are at risk for or who have a documented history of a systemic embolic event.

REFERENCES

1. Dines DE, Arms RA, Bernatz PE, et al. Pulmonary AV fistula. Mayo Clin Proc 1974;49:460–5.

2. Hodgson CH, Kaye RL. Pulmonary arteriovenous fistula and hereditary hemorrhagic telangiectasia: a review and report of 35 cases of fistula. Dis Chest 1963;43:449–55.

3. Amin H, Friere A, Lal C, et al. Pulmonary arteriovenous malformations and Osler Weber Rendu syndrome: an unusual cause of dyspnea. Internet J Pulm Med 2004;5(2):1–5.

4. Khurshid I, Downie GH. Pulmonary arteriovenous malformation. Postgrad Med J 2002;78(918):191–7.

5. Duncan BW, Desai S. Pulmonary arteriovenous malformations after cavopulmonary anastomosis. Ann Thorac Surg 2003;76(5):1759–66.

6. Gossage JR, Kanj G. Pulmonary arteriovenous malformations. A state of the art review. Am J Respir Crit Care Med 1998;158(2):643–61.

7. Will PM, Serrian JL, Dawson JT. An unusual case of cyanotic heart disease in a patient with patent foramen ovale and right ventricular hypertrophy. Clin Cardiol 1996;19(5):429–32.

8. Barzilai B, Waggoner AD, Spessert C, et al. Two-dimensional contrast echocardiography in the detection and follow-up of congenital pulmonary arteriovenous malformations. Am J Cardiol 1991; 68(15):1507–10.

9. Cottin V, Chinet T, Lavole A, et al. Pulmonary arteriovenous malformations in hereditary hemorrhagic telangiectasia: a series of 126 patients. Medicine 2007;86(1):1–17.

10. Cottin V, Plauchu H, Bayle JY, et al. Pulmonary arteriovenous malformations in patients with hereditary hemorrhagic telangiectasia. Am J Respir Crit Care Med 2004;169(9):994–1000.

11. Anticoli S, Pezzella FR, Siniscalchi A, et al. Pulmonary arteriovenous malformation as a cause of embolic stroke: case report and review of the literature. Interv Neurol 2015;3(1):27–30.

12. Parees I, Horga A, Santamarina E, et al. Stroke after prolonged air travel associated with a pulmonary arteriovenous malformation. J Neurol Sci 2010; 292(1–2):99–100.

13. Rao SC, Main ML. Transoesophageal echocardiographic diagnosis of pulmonary arteriovenous malformation in a patient with ischaemic stroke. Eur J Echocardiogr 2009;10(2):347–9.

14. Retnakaran RR, Faughnan ME, Chan RP, et al. Pulmonary arteriovenous malformation: a rare, treatable cause of stroke in young adults. Int J Clin Pract 2003;57(8):731–3.

15. Sladden D, Casha A, Azzopardi C, et al. A large pulmonary arteriovenous malformation causing cerebrovascular accidents. BMJ Case Rep 2015;2015. pii:bcr2014207786.

16. Todo K, Moriwaki H, Higashi M, et al. A small pulmonary arteriovenous malformation as a cause of recurrent brain embolism. AJNR Am J Neuroradiol 2004; 25(3):428–30.

17. Al-Saleh S, Mei-Zahav M, Faughnan ME, et al. Screening for pulmonary and cerebral arteriovenous malformations in children with hereditary haemorrhagic telangiectasia. Eur Respir J 2009;34(4): 875–81.

18. Chowdhury UK, Kothari SS, Bishnoi AK, et al. Successful lobectomy for pulmonary arteriovenous malformation causing recurrent massive haemoptysis. Heart Lung Circ 2009;18(2):135–9.

19. Metin K, Karacelik M, Yavaccan O, et al. Surgical treatment of pulmonary arteriovenous malformation: report of two cases and review of the literature. J Int Med Res 2005;33(4):467–71.

20. Yamada S, Masuda D, Inoue H. Video-assisted simultaneously stapled segmentectomy for pulmonary arteriovenous malformation located in the pulmonary hilum. Jpn J Thorac Cardiovasc Surg 2006;54(12):543–6.

21. Feltes TF, Bacha E, Beekman RH 3rd, et al. Indications for cardiac catheterization and intervention in pediatric cardiac disease: a scientific statement from the American Heart Association. Circulation 2011;123(22):2607–52.

22. van Gent MW, Post MC, Luermans JG, et al. Screening for pulmonary arteriovenous malformations using transthoracic contrast echocardiography: a prospective study. Eur Respir J 2009;33(1): 85–91.

23. van Gent MW, Post MC, Snijder RJ, et al. Real prevalence of pulmonary right-to-left shunt according to genotype in patients with hereditary hemorrhagic telangiectasia: a transthoracic contrast echocardiography study. Chest 2010;138(4):833–9.

24. Wallace S, Gianturco C, Anderson JH, et al. Therapeutic vascular occlusion utilizing steel coil technique: clinical applications. AJR Am J Roentgenol 1976;127(3):381–7.

25. Meek ME, Meek JC, Beheshti MV. Management of pulmonary arteriovenous malformations. Semin Intervent Radiol 2011;28(1):24–31.

26. Veeram Reddy SR, Patel VG, Gualano SK. Amplatzer vascular plug IV for occlusion of pulmonary arteriovenous malformations in a patient with cryptogenic stroke. Ann Pediatr Cardiol 2014;7(2):145–7.

Congenital Malformations Leading to Paradoxical Embolism

Elchanan Bruckheimer, MBBS

KEYWORDS

- Paradoxical embolism • Congenital defects • Cyanosis • Shunt

KEY POINTS

- Any congenital cardiovascular malformation affording a bypass of the filtration of blood by the pulmonary circulation, a right-to-left shunt, can be associated with paradoxical embolism.
- The formation of the systemic venous system and the septation of the heart are complex embryologic processes that, when aberrant, create unusual connections and pathways.
- After correction or palliation, potential or residual right-to-left shunts may develop owing to leaks, changes in physiology, collateral formation, or pulmonary arteriovenous fistulae.
- Anticoagulation is essential to prevent paradoxical emboli; however, the hematologic disturbances and the most appropriate anticoagulation therapy in these patients require further evaluation.
- Surgery and transcatheter interventions are a major cause of stroke/paradoxical emboli in patients with congenital heart defects and preventive actions are of major importance.

INTRODUCTION

The role of the lungs and the pulmonary circulation as both oxygenator and filter of the systemic venous return was first described by *Ibn Nafis Damashqi* in his 'Commentary on the Anatomy of Canon of Avicenna' written in 1242.[1] A translation from the Arabic has been published as follows:

> … after the blood has been refined in the right ventricle of the heart, it must reach the left ventricle where in it is impregnated with the vital spirit (pneuma) but there is no opening between these two ventricles as the septum between them is thick and solid and in contrast to what some people have imagined, there is no visible pores and also contrary to what Galen has said there are no invisible pores connecting them. And thus this blood after it is refined must flow via the vena arteriosa (pulmonary artery) to the lungs where it

> must spread and be mingled with air and its most delicate substance be refined and then flow through the arteria venosa (pulmonary vein) so that the blood that has been mixed with air and is ready to receive the vital spirit reaches the left chamber of the heart.

This absolute separation of the right and left circulations and the *"refinement"* of blood in the pulmonary circulation are essential to prevent the passage of thrombotic material from the systemic venous system in to the systemic arterial circulation. Any breach of the intracardiac septae or circumvention of the pulmonary capillary network has the potential to cause a paradoxical embolus.[2,3] The most common causes are a patent foramen ovale (PFO), atrial septal defects (ASDs), and pulmonary arteriovenous malformations, which are discussed extensively in other sections of this issue (see Suradi HS, Hijazi ZM: Patent Foramen Ovale: Stroke and device Closure, in

Conflicts of Interest: None.
Cardiac Catheterization, Section of Pediatric Cardiology, Schneider Children's Medical Center Israel, Kaplan 14, Petach Tikva 42902, Israel
E-mail address: elchananb@bezeqint.net

Cardiol Clin 34 (2016) 247–254
http://dx.doi.org/10.1016/j.ccl.2015.12.005
0733-8651/16/$ – see front matter © 2016 Elsevier Inc. All rights reserved.

this issue; Leppert M, Poisson NS, Carroll JD: Atrial Septal Defects and Cardioembolic Strokes, in this issue; and Holzer RJ, Cua C: Pulmonary Arteriovenous Malformations and Risk of Stroke, in this issue). The purpose of this article is to discuss other forms of congenital cardiovascular malformations that are associated with paradoxical emboli and the possible pathophysiology in both untreated and corrected or palliated defects.

ISOLATED SYSTEMIC VENOUS ABNORMALITIES AND PARADOXICAL EMBOLI

The complex embryology of the systemic veins in the developing fetus affords many unusual malformations.[4] Three different paired venous systems—the cardinal, vitelline, and umbilical systems—undergo a series of staged organized processes of involution and attachment to each other, the sinus venosus, and other developing organs so that after birth the systemic venous return from the upper body drains via a right-sided superior vena cava (SVC) to the right atrium and a right-sided inferior vena cava (IVC) drains the lower body similarly.[5]

Persistent Left Superior Vena Cava

The most common form of isolated systemic venous abnormality is the persistence of the left SVC (LSVC) owing the failure of involution of the left common cardinal vein, which occurs in 0.3% of the population.[6] The persistent LSVC drains to the coronary sinus, which runs behind the left atrium to drain normally in to the right atrium and is, therefore, asymptomatic. However, rarely, there is partial or complete unroofing of the coronary sinus and the systemic venous return drains directly in to the left atrium. Persistent LSVC to the left atrium has been described as a cause of paradoxical emboli causing stroke after upper extremity trauma and there are a number of case reports of brain abscesses.[7,8] A connection between the innominate vein and the left upper pulmonary vein has also been described as a cause for transient ischemic attacks as have collaterals that have developed after right SVC obstruction.[9–13] These are probably not true LSVC, but a different persistent embryonic connections such as a vertical vein or levoatrial cardinal vein.

Right Superior Vena Cava Draining to the Left Atrium

This is a very rare anomaly, especially when it appears as an isolated finding, and may be owing to a sinus venosus defect of the RSVC in fetal life causing preferential flow to the left atrium with hypoplasia or involution of the proximal RSVC.[14] The right SVC, therefore, may drain solely to the left atrium or to both atria and is a very uncommon cause of cyanosis and paradoxical embolus.[15]

Inferior Vena Cava "Draining to the Left Atrium"

The formation of the IVC is more complex than the SVC and depends on 5 different segments, of which 4 have a bilateral presence, to connect and involute appropriately.[4,16] Even though multiple abnormalities of the IVC have been described there is no proven case of an IVC connecting directly to the left atrium.[5] In the fetus, oxygenated blood from the placenta flows through the IVC to the right atrium and is deflected across the foramen ovale, by the Eustachian valve, to the left atrium. The persistence of a large Eustachian valve associated with a patent foramen ovale after birth can similarly deflect some systemic venous blood to the left atrium, giving the impression that the IVC is directly connected.[4,5] Lampropoulos and colleagues[16] described a right-sided dual IVC drainage with anterior IVC draining to the right atrium and the posterior channel draining via a venous collateral to a right pulmonary vein into the left atrium. The patient presented with cyanosis and a transient ischemic attack and had had a cerebellar infarct documented on MRI 6 months previously. The pathologic specimen of a case report by Gardner and Cole[17] of a woman with cyanosis and an IVC directly connected to the left atrium was reevaluated by Geva[5] and demonstrated to be the incorrect diagnosis.

In situs solitus and situs inversus totalis, the anatomic relationships of the systemic veins are typically intact. However, in visceral heterotaxy–atrial isomerism the systemic, and pulmonary, venous connections can be anomalous and often are associated with complex intracardiac defects. The drainage of the IVC to the "left-sided" atrium has been described, but this is in fact a morphologic right atrium with or without anomalous pulmonary venous return.[4,5]

Ductus Venosus

The ductus venosus forms in the fetal liver and connects the (left) umbilical vein to the right hepatic vein to the suprahepatic segment of the IVC to deliver the oxygenated blood from the placenta to the right atrium.[4] The ductus venosus acts as a sphincter of the low resistance placental circuit to prevent excessive shunting and fetal cardiac volume overload and also directs blood in to the developing portal venous system.[4,18]

After birth, the ductus venosus involutes after a few days. In rare circumstances, the ductus venosus remains patent and presents a congenital portosystemic shunt. The umbilical vein–ductus venosus is used commonly in the neonatal intensive care unit for central venous catheter placement. Unfortunately, the catheter can cause portal vein thrombosis and has been reported as a cause for paradoxical embolism in neonates with and without congenital heart disease,[19] the latter owing to the flow being directed across a PFO as in the fetus.

Many abnormalities of the ductus venosus and umbilical venous drainage have been described since Abernethy's original description and are often associated with congenital abnormalities of the IVC, polyspenia, visceral heterotaxy, and atrial isomerism.[20] A congenital portosystemic shunt can cause the hepatopulmonary syndrome (HPS) with the development of diffuse pulmonary arteriovenous malformations leading to severe hypoxemia.[18,20] This can be reversed by closure of the shunt or liver transplantation with regression of the pulmonary arterial venous malformations (PAVMs). The high prevalence of portosystemic shunts in patients with polysplenia, interrupted IVC, or isomerism is of particular interest because these patients have a tendency to develop PAVMs spontaneously or after a cavopulmonary anastomosis.[20]

Although PAVMs are a well-recognized cause of stroke and paradoxical emboli in patients with and without hereditary hemorrhagic telangiectasia, there are no reports of paradoxical embolism specifically related to PAVM development associated with HPS.[21] Rare case reports of brain abscess have been described in HPS and this may be owing to the small and diffuse nature of the PAVMs in this setting, which only allow for passage of infected microemboli.[22] There are, of course, reports of neurologic impairment related to hyperammonemia and hepatic encephalopathy owing to congenital portosystemic shunts,[23] but the cause is metabolic and not embolic. In elderly patients, stroke may be from other causes.

An unusual pulmonary arteriovenous malformation causing a paradoxical embolus is the report of a young lady[24] who suffered from a splenic infarct owing to a right pulmonary artery to left atrial fistula causing a right-to-left shunt.

Diagnosis of right to left shunts whether or not associated with paradoxical emboli should be systematic and straightforward and is extensively covered in another section of this issue (see Holzer RJ, Cua C: Pulmonary Arteriovenous Malformations and Risk of Stroke, in this issue). Here are listed a few additional suggestions relating to the anatomies as described:

- Pulse oximetry less than 96% should raise suspicion in the absence of known cardiac or respiratory disease.
- Color Doppler echocardiography can often visualize abnormal systemic connections but, importantly, cannot rule them out. A sensitive test is "bubble-contrast" echocardiography, which should be injected in the left arm to rule out abnormalities of a LSVC. Injection in the right arm can miss an anomalous LSVC if there is no bridging vein.
- The passage of bubbles via the pulmonary veins to the left atrium raises the suspicion of PAVMs. A detailed history, including family history, to assess for hemorrhagic telangiectasia is essential. In the absence of such history and the absence of known liver disease a postprandial blood ammonia level should be taken to evaluate for a portosystemic shunt and HPS.
- Noninvasive imaging with Duplex ultrasonography, computed tomography angiography, and MRI are useful, but abnormal venous flows can be missed or difficult to interpret owing to lack of opacification by contrast determined by flow patterns. In specific cases, especially of the IVC and portal systems, selective venography with balloon occlusion or selective arteriography to image the venous phase is required.

Treatment is lesion specific and often abnormal venous pathways can be surgically redirected or undergo transcatheter occlusion if there is an alternative normal drainage pathway.

UNIVENTRICULAR HEARTS AND PARADOXICAL EMBOLI

Congenital heart defects involving the intracardiac septae can be classified into 2 groups, namely, biventricular and univentricular hearts. A biventricular heart with a septal defect can usually be repaired so that the separation of the pulmonary and systemic circulations is complete with each circulation supported by a ventricle. Examples of these include forms of ASDs, ventricular septal defects, balanced atrioventricular canals, tetralogy of Fallot, and transposition of the great vessels.

Univentricular defects include tricuspid atresia, hypoplastic left heart syndrome, and unbalanced atrioventricular canals. Univentricular hearts have a degree of intracardiac right-to-left shunt from birth until separation of the circulations. This separation requires a series of interventions in which the SVC and subsequently IVC venous returns are connected directly to the pulmonary arteries, bypassing the right heart. The former is the Glenn shunt and the latter is the Fontan circulation. The Fontan procedure has undergone a number of versions; however, in nearly all of them the flow is passive and the pulmonary venous blood returns to an atrium and a ventricle that supports only the systemic circulation.[25] Even after the Fontan completion, a right-to-left shunt may be present either from an intended surgical fenestration, an unintended leak, a venous collateral to the pulmonary venous circulation, or PAVMs.[25–27] As mentioned,[20] PAVMs often develop in patients with cavopulmonary connections especially when hepatic venous blood flow is excluded from the pulmonary circulation (e.g., Glenn or Kawashima, a Glenn procedure in a patient with interrupted IVC and azygos continuation). Venous collaterals can develop between the relatively high-pressure Fontan to the lower pressure pulmonary venous atrium, or directly, or via complex connections including the portal system and anomalous hepatic veins especially in cases of visceral heterotaxy and atrial isomerism.[25–27]

The continuous presence of a right-to-left shunt in conjunction with passive, often sluggish, flow, arrhythmias, and prosthetic material exposes these patients to a continuing risk for paradoxical emboli.[28–31] Thromboembolism and paradoxical emboli in Fontan patients have been well-documented. Rosenthal and colleagues[25] reported a retrospective series of 70 patients with different forms of Fontan, of whom 14 patients (20%) developed a thromboembolic complication during a mean follow-up of 5.2 ± 4.7 years. Twelve patients had thrombi in the venous circulation. Six of the patients were asymptomatic, 5 had various symptoms, and 3 presented with cerebrovascular events, of which at least one was from a paradoxical embolus via a venous collateral. None of the patients were on anticoagulation therapy. Potter and colleagues[32] reported on 210 patients with a Fontan circulation of whom 50% were not prescribed thromboembolic prophylaxis; 24.3% received aspirin and 25.7% received warfarin. In multivariate analyses, lack of aspirin or warfarin was associated with a significantly higher thromboembolic event rate when compared with therapy. Twenty-year freedom from thromboemboli was 86% versus 52% in patients with and without thromboprophylaxis, respectively, with no difference in thromboembolism between aspirin or warfarin. A controlled study by Monagle and colleagues[29] randomized patients to heparin/warfarin or aspirin in the first 2 years after Fontan surgery also did not find a significant difference between the 2 therapies in preventing thromboembolism. Idorn and colleagues[26] retrospectively evaluated a different group of 210 patients in Denmark with a Fontan circulation, of whom 8.1% had thromboembolism with 9 patients suffering from cerebrovascular accidents. Whole blood assays of global hemostasis, clot strength, and platelet aggregation were analyzed prospectively in 112 patients and in a subset plasma was analyzed for biomarkers reflecting endothelial and platelet function. The authors did not find a significant difference in hemostatic function between patients with or without thromboembolism. Indeed, global hemostasis was normal in both groups without hypercoagulability being demonstrated.

In these, and in additional reports and reviews,[25–34] a significant proportion of thromboembolism was clinically silent and discovered on routine imaging; therefore, the prevalence is probably higher than reported. The mechanisms of thromboembolism in congenital heart disease in general, and in the Fontan circulation in particular, are not fully understood. The appropriate anticoagulation regimens remain to be defined and there are no clear recommendations, although the use of anticoagulation is reasonable.[30] The surgical or transcatheter closure of residual shunts, fenestrations, and venous collaterals has to be evaluated for each patient's current condition and hemodynamics of the specific Fontan circulation.

BIVENTRICULAR HEARTS AND PARADOXICAL EMBOLI

All congenital defects of the intracardiac septae can be associated with paradoxical emboli before closure.[2,35,36] An ASD or PFO in an otherwise normal heart will typically shunt left-to-right during diastole because the filling pressures and resistance of the right ventricle are less than that of the left ventricle. However, this shunt can be reversed temporarily by a hemodynamic change caused by a Valsalva maneuver, sneezing, or similar action. Functional changes of the right ventricle can occur after an inferior wall myocardial infarction, reducing the diastolic compliance of the ventricle causing a significant right-to-left interatrial shunt. Pericardial disease such as a pericardial effusion or constrictive pericarditis can also reverse the shunt to be right to left.[2]

In addition to these hemodynamic causes, the right-to-left shunt across a PFO or ASD may be caused by functional/anatomic changes, which are exacerbated by orthostatism. The platypnoea–orthodeoxia syndrome[37] is a relatively rare condition of breathlessness and cyanosis occurring on standing in association with an ASD or PFO. Proposed mechanisms causing this phenomenon include elongation or dilation of the aorta, which influence the position and shape of a PFO or ASD so that the venous return from the IVC is channeled directly toward the defect and this may be further facilitated by the presence of a prominent Eustachian valve or Chiari network. On standing the ASD/PFO is stretched open and the right-to-left shunt is exacerbated causing the symptoms of breathlessness and cyanosis.[37]

In Ebstein's anomaly, apical displacement of a dysplastic tricuspid valve, there is an associated PFO or ASD in 80% to 90% of cases.[38] In its more severe forms, cyanosis develops owing to a combination of tricuspid regurgitation and limited right ventricular volume and compliance, increasing the right atrial pressure resulting in a right-to-left shunt. Recently, a report[38] described a series of 128 patients with Ebstein's anomaly of whom 23% had a history of at least 1 possible paradoxical embolic event, including a stroke or transient ischemic attack, brain abscess, or myocardial infarction. The median age at occurrence of the embolic event was 49 years with the best predictors of an embolic event being the presence of an ASD and older age at surgery. There was no association with classic cardiovascular risk factors for stroke. The authors noted that none of the patients suffered from a recurrent event after closure of the ASD or PFO and, therefore, suggested that earlier intervention should be considered in these patients. Some patients with Ebstein's anomaly with a moderate or lesser degree of tricuspid regurgitation, which does not require surgical repair, may benefit from transcatheter closure of the interatrial shunt with a device.[39]

Ventricular septal defects of all types (perimembranous, muscular, atrioventricular septal defects/canal), in otherwise structurally normal hearts. will shunt left to right during systole because the pulmonary vascular resistance is usually lower than that of the systemic vasculature. However, in the presence of increased pulmonary vascular resistance or right ventricular outflow obstruction, a right-to-left shunt can occur. Well-known examples include tetralogy of Fallot and the Eisenmenger syndrome.

In tetralogy of Fallot, there is a large subarterial VSD and subpulmonic, pulmonic, and often supravalvar pulmonic stenosis. The degree of obstruction in the right ventricular outflow worsens during infancy and cyanosis becomes more pronounced after 6 months of age. "Cyanotic" or "tet" spells are typical of untreated tetralogy of Fallot and are owing to a sudden and acute increase in the severity of outflow obstruction and the ensuing severe hypoxia can cause brain damage or even death. Untreated tetralogy of Fallot is associated with paradoxical emboli and cerebral abscesses, which usually parallel the degree of cyanosis.[40]

Prolonged exposure of the low-resistance pulmonary vasculature to increased blood flow and pressure from a left-to-right shunt, as with a large unrestrictive ventricular septal defect, causes a series of changes to pulmonary endothelial function and the ultrastructure of the pulmonary arterial wall.[41] These functional and structural changes are eventually irreversible and the pulmonary vascular resistance exceeds that of the systemic vasculature with reversal of the shunt to be right to left. This progression of events is termed the Eisenmenger syndrome.[41,42] The right-to-left shunt and consequent cyanosis and systemic hypoxia lead to a series of hematologic changes including erythrocytosis, hyperviscosity, and alterations in coagulability.[33,35,43]

A recent report by Jensen and colleagues[34] found a prevalence of 47% of cerebral infarcts on brain MRI in adult patients with cyanotic congenital heart disease of whom 80% had biventricular hearts, with the majority of those having Eisenmenger syndrome. This is a higher prevalence than previously reported and may be related to the extensive scanning performed with "silent" infarcts demonstrated on MRI despite the absence of clinical findings. The report did not find a significant difference in erythrocytosis, iron stores, platelet counts, and thromboelastography between patients with and without thrombosis. The high prevalence of white matter hyperintensity lesions on the MRI scans, which are suggestive of ischemic lesions, could imply that the infarcts were not thromboembolic. On the other hand, there was a trend of iron deficiency and infarction and previous studies have reported that iron deficiency causing microcytosis is an independent factor associated with stroke. The relationship between the hematologic findings and cerebral thrombosis is unclear and requires further definition, as do the relationships between iron repletion/depletion, viscosity, and coagulability before recommendations for anticoagulation protocols can be made.[30,31,33,44–46]

A further risk factor for paradoxical emboli in patients with intracardiac shunts is the presence of transvenous pacing leads. Khairy and colleagues[47] reported on a cohort of 202 patients with intracardiac shunts, of whom 64 had transvenous pacing leads, 56 had epicardial leads, and 82 had a right-to-left shunt with no pacing leads. Of the transvenous group, 15.6% had at least 1 systemic thromboembolic episode compared with 8.9% of the epicardial group and 11% of those with no pacemaker leads. In multivariate, stepwise regression analyses, transvenous leads remained an independent predictor of systemic thromboemboli incurring a greater than 2-fold increased risk in patients with intracardiac shunts. Of note is that, although the majority of patients with transvenous leads had right-to-left shunts, 2 patients did not; therefore, the authors recommend avoiding transvenous lead placement with any intracardiac shunt.

Pediatric stroke from all causes is a topic of increasing interest with the recent formation of tasks forces and committees[44–46] to study the causes and appropriate treatment. Prevention is of course of paramount importance and although this topic is beyond the scope of this review, it is of note that many cases of stroke occur periprocedurally, particularly in children with cyanotic heart disease suggesting that many of these cases are from paradoxical emboli.[44]

SUMMARY

Paradoxical embolism in cardiovascular malformations has become a topic of major interest, particularly concerning cryptogenic stroke, its association with a PFO, and appropriate management with anticoagulation therapy and device closure. Other forms of congenital defects associated with paradoxical embolism are less common and often involve unusual connections and pathways either owing to the complex embryologic processes or after correction or palliation of the defects. Potential or residual right-to-left shunts may still develop after intervention owing to leaks, changes in physiology, collateral formation, or the development of pulmonary arteriovenous fistulae. The combination of abnormal structure, abnormal flow, and coagulation, polycythemia, prosthetic materials and pacing leads, arrhythmias, and multiple interventions contribute to the occurrence of paradoxical emboli in patients with congenital malformations. Although anticoagulation in patients with untreated or palliated cyanotic heart defects and Eisenmenger syndrome is necessary to prevent paradoxical emboli, the hematologic disturbances and the most appropriate anticoagulation therapy in these patients still warrant further investigation.

REFERENCES

1. Azizi MH, Nayernouri T, Azizi F. A brief history of the discovery of the circulation of blood in the human body. Arch Iran Med 2008;11:345–50.

2. Windecker S, Stortecky S, Meier B. Paradoxical embolism. J Am Coll Cardiol 2014;64:403–15.

3. Ammash N, Warnes CA. Cerebrovascular events in adult patients with cyanotic congenital heart disease. J Am Coll Cardiol 1996;28:768–72.

4. Yagel S, Kivilevitch Z, Cohen SM, et al. The fetal venous system, part I: normal embryology, anatomy, hemodynamics, ultrasound evaluation and Doppler investigation. Ultrasound Obstet Gynecol 2010;35:741–50.

5. Geva T. Abnormal systemic venous connections. In: Allen HD, Driscoll DJ, Shaddy RE, et al, editors. Moss and Adams' heart disease in infants, children, and adolescents. 8th edition. Baltimore (MD): Lippincott Williams & Wilkins; 2013. p. 841–63.

6. van Praagh S, Geva T, Lock JE, et al. Biatrial or left atrial drainage of the right superior vena cava: anatomic, morphogenetic, and surgical considerations–report of three new cases and literature review. Pediatr Cardiol 2003;24:350–63.

7. Ch'ng JK, Soon JL, Lim CH. Paradoxical emboli from left superior vena cava causing recurrent brain abscess. Singapore Med J 2012;53:e21–3.

8. Troost E, Gewillig M, Budts W. Percutaneous closure of a persistent left superior vena cava connected to the left atrium. Int J Cardiol 2006;106:365–6.

9. Recto MR, Sadlo H, Sobczyk WL. Rare case of persistent left superior vena cava to left upper pulmonary vein: pathway for paradoxical embolization and development of transient ischemic attack and subsequent occlusion with an Amplatzer vascular plug. J Invasive Cardiol 2007;19:E313–6.

10. Hutyra M, Skala T, Sanak D, et al. Persistent left superior vena cava connected through the left upper pulmonary vein to the left atrium: an unusual pathway for paradoxical embolization and a rare cause of recurrent transient ischaemic attack. Eur J Echocardiogr 2010;11:E35.

11. Saremi F, Vojdani E, Vorobiof G, et al. Right to left shunting through communications between the left superior intercostal vein tributaries and the left atrium: a potential cause of paradoxical embolism. Int J Cardiol 2013;167:2867–74.

12. Tsang W, Boulos M, Moody AR, et al. An unusual cause of stroke–the importance of saline contrast echocardiography. Echocardiography 2008;25:908–10.

13. Nascimbene A, Angelini P. Superior vena cava thrombosis and paradoxical embolic stroke due to collateral drainage from the brachiocephalic vein to the left atrium. Tex Heart Inst J 2011;38:170–3.

14. Baggett C, Skeen SJ, Gantt DS, et al. Isolated right superior vena cava drainage into the left atrium diagnosed noninvasively in the peripartum period. Tex Heart Inst J 2009;36:611–4.

15. Shapiro EP, Al-Sadir J, Campbell NP, et al. Drainage of right superior vena cava into both atria. Review of the literature and description of a case presenting with polycythemia and paradoxical embolization. Circulation 1981;63:712–7.

16. Lampropoulos K, Gewillig M, Budts W. Unusual right-to-left shunt by single-sided bilateral inferior vena cava. Congenit Heart Dis 2011;6:484–7.

17. Gardner DL, Cole L. Long survival with inferior vena cava draining into left atrium. Br Heart J 1955;17:93–7.

18. Bruckheimer E, Dagan T, Atar E, et al. Staged transcatheter treatment of portal hypoplasia and congenital portosystemic shunts in children. Cardiovasc Intervent Radiol 2013;36:1580–5.

19. Rambaud J, Grévent D, Bergounioux J. Portal vein thrombosis and stroke in a patient with tetralogy of Fallot. J Pediatr Gastroenterol Nutr 2015;60:e12–4.

20. McElhinney DB, Marx GR, Newburger JW. Congenital portosystemic venous connections and other abdominal venous abnormalities in patients with polysplenia and functionally univentricular heart disease: a case series and literature review. Congenit Heart Dis 2011;6:28–40.

21. Cartin-Ceba R, Swanson KL, Krowka MJ. Pulmonary arteriovenous malformations. Chest 2013; 144:1033–44.

22. Salerno D. CNS complications in pulmonary arteriovenous malformations. Chest 2014;145:426.

23. Takahashi S, Yoshida E, Sakanishi Y, et al. Congenital multiple intrahepatic portosystemic shunt: an autopsy case. Int J Clin Exp Pathol 2013;7(1):425–31.

24. Kavarana MN, Devaney EJ, Torres ML, et al. Right pulmonary artery to left atrial fistula: a rare presentation. World J Pediatr Congenit Heart Surg 2012;3: 382–4.

25. Rosenthal DN, Friedman AH, Kleinman CS, et al. Thromboembolic complications after Fontan operations. Circulation 1995;92(9 Suppl):II287–93.

26. Idorn L, Jensen AS, Juul K, et al. Thromboembolic complications in Fontan patients: population-based prevalence and exploration of the etiology. Pediatr Cardiol 2013;34:262–72.

27. Monagle P, Cochrane A, McCrindle B, et al. Thromboembolic complications after Fontan procedures–the role of prophylactic anticoagulation. J Thorac Cardiovasc Surg 1998;115:493–8.

28. McCrindle BW, Manlhiot C, Cochrane A, et al, Fontan Anticoagulation Study Group. Factors associated with thrombotic complications after the Fontan procedure: a secondary analysis of a multicenter, randomized trial of primary thromboprophylaxis for 2 years after the Fontan procedure. J Am Coll Cardiol 2013;61:346–53.

29. Monagle P, Cochrane A, Roberts R, et al, Fontan Anticoagulation Study Group. A multicenter, randomized trial comparing heparin/warfarin and acetylsalicylic acid as primary thromboprophylaxis for 2 years after the Fontan procedure in children. J Am Coll Cardiol 2011;58:645–51.

30. Giglia TM, Massicotte MP, Tweddell JS, et al, American Heart Association Congenital Heart Defects Committee of the Council on Cardiovascular Disease in the Young, Council on Cardiovascular and Stroke Nursing, Council on Epidemiology and Prevention, and Stroke Council. Prevention and treatment of thrombosis in pediatric and congenital heart disease: a scientific statement from the American Heart Association. Circulation 2013;128:2622–703.

31. McCrindle BW, Li JS, Manlhiot C, et al. Challenges and priorities for research: a report from the National Heart, Lung, and Blood Institute (NHLBI)/National Institutes of Health (NIH) working group on thrombosis in pediatric cardiology and congenital heart disease. Circulation 2014; 130:1192–203.

32. Potter BJ, Leong-Sit P, Fernandes SM, et al. Effect of aspirin and warfarin therapy on thromboembolic events in patients with univentricular hearts and Fontan palliation. Int J Cardiol 2013; 168:3940–3.

33. Jensen AS, Johansson PI, Idorn L, et al. The haematocrit–an important factor causing impaired haemostasis in patients with cyanotic congenital heart disease. Int J Cardiol 2013;167: 1317–21.

34. Jensen AS, Idorn L, Thomsen C, et al. Prevalence of cerebral and pulmonary thrombosis in patients with cyanotic congenital heart disease. Heart 2015;101: 1540–6.

35. Perloff JK, Marelli AJ, Miner PD. Risk of stroke in adults with cyanotic congenital heart disease. Circulation 1993;87:1954–9.

36. Hoffmann A, Chockalingam P, Balint OH, et al. Cerebrovascular accidents in adult patients with congenital heart disease. Heart 2010;96:1223–6.

37. Cheng TO. Platypnea-orthodeoxia syndrome: etiology, differential diagnosis, and management. Catheter Cardiovasc Interv 1999;47:64–6.

38. Attenhofer Jost CH, Connolly HM, Scott CG, et al. Increased risk of possible paradoxical embolic events in adults with Ebstein anomaly and severe tricuspid regurgitation. Congenit Heart Dis 2014;9:30–7.

39. Jategaonkar SR, Scholtz W, Horstkotte D, et al. Interventional closure of atrial septal defects in adult patients with Ebstein's anomaly. Congenit Heart Dis 2011;6:374–81.

40. Yang MC, Chiu SN, Wang JK, et al. Natural and unnatural history of tetralogy of Fallot repaired during adolescence and adulthood. Heart Vessels 2012; 27(1):65–70.

41. Frank DB, Hanna BD. Pulmonary arterial hypertension associated with congenital heart disease and Eisenmenger syndrome: current practice in pediatrics. Minerva Pediatr 2015;67:169–85.

42. Krieger EV, Leary PJ, Opotowsky AR. Pulmonary hypertension in congenital heart disease: beyond

Eisenmenger syndrome. Cardiol Clin 2015;33: 599–609.

43. Broberg CS, Bax BE, Okonko DO, et al. Blood viscosity and its relationship to iron deficiency, symptoms, and exercise capacity in adults with cyanotic congenital heart disease. J Am Coll Cardiol 2006; 48:356–65.

44. Asakai H, Cardamone M, Hutchinson D, et al. Arterial ischemic stroke in children with cardiac disease. Neurology 2015;85:1–7.

45. Sinclair AJ, Fox CK, Ichord RN, et al. Stroke in children with cardiac disease: report from the international pediatric stroke study group symposium. Pediatr Neurol 2015;52:5–15.

46. Dowling MM, Hynan LS, Lo W, et al, International Paediatric Stroke Study Group. International paediatric stroke study: stroke associated with cardiac disorders. Int J Stroke 2013;8(Suppl A100):39–44.

47. Khairy P, Landzberg MJ, Gatzoulis MA, et al, Epicardial Versus ENdocardial pacing and Thromboembolic events Investigators. Transvenous pacing leads and systemic thromboemboli in patients with intracardiac shunts: a multicenter study. Circulation 2006;113:2391–7.

The Epidemiology of Atrial Fibrillation and Stroke

Francesca Pistoia, MD, PhD*, Simona Sacco, MD,
Cindy Tiseo, MD, Diana Degan, MD, Raffaele Ornello, MD,
Antonio Carolei, MD, FAHA

KEYWORDS

- Epidemiology • Atrial fibrillation • Stroke • Cardioembolic stroke • Cryptogenic stroke

KEY POINTS

- The incidence of atrial fibrillation and stroke are expected to increase worldwide in the next decades as a result of the progressive aging of the population and the growing diffusion of unhealthy cardiovascular habits.
- The contribution of atrial fibrillation to the incidence and outcome of ischemic stroke is huge, as shown by the fivefold increased risk of stroke in patients with the arrhythmia.
- Atrial fibrillation is commonly responsible for cardioembolic stroke, which is particularly severe in terms of mortality and residual disability.
- Atrial fibrillation may be underdiagnosed in some cases and be responsible for a high proportion of cryptogenic strokes.

INTRODUCTION

Atrial fibrillation (AF) is one of the major cardiac rhythm disturbances, responsible for a high rate of cardiovascular and cerebrovascular morbidity and mortality, resulting in a high health care cost and public health burden. It is defined as a supraventricular tachyarrhythmia with uncoordinated atrial activation and consequently ineffective atrial contraction.[1] It is commonly classified according to the duration of single episodes.[1] Specifically, an episode that terminates spontaneously or with intervention within 7 days from onset is classified as paroxysmal AF, whereas a more sustained disease, lasting more than 7 days or more than 12 months, is defined as persistent AF or long-standing persistent AF, respectively. Moreover, paroxysmal episodes may recur with a variable frequency along the life span and both paroxysmal and persistent episodes may coexist in the same individual. On the other hand, the term permanent AF implies a condition of irreversibility, which is mainly deduced by clinical findings and refers to patients in whom a consensus to stop further attempts to restore and/or maintain sinus rhythm has been reached.[1] Finally, depending on the underlying pathophysiology, the AF may be classified as valvular or nonvalvular, the latter denoting a form characterized by the absence of rheumatic mitral stenosis, mechanical or bioprosthetic heart valve, or mitral valve repair. AF may be asymptomatic or present with a wide spectrum of symptoms, including fatigue, palpitations, dyspnea, hypotension, and syncope.[1,2] It may coexist with many other comorbidities, such as hypertension, hyperlipidemia, ischemic heart disease, heart failure, anemia, diabetes mellitus, arthritis, and chronic obstructive pulmonary disease. Finally, it is a

Authors have no commercial or financial conflicts of interest or funding sources to be disclosed.
Department of Biotechnological and Applied Clinical Sciences, Neurological Institute, University of L'Aquila, Via Vetoio, L'Aquila 67100, Italy
* Corresponding author.
E-mail address: francesca.pistoia@univaq.it

Cardiol Clin 34 (2016) 255–268
http://dx.doi.org/10.1016/j.ccl.2015.12.002
0733-8651/16/$ see front matter © 2016 Elsevier Inc. All rights reserved.

cardiology.theclinics.com

well-known risk factor for ischemic stroke, which, in some cases, may represent the first manifestation of the arrhythmia, and for myocardial infarction, and heart failure.[3]

EPIDEMIOLOGY OF ATRIAL FIBRILLATION

The frequency of AF in the general population is progressively increasing as a result of greater life expectancy, increased prevalence of risk factors for AF, and improved survival after myocardial infarction. The worldwide age-adjusted prevalence of AF, as estimated in the 2010 Global Burden of Disease Study, is 5.96 per 1000 in men and 3.73 per 1000 in women, accounting for approximately 33 million people.[4] In the United States, AF affects about 3 to 5 million individuals and it is expected to affect greater than 8 million people by 2050.[5] In Europe, AF affects about 8 million people and it is expected to rise dramatically to 18 million by 2060.[6] The prevalence of AF in the general population is about 3%. Prevalence may vary across different countries: the highest prevalence rates have been found in United Kingdom (7.2%), followed by Spain (6.1%), Netherlands (5.5%), and Australia (4%). The lowest rates have been reported in Iran (2.8%), Portugal (2.5%), Brazil (2.4%), Germany (2.2%), Sweden (2%), France (1.6%), United States (1.1%), Switzerland (0.9%), China (0.9%), Kenia (0.7%), Thailand (0.4%), and India (0.1%).[7–21] Discrepancies in prevalence rates across different countries can be attributed to differences in study design, and to genetics and environmental factors. Moreover, the prevalence of AF is significantly higher in white individuals (8.0%) compared with black (3.8%), Hispanic (3.6%), and Asian (3.9%) ethnic groups.[22,23] Prevalence progressively increases with the advancing age, reaching almost 6% to 8% in patients aged 75 years and 10% in the oldest old.[24,25] In this respect, the Screening for Atrial Fibrillation in the Elderly (SAFE) study recently reported a prevalence of 7.2% in patients aged 65 years and older and a prevalence of 10.3% in those age 75 years and older.[26] The age distribution also shows some geographic variations as highlighted by the Randomized Evaluation of Long-term anticoagulant therapY (RE-LY) Atrial Fibrillation Registry showing that patients with AF in Africa, India, and the Middle East are on average 10 to 12 years younger than patients from other regions of the world.[25] The prevalence is higher in men than in women across all the age groups and in all countries with the exception of China.[27] Moreover, paroxysmal AF is more common than persistent AF in young patients and in women.[28]

Recent evidences suggest that AF is often underdiagnosed and its real prevalence may be higher than that reported.[29,30] The reason for missed diagnoses is that spot electrocardiograms (ECGs), compared with continuous ECG monitoring are at risk of underestimating the incidence of paroxysmal silent AF. In this respect, a recent study in a Swedish 75 to 76-year-old population found that a stepwise screening program for AF, based on the combination of a 12-lead ECG recording, followed by a 2-weeks continuous ECG recording, significantly improved the recognition of silent AF especially in subjects with vascular risk factors.[29] Specifically, after including the share of patients who underwent a 2-week continuous ECG recording, the baseline prevalence of AF increased from 9.6% to 14%, thus confirming that isolated ECG recordings may fail to capture paroxysmal AF and that AF screening programs may have useful implications for stroke prevention.[29] Similarly, systematic screening programs based on intermittent ECG recordings showed that mass screening for AF in an elderly population is able to identify a significant proportion of participants with untreated AF.[30] Finally, other studies and meta-analyses evaluated whether screening programs are really cost-effective in the framework of stroke prevention.[31,32] These studies suggested that opportunistic rather than systematic screening, based on pulse taking, followed by invitation for ECG in the presence of an irregular pulse, may be the most cost-effective method for AF screening.[31,32] In the light of these evidences, both the American Heart Association and the American Stroke Association Primary Prevention of Stroke Guidelines, and the 2012 Focused Update of AF Guidelines from the European Society of Cardiology, recommended this opportunistic screening in the primary care setting of patients 65 years and older.[33,34] However, further research is needed to ascertain which screening method is most suitable to detect new cases of AF compared with routine practice and which patients may benefit from prophylactic anticoagulation following the detection of a silent AF.

Risk factors associated with the development of AF include obesity, smoking, hypertension, diabetes, and the presence of cardiac diseases such as coronary artery disease, heart failure, rheumatic heart disease, and valvular heart disease. Hypertension and diabetes are the most common medical conditions associated with AF worldwide, being present in greater than 70% and in greater than 19% of the patients with AF, respectively.[35,36] A close link between an elevated body mass index (BMI) and the development of AF has also been reported, suggesting that the risk of

AF among obese individuals is 1.6 greater than that recognized in subjects with a normal BMI.[37] Besides, coronary artery disease, as well as heart failure and valvular heart disease, strongly contribute to the development of AF worldwide. Given the progressive aging of the population and the wide diffusion of unhealthy lifestyles, their contribution is expected to further grow in the next decades.[27] Finally, the relationship between physical activity and the development of AF is quite controversial. The high prevalence of AF found among highly trained athletes suggests the presence of a U-shaped relationship between the exercise dose and the relative risk of developing AF.[38] However, a recent retrospective cohort study found an inverse relationship between AF and cardiorespiratory fitness that was more evident in obese compared with normal weight subjects.[39]

EPIDEMIOLOGY OF STROKE

Stroke is the second leading cause of death worldwide and the third in most Western countries. It also represents the main cause of disability among adult people, being responsible for a relevant economic burden in terms of health care direct costs and indirect costs linked to missed productivity. Data from the European Union show that stroke is responsible for 14% of all annual deaths and that there are approximately 8 million stroke survivors with a financial burden for stroke of about €62 billion per year.[40] Time trends of stroke suggest that the number of new cases is predicted to decrease in high-income countries as a result of more effective prevention and advances in stroke care and life support procedures. In contrast, cases of stroke are expected to increase in low to middle-income countries as a consequence of the progressive aging of the population and the diffusion of unhealthy habits.[41] Ischemic stroke accounts for about 67% to 81% of all cases of stroke, whereas intracerebral hemorrhage and subarachnoid hemorrhage account for 7% to 20%, and 1% to 7%, of cases, respectively.[42] Undefined strokes are responsible for a variable proportion of cases, ranging from 2% to 15% of all strokes.[42] In population-based studies, incidence rates of stroke range from 1.3 per 1000 to 4.1 per 1000 with the lowest incidence rates being found in the United Kingdom and the highest ones in Japan[41,43–47] (**Table 1**). Moreover, incidence rates are higher in the oldest age groups, in men compared with women, and in black compared with white populations.[43–48] In accordance with the aforementioned evidence from high-income countries, preliminary data from the L'Aquila Stroke Registry show a decreasing trend in the

incidence of stroke: the crude incidence rate for first-ever stroke decreased from 2.92 per 1000 in the years 1994 to 1998, to 1.44 per 1000 in the years 2011 to 2012 (unpublished data). A similar significant decrease in 30-day and 1-year case fatality rates was also observed (unpublished data).

Prevalence rates range from 1.7 per 1000 in the Philippines to 10.2 per 1000 in New Zealand, with few geographic variations.[43,48] Mortality at 1 month from stroke onset is about 23% and it is higher for intracerebral hemorrhage (42%) and subarachnoid hemorrhage (32%) than for ischemic stroke (16%).[43,44] Modifiable risk factors for ischemic stroke include arterial hypertension, smoking, obesity, unhealthy cardiovascular diet, sedentary lifestyle, diabetes mellitus, atrial fibrillation, alcohol intake, psychosocial stress, and depression, whereas significant risk factors for intracerebral hemorrhagic stroke include hypertension, smoking, obesity, unhealthy diet, and alcohol intake.[49]

EPIDEMIOLOGY OF ISCHEMIC STROKE SUBTYPES AND LINK WITH ATRIAL FIBRILLATION

Ischemic stroke may be classified according to the Oxford Community Stroke Project (OCSP) classification, which defines stroke based on the involved vascular territory[50] (**Table 2**), and to the Trial of Org 10172 in Acute Stroke Treatment (TOAST) classification, which is focused on the underlying pathophysiology[51] (**Table 3**).

As previously discussed, AF is a well-known risk factor for ischemic stroke, causing a fivefold increased risk of stroke.[3,52] Data from the L'Aquila Stroke Registry (1994–1998) reported a prevalence of AF in patients with ischemic stroke of about 24.6%.[3] In the same registry, the prevalence increased with age in both sexes, the presence of AF was more frequently associated with total anterior circulation infarcts, and it was responsible for a worst outcome in terms of 30-day and 1-year mortality and rate of stroke recurrences within the first year of follow-up.[3] These data are in line with those from other studies showing that AF is present in 25% to 30% of patients with an acute ischemic stroke.[29] The heterogeneity of findings depends on the age of the included patients and the modalities and timing for AF detection. Interestingly, a recent study, which investigated the prevalence of AF in patients with ischemic stroke or transient ischemic attack (TIA), found an overall prevalence of AF of about 28.6%, with a previously documented history of AF in 19.7% of patients, a newly diagnosed AF in the emergency room in 3.8% of patients, and a newly diagnosed AF during a 3-month period following the acute event in

Table 1
Crude incidence rates (per 1000) of stroke in population-based studies

Study Location	Years	Incidence Rate (95% CI)
Oyabe, Japan	1987–1991	4.1 (3.8–4.4)
Frederiksberg, Denmark	1989–1990	3.1 (2.7–3.4)
Espoo-Kauniainen, Finland	1989–1991	2.2 (2.0–2.4)
Auckland, New Zealand	1991–1992	1.4 (1.3–1.5)
Novosibirsk, Russia	1992	2.3 (2.1–2.5)
Belluno, Italy	1992–1993	2.2 (2.0–2.4)
Arcadia, Greece	1993–1995	3.4 (3.1–3.7)
Innherred, Norway	1994–1996	3.1 (2.8–3.4)
Erlangen, Germany	1994–1998	1.3 (1.2–1.4)
L'Aquila, Italy	1994–1998	2.9 (2.9–3.0)
Perth, Australia	1995–1996	1.6 (1.4–1.8)
South London, UK	1995–1996	1.3 (1.2–1.4)
Melbourne, Australia	1996–1997	2.1 (1.8–2.3)
Martinique, Caribbean	1998–1999	1.6 (1.5–1.8)
Uzhgorod, Ovest Ucraina	1999–2001	2.8 (2.5–3.1)
Perth, Australia	2000–2001	1.2 (1.0–1.4)
Dijon, France	2000–2006	1.1 (1.0–1.2)
Lund-Orup, Sweden	2001–2002	1.9 (1.7–2.1)
Tartu, Estonia	2001–2003	2.2 (2.0–2.4)
Auckland, New Zealand	2002–2003	1.5 (1.5–1.6)
Oxfordshire, UK	2002–2004	1.4 (1.2–1.6)
Valle d'Aosta, Italy	2004–2005	2.2 (2.0–2.5)
Mumbai, India	2005–2006	1.4 (1.3–1.5)
Martinique, Caribbean	2007–2008	1.5 (1.3–1.6)
Kurashiki, Japan	2009–2010	1.6 (1.5–1.7)
Dublin, Ireland	2012	1.7 (1.5–1.8)

Data from Refs.[41,43–47]

Table 2
Definition of subtypes of ischemic stroke according to the Oxford Community Stroke Project classification

OCSP Subtypes	Definition
Lacunar Infarct (LACI)	One of the 4 classic clinical lacunar syndromes (the pure motor stroke, the pure sensory stroke, the sensorimotor stroke, the ataxic hemiparesis that includes the dysarthria- clumsy hand syndrome). Patients with faciobrachial or brachiocrural deficits are included, but more restricted deficits are not.
Total anterior circulation infarct (TACI)	Combination of new higher cerebral dysfunction (eg, dysphasia, dyscalculia, visuospatial disorders), homonymous visual field defect and ipsilateral motor and/or sensory deficit of a least 2 areas of the face, arm, and leg.
Partial anterior circulation infarct	Only 2 of the 3 components of the TACI syndrome, with higher dysfunction alone, or with a motor/sensory deficit more restricted than those classified as LACI (eg, confined to 1 limb, or to the face and hand, but not the whole arm).
Posterior circulation infarct	Any of the following: ipsilateral cranial nerve palsy with contralateral motor and/or sensory deficit, bilateral motor and/or sensory deficit, disorder of conjugate eye movement, cerebellar dysfunction without ipsilateral long-tract deficit, or isolated homonymous visual field defect.

Data from Bogousslavsky J, Cachin C, Regli F, et al. Cardiac sources of embolism and cerebral infarction—clinical consequences and vascular concomitants: the Lausanne Stroke Registry. Neurology 1991;41:855–9.

Table 3
Definition of subtypes of ischemic stroke according to the Trial of Org 10172 in Acute Stroke Treatment criteria

TOAST Subtypes	Definition
Large-artery atherosclerosis	These patients have clinical and brain imaging findings of either significant (>50%) stenosis or occlusion of a major brain artery or branch cortical artery, presumably due to atherosclerosis. Clinical findings include those of cerebral cortical impairment (eg, aphasia, neglect, restricted motor involvement) or brainstem or cerebellar dysfunction. A history of intermittent claudication, transient ischemic attacks (TIAs) in the same vascular territory, a carotid bruit, or diminished pulses supports the clinical diagnosis. Cortical or cerebellar lesions and brainstem or subcortical hemispheric infarcts >1.5 cm in diameter on computed tomography (CT) or MRI are considered to be of potential large-artery atherosclerotic origin. Supportive evidence by duplex imaging or arteriography of a stenosis of >50% of an appropriate intracranial or extracranial artery is needed. Diagnostic studies should exclude potential sources of cardiogenic embolism. The diagnosis of stroke secondary to large-artery atherosclerosis cannot be made if duplex or arteriographic studies are normal or show only minimal changes.
Cardioembolism	This category includes patients with arterial occlusions presumably due to an embolus arising in the heart. Cardiac sources are divided into high-risk and medium-risk groups based on the evidence of their relative propensities for embolism. At least one cardiac source for an embolus must be identified for a possible or probable diagnosis of cardioembolic stroke. Clinical and brain imaging findings are similar to those described for large-artery atherosclerosis. Evidence of a previous TIA or stroke in more than one vascular territory or systemic embolism supports a clinical diagnosis of cardiogenic stroke. Potential large-artery atherosclerotic sources of thrombosis or embolism should be eliminated. A stroke in a patient with a medium-risk cardiac source of embolism and no other cause of stroke is classified as a possible cardioembolic stroke.
Small-artery occlusion (lacune)	This category includes patients whose strokes are often labeled as lacunar infarcts in other classifications. The patient should have one of the traditional clinical lacunar syndromes and should not have evidence of cerebral cortical dysfunction. A history of diabetes mellitus or hypertension supports the clinical diagnosis. The patient should also have a normal CT or MRI examination or a relevant brain stem or subcortical hemispheric lesion with a diameter of <1.5 cm demonstrated. Potential cardiac sources for embolism should be absent and evaluation of the large extracranial arteries should not demonstrate a stenosis of >50% in an ipsilateral artery.
Other determined cause	This category includes patients with rare causes of stroke, such as nonatherosclerotic vasculopathies, hypercoagulable states, or hematologic disorders. Patients in this group should have clinical and CT or MRI findings of an acute ischemic stroke, regardless of the size or location. Diagnostic studies such as blood tests or arteriography should reveal one of these unusual causes of stroke. Cardiac sources of embolism and large-artery atherosclerosis should be excluded by other studies.
Undetermined cause	In several instances, the cause of a stroke cannot be determined with any degree of confidence. Some patients have no likely cause determined despite an extensive evaluation. In others, no cause is found but the evaluation was cursory. This category also includes patients with 2 or more potential causes of stroke so that the physician is unable to make a final diagnosis.

Data from Palacio S, Hart RG. Neurologic manifestations of cardiogenic embolism: an update. Neurol Clin 2002;20:179–93.

5.2%.[28] Moreover, in the same group of patients, paroxysmal AF was more commonly associated with stroke and TIA compared with persistent AF.[28] Similarly, a recent meta-analysis comparing the results of different studies showed that poststroke AF is commonly diagnosed in the emergency room in 7.7% of cases, in the hospital in 5.1% of cases, in the first ambulatory period in 10.7% of cases, and in second ambulatory period in 16.9% of cases, thus confirming that the

Table 4
Trial of Org 10172 in Acute Stroke Treatment distribution in different population-based studies

Study	Country	Inclusion Period	Study Design	Age Limits	Cases	CT	MRI	ECG	Holter ECG	TTE	TEE	Intracranial Vascular Imaging: TDS, MRA, CTA, CA	Carotid Imaging: DS, MRA, CTA, CA	LAA	CE	SAO	OC	UND
Alzamora et al,[57] 2008	Spain	January 1, 2003-December 31, 2003	Population	All	247	100	46	98	n.r.	44	n.r.	81	81	18	27	29	0	26
Aquil et al,[58] 2011	Pakistan	January 2007-December 2007	Hospital	>18	100	100		nr	nr	100	nr	100 MRA	100 DS	31	8	43	1	18
Bejot et al,[59] 2008	France	January 1, 2005-December 31, 2006	Population	All	332	100 (99 CT; 27 MRI)		100		67		n.r.	84%	36	24	27		13
Biswas et al,[60] 2009	USA	July 1, 2005-June 30, 2008	Hospital	All	31 347	100	100	100	100	100	n.r.	100 MRA	100 MRA; 100 DS	22 35	10 24	45 23	0 3	23 15
Carod-Artal et al,[61] 2014	Brazil, Spain	2009–2010	Hospital	All	500	100		100	n.r.	100	n.r.	100	100	12	17	19	7	45
Consoli et al,[62] 2015	Italy	November 2011 - February 2013	Hospital	All	1130	100		100	n.r.	n.r.	n.r.	100	100	18	28	22	3	29
D'Anna et al,[63] 2015	Italy	April 1, 2007 - March 31, 2009	Hospital	All	429	99	7	100	n.r.	100	n.r.	100	100	12	21	17	2	48
Feigin et al,[64] 2006	New Zealand	March 1, 2002- February 28, 2003	Hospital	≥15	1032	n.r. (91% of total pop 1423)		98	n.r.	13	n.r.	4 MRA; 13 carotid DS		6	29	11	3	51
Goldstein et al,[65] 2003	USA	April 1995 - March 1997	Hospital	All	520 255	91 92	36 52	82 74	3 2	53 54	10 11	3 CA 9 CA	62 62	13 13	17 18	26 27	1 2	43 40
Grau et al,[66] 2001	Germany	January 1998- December 1999	Hospital	All	5017	97	29	n.r.	n.r.	63		90 DS; 20 CTA or MRA or CA	83	21	25	21	3	30

Study	Country	Study period	Setting	Age	N													
Gutierrez et al,[67] 2014	USA	November 2008 - February 2011	Hospital	All	389	95	83	n.r.	n.r.	93	34	52 DS, 80 MRA, 86 26 CTA, 22 CA	86	22	34	21	10	13
Hajsadeghi et al,[68] 2013	Iran	September 2010- September 2011	Hospital	All	125	100		n.r.	n.r.	n.r.	n.r.	n.r.	n.r.	26	45	15		14
Jung et al,[69] 2012	Korea	January 2002- November 2010	Hospital	≥16	36,191	n.r. (64% of total pop 46,098)	n.r. (92% of total pop)	n.r.	n.r. (20% of tot pop)	n.r. (64% of tot pop)	n.r. (11% of n.r. tot pop)	n.r. (MRA 81% of tot pop; CA 9% of tot pop; TDS 54% of tot pop)	n.r.	36	17	25	2	20
Kaul et al,[70] 2002	India	February 1, 2000- January 31, 2001	Hospital	All	392	100	n.r.	n.r.	n.r.	82	n.r.	64	82	41	10	18	4	27
Kolominsky-Rabas et al,[71] 2001	Germany	1994–1998	Population	All	531	n.r.	n.r.	n.r.	n.r.	62	n.r.	89 carotid DS or TDS; 15 cerebral CA		13	27	23	2	35
Lang et al,[72] 2013	China	December 2008 - December 2010	Hospital	All	577	n.r.	n.r.	n.r.	n.r.	n.r.	n.r.	n.r.	n.r.	32	22	37	4	5
Lange et al,[73] 2015	Brazil	January 1, 2005 - December 31, 2006	Population	All	608	100	n.r.	100	n.r.	100	n.r.	100	100	25	15	28	3	29
Lavados et al,[74] 2007	Chile	July 1, 2000- June 30, 2002	Population	All	185	100	n.r.	76	1	36	3	—	25	4	27	31	1	37
Leyden et al,[75] 2013	Australia	July 15, 2009- July 15 2010	Population	All	258	94 (62 CT only; 33 both)	94 (62 CT only; 5 MRI only; 33 both)	n.r.	n.r.	n.r.	n.r.	86	86	16	42	11	6	25
Liu et al,[76] 2006	China	from July 2002	Hospital	≥18	610	100		100	n.r.	100	n.r.	n.r.	100	20	26	20		34
Markus et al,[77] 2007	UK	1999–2005	Hospital	All	525	65	8	n.r.	n.r.	57	n.r.	25	97	9	19	38	3	31
					523			n.r.	n.r.			15		16	33	16	3	32

(continued on next page)

Table 4
(continued)

Study	Country	Inclusion Period	Study Design	Age Limits	Cases	CT	MRI	ECG	Holter ECG	TTE	TEE	Intracranial Vascular Imaging: TDS, MRA, CTA, CA	Carotid Imaging: DS, MRA, CTA, CA	LAA	CE	SAO	OC	UND
														TOAST Distribution %				
Marnane et al,[78] 2010	Ireland	December 1, 2005-November 30, 2006	Population	All	381	99		94		75		29 MRA	82	9	34	15	3	39
Medic et al,[79] 2013	Serbia	March 2008	Hospital	All	300	100		n.r.	17	37		67 DS; 37 CTA or MRA	97; 37 CTA or MRA	36	26	23	1	14
Nacu et al,[80] 2015	Norway	2006–2012	Hospital	15–100	2484	Full assessment: 32%								12	33	12	3	40
Nam et al,[81] 2012	Korea	1997–2007	Hospital	All	3278	100		100	52	51		92		24	21	15	3	37
Ntaios et al,[82] 2014	Greece	January 1, 1993-December 31, 2010	Hospital	All	2730	100	27	100	11	54	9	33	71	18	36	24	2	20
Paciaroni et al,[83] 2003	Italy	started in 1998	Population	All	1284	100	58	100	n.r.	41	22	58 MRA; 30 CA; 40 TDS	100	21	20	37	6	16
Pikija et al,[84] 2012	Croatia	July 1, 2007-June 30, 2009	Population	All	748	n.r. (87% of tot pop 1017)	n.r. (1% of tot pop)	100	n.r.	n.r. (2% of tot pop)		n.r. (CA 2% of tot pop; CTA 1%)	n.r. (31% of tot pop)	33	15			43
Porcello Marrone et al,[85] 2013	Brazil	January 2006-December 2009	Hospital	All	688	100		100		n.r.		n.r.	n.r.	32	28	19	4	17
Renjen et al,[86] 2015	India	January 1, 2004-December 31, 2006	Hospital	All	244	n.r.	n.r.	n.r.	n.r.	n.r.		n.r.	n.r.	57	5	8	3	27
Saposnik et al,[87] 2000	USA Argentina	July 1997 - March 1999	Hospital	All	479 361	n.r.	n.r.	n.r.	n.r.	n.r.		n.r.	n.r.	25 12	34 21	27 42	6 6	8 18

Source	Country	Study period	Setting	Age	No.	Diagnostic investigations (%)							LAA	CE	SAO	OC	UND
Schulz & Rothwell,[88] 2003	UK	November 1981–October 1986 from 2002	All		545	n.r.	n.r.	n.r.	n.r.	n.r.	n.r.	n.r.	14	23	22	6	35
					102								17	19	19	3	42
Sciolla et al,[89] 2005	Italy	May 1, 1999–July 31, 1999	Hospital	>25	443	96	100	5	19	25	12	70	33	17	30	3	17
Sen et al,[90] 2013	USA	2000–2009	Hospital	>18	1069	100	100	100	100	100	n.r.	100	17	24	15	6	38
Shibazaki et al,[91] 2009	Japan	March 2006–May 2007	Hospital	All	200	100							9	41	16		34
Song et al,[92] 2012	USA	October 2004–July 2007	Hospital	All	261	100 (95 DWI)	100	n.r.	n.r.	100	n.r.	100	8	31	11	7	44
					89								10	30	10	15	35
Stead et al,[93] 2011	USA	December 2001–March 2004	Hospital	All	500	100	n.r.	n.r.	65 (92% of which were TE)	n.r. n.r.	vascular imaging: 85% (65% of these having CTA or MRA)		19	29	15	4	33
Syed et al,[94] 2003	Pakistan	August 1999–June 2001	Hospital	>4	393	100	100	n.r.	100	100	n.r.	100	27	6	43	4	20
Toso et al,[95] 2006	Italy	January 2005–October 2005	Hospital	≥18	2573	100; 24 both	n.r.	n.r.	42	12 TDS;	77		29	25	26	7	13
van den Herik et al,[96] 2012	The Netherlands	December 2005–February 2009	Hospital	All	660	100	100	n.r.	n.r.	CTA n.r.	CTA n.r	CTA n.r.	17	15	16	6	47
Zecca et al,[97] 2014	Italy	December 2003–June 2008	Hospital	18–90	114	100	100	n.r.	n.r.	100	n.r.	100	23	30	17	0	30

Abbreviations: CA, conventional angiography; CE, cardioembolic; CTA, CT angiography; DS, duplex sonography; LAA, large-artery atherosclerosis; MRA, MR angiography; n.r., not reporting % but examination was done in some cases; OC, other cause; SAO, small-artery occlusion; TDS, transcranial Doppler sonography; TEE, transesophageal echocardiography; TTE, transthoracic echocardiography; UND, undetermined cause.

diagnosis of AF is not even immediate and its real prevalence in stroke patients may be seldom underestimated.[53]

Stroke associated with the presence of AF is commonly cardioembolic and it is characterized by large, multiple, and often bilateral infarcts, which may involve different vascular territories.[54] Cardioembolic stroke typically accounts for approximately 15% to 20% of all ischemic strokes.[55,56] However, a trend toward a higher prevalence of cardioembolic stroke compared with stroke related to large-artery atherosclerosis has been recently reported in high-income countries, probably as a result of an improved control of hypertension, hyperlipidemia, and hyperglycemia[57–97] **(Table 4)**. Data from the L'Aquila Stroke Registry (2011–2012) are in line with this trend, showing a higher proportion of cardioembolic stroke (34.7%) with respect to stroke due to large-artery atherosclerosis (11.5%) and small-artery occlusion (14.5%). In the same registry, the most common risk factors associated with cardioembolic stroke were arterial hypertension, AF and coronary heart disease. The proportion of AF increased from 24.2% in the 1994 to 1998 registry to 31.5% in the 2011 to 2012 period, and it was significant in patients 85 years and older, whereas there was a reduction of hypercholesterolemia, and cigarette smoking (unpublished data). Moreover, cardioembolic stroke caused by AF is particularly severe and shows the highest rates of mortality and permanent disability.[3,29] Specifically, patients with AF-related stroke show a 50% likelihood of death within 1 year, compared with 27% for strokes not related to AF.[40] Long-term outcomes are also poor, as reported by a recent study showing in patients with AF-related stroke, a 5-year survival of 39%, a 5-year recurrence rate of 21.5%, and a nursing home requirement rate of 26%.[98] In the same study, the CHA2DS2-VASc (congestive heart failure, hypertension, age ≥75 years, diabetes mellitus, stroke or transient ischemic attack, vascular disease, age 65–74 years, female sex) and the CHADS2 (congestive heart failure, hypertension, age =75 years, diabetes mellitus, stroke or transient ischemic attack) scores were strong independent predictors of late fatality and disability, suggesting the usefulness of these scores for both stroke risk prediction in AF and outcome assessment after a stroke due to AF.[97]

Finally, it should be highlighted that AF may be significantly associated with cryptogenic strokes, which represent about a third of all ischemic brain events. In fact, paroxysmal AF may go undetected with short periods of ECG monitoring, thus contributing to the increase the proportion of strokes with a missed etiologic diagnosis. In this respect, the CRYptogenic STroke And underLying AF (CRYSTAL AF) trial recently investigated whether a long-term cardiac monitoring through an implantable cardiac monitor was able to improve the rate of AF detection in subjects with cryptogenic stroke.[99] Results showed that this monitoring was more effective than conventional follow-up in detecting AF after cryptogenic stroke.[99] Similarly, the 30-Day Cardiac Event Monitor Belt for Recording Atrial Fibrillation after a Cerebral Ischemic Event (EMBRACE) trial found an AF incidence of 16% along a 30-day monitoring period compared with the incidence of 3.2% in the control group receiving a 24-hour Holter monitoring.[100] All together, these data confirm that a more careful assessment is essential to recognize the presence of AF in patients with stroke, to better define ischemic stroke subtypes and to orientate therapeutic options.

REFERENCES

1. January CT, Wann LS, Alpert JS, et al. Yancy CW for the ACC/AHA task force members. 2014 AHA/ACC/HRS guideline for the management of patients with atrial fibrillation: a report of the American College of Cardiology/American Heart Association Task Force on Practice Guidelines and the Heart Rhythm Society. Circulation 2014;130:e199–267.
2. Lip GY, Tse HF, Lane DA. Atrial fibrillation. Lancet 2012;379:648–61.
3. Marini C, De Santis F, Sacco S, et al. Contribution of atrial fibrillation to incidence and outcome of ischemic stroke: results from a population-based study. Stroke 2005;36:1115–9.
4. Chugh SS, Havmoeller R, Narayanan K, et al. Worldwide epidemiology of atrial fibrillation: a global burden of disease 2010 study. Circulation 2014;129:837–47.
5. Colilla S, Crow A, Petkun W, et al. Estimates of current and future incidence and prevalence of atrial fibrillation in the U.S. adult population. Am J Cardiol 2013;112:1142–7.
6. Stefansdottir H, Aspelund T, Gudnason V, et al. Trends in the incidence and prevalence of atrial fibrillation in Iceland and future projections. Europace 2011;13:1110–7.
7. Majeed A, Moser K, Carroll K. Trends in the prevalence and management of atrial fibrillation in general practice in England and Wales, 1994–1998: analysis of data from the general practice research database. Heart 2001;86:284–8.
8. Barrios V, Calderón A, Escobar C, et al, for the Primary Care Group in the Clinical Cardiology Section of the Spanish Society of Cardiology. Patients with atrial fibrillation in a primary care setting: Val-FAAP study. Rev Esp Cardiol 2012;65:47–53.

9. Heeringa J, van der Kuip DA, Hofman A, et al. Prevalence, incidence and lifetime risk of atrial fibrillation: the Rotterdam study. Eur Heart J 2006; 27:949–53.

10. Sturm JW, Davis SM, O'Sullivan JG, et al. The avoid stroke as soon as possible (ASAP) general practice stroke audit. Med J Aust 2002;176:312–6.

11. Habibzadeh F, Yadollahie M, Roshanipoor M, et al. Prevalence of atrial fibrillation in a primary health care centre in Fars province, Islamic republic of Iran. East Mediterr Health J 2004;10:147–51.

12. Bonhorst D, Mendes M, Adragão P, et al. Prevalence of atrial fibrillation in the Portuguese population aged 40 and over: the FAMA study. Rev Port Cardiol 2010;29:331–50.

13. Kawabata-Yoshihara LA, Benseñor IM, Kawabata VS, et al. Prevalence of electrocardiographic findings in elderly individuals: the São Paulo aging & health study. Arq Bras Cardiol 2009;93:602–7.

14. Wilke T, Groth A, Mueller S, et al. Oral anticoagulation use by patients with atrial fibrillation in Germany. Adherence to guidelines, causes of anticoagulation under-use and its clinical outcomes, based on claims-data of 183,448 patients. Thromb Haemost 2012;107:1053–65.

15. Friberg L, Rosenqvist M, Lip GY. Net clinical benefit of warfarin in patients with atrial fibrillation: a report from the Swedish atrial fibrillation cohort study. Circulation 2012;125:2298–307.

16. Charlemagne A, Blacher J, Cohen A, et al. Epidemiology of atrial fibrillation in France: extrapolation of international epidemiological data to France and analysis of French hospitalization data. Arch Cardiovasc Dis 2011;104:115–24.

17. Naccarelli GV, Varker H, Lin J, et al. Increasing prevalence of atrial fibrillation and flutter in the United States. Am J Cardiol 2009;104:1534–9.

18. Schmutz M, Beer-Borst S, Meiltz A, et al. Low prevalence of atrial fibrillation in asymptomatic adults in Geneva, Switzerland. Europace 2010; 12:475–81.

19. Chen X, Wang H, Zhang H, et al. The prevalence survey and influential factors of atrial fibrillation in Taiyuan. Heart 2011;97:A91–2.

20. Shavadia J, Yonga G, Mwanzi S, et al. Clinical characteristics and outcomes of atrial fibrillation and flutter at the Aga Khan University Hospital, Nairobi: cardiovascular topics. Cardiovasc J Afr 2013;24:6–9.

21. Kiatchoosakun S, Pachirat O, Chirawatkul A, et al. Prevalence of cardiac arrhythmias in Thai community. J Med Assoc Thai 1999;82:727–33.

22. Hernandez MB, Asher CR, Hernandez AV, et al. African American race and prevalence of atrial fibrillation: a meta-analysis. Cardiol Res Pract 2012; 2012:275624.

23. Dewland TA, Olgin JE, Vittinghoff E, et al. Incident atrial fibrillation among Asians, Hispanics, blacks, and whites. Circulation 2013;128:2470–7.

24. Go AS, Hylek EM, Phillips KA, et al. Prevalence of diagnosed atrial fibrillation in adults: national implications for rhythm management and stroke prevention: the anticoagulation and risk factors in atrial fibrillation (ATRIA) study. JAMA 2001; 285:2370–5.

25. Oldgren J, Healey JS, Ezekowitz M, et al, for the RE-LY Atrial Fibrillation Registry Investigators. Variations in cause and management of atrial fibrillation in a prospective registry of 15,400 emergency department patients in 46 countries: the RE-LY atrial fibrillation registry. Circulation 2014;129: 1568–76.

26. Hobbs FD, Fitzmaurice DA, Mant J, et al. A randomised controlled trial and cost-effectiveness study of systematic screening (targeted and total population screening) versus routine practice for the detection of atrial fibrillation in people aged 65 and over. The SAFE study. Health Technol Assess 2005;9:1–74.

27. Rahman F, Kwan GF, Benjamin EJ. Global epidemiology of atrial fibrillation. Nat Rev Cardiol 2014;11: 639–54.

28. Rizos T, Wagner A, Jenetzky E, et al. Paroxysmal atrial fibrillation is more prevalent than persistent atrial fibrillation in acute stroke and transient ischemic attack patients. Cerebrovasc Dis 2011; 32:276–82.

29. Engdahl J, Andersson L, Mirskaya M, et al. Stepwise screening of atrial fibrillation in a 75-year-old population: implications for stroke prevention. Circulation 2013;127:930–7.

30. Svennberg E, Engdahl J, Al-Khalili F, et al. Mass screening for untreated atrial fibrillation: the STROKESTOP study. Circulation 2015;131:2176–84.

31. Fitzmaurice DA, Hobbs FD, Jowett S, et al. Screening versus routine practice in detection of atrial fibrillation in patients aged 65 or over: cluster randomised controlled trial. BMJ 2007;335:83.

32. Moran PS, Flattery MJ, Teljeur C, et al. Effectiveness of systematic screening for the detection of atrial fibrillation. Cochrane Database Syst Rev 2013;(4):CD009586.

33. Goldstein LB, Bushnell CD, Adams RJ, et al, American Heart Association Stroke Council, Council on Cardiovascular Nursing, Council on Epidemiology and Prevention, Council for High Blood Pressure Research, Council on Peripheral Vascular Disease, Interdisciplinary Council on Quality of Care and Outcomes Research. Guidelines for the primary prevention of stroke: a guideline for healthcare professionals from the American Heart Association/American Stroke Association. Stroke 2011;42:517–84.

34. Camm AJ, Lip GY, De Caterina R, et al, for the ESC Committee for Practice Guidelines (CPG). 2012 focused update of the ESC guidelines for the management of atrial fibrillation: an update of the 2010 ESC guidelines for the management of atrial fibrillation. Developed with the special contribution of the European Heart Rhythm Association. Eur Heart J 2012;33:2719–47.

35. Kakkar AK, Mueller I, Bassand JP, et al, for the GARFIELD Registry Investigators. Risk profiles and antithrombotic treatment of patients newly diagnosed with atrial fibrillation at risk of stroke: perspectives from the international, observational, prospective GARFIELD registry. PLoS One 2013; 8:e63479.

36. Chiang CE, Naditch-Brûlé L, Murin J, et al. Distribution and risk profile of paroxysmal, persistent, and permanent atrial fibrillation in routine clinical practice: insight from the real-life global survey evaluating patients with atrial fibrillation international registry. Circ Arrhythm Electrophysiol 2012;5:632–9.

37. Wanahita N, Messerli FH, Bangalore S, et al. Atrial fibrillation and obesity–results of a meta-analysis. Am Heart J 2008;155:310–5.

38. La Gerche A, Schmied CM. Atrial fibrillation in athletes and the interplay between exercise and health. Eur Heart J 2013;34:3599–602.

39. Qureshi WT, Alirhayim Z, Blaha MJ, et al. Cardiorespiratory fitness and risk of incident atrial fibrillation: results from the henry ford exercise testing (FIT) project. Circulation 2015;131:1827–34.

40. Knight E. How can we avoid a stroke crisis? Working group report: stroke prevention in patients with atrial fibrillation. Available at: www.stopafib.org/newsitem.cfm. Accessed October 27, 2015.

41. Feigin VL, Krishnamurthi RV, Parmar P, et al, for the GBD 2013 Writing Group and the GBD 2013 Stroke Panel Experts Group. Update on the global burden of ischemic and hemorrhagic stroke in 1990-2013: the GBD 2013 study. Neuroepidemiology 2015;45: 161–76.

42. Pistoia F, Sacco S, Degan D, et al. Hypertension and stroke: epidemiological aspects and clinical evaluation. High Blood Press Cardiovasc Prev 2015. [Epub ahead of print].

43. Feigin VL, Lawes CM, Bennett DA, et al. Stroke epidemiology: a review of population-based studies of incidence, prevalence, and case-fatality in the late 20th century. Lancet Neurol 2003;2:43–53.

44. Sacco S, Di Gianfilippo G, Di Napoli M, et al. Stroke in Italy: five-year results of the L'Aquila stroke registry (1994–1998) and comparison with comparable national and international population studies. Riv Ital Neurobiol 2006;2:109–36.

45. Olindo S, Chausson N, Mejdoubi M, et al. Trends in incidence and early outcomes in a Black Afro-Caribbean population from 1999 to 2012: Etude Réalisée en Martinique et Centrée sur L'Incidence des Accidents Vasculaires Cérébraux II Study. Stroke 2014;45:3367–73.

46. Iguchi Y, Kimura K, Sone K, et al, Kurashiki Stroke Registry Investigators. Stroke incidence and usage rate of thrombolysis in a Japanese urban city: the Kurashiki stroke registry. J Stroke Cerebrovasc Dis 2013;22:349–57.

47. Kelly PJ, Crispino G, Sheehan O, et al. Incidence, event rates, and early outcome of stroke in Dublin, Ireland. The North Dublin population stroke study. Stroke 2012;43:2042–7.

48. Carolei A, Sacco A, De Santis F, et al. Epidemiology of stroke. Clin Exp Hypertens 2002;24: 479–83.

49. O'Donnell MJ, Xavier D, Liu L, et al, for the INTERSTROKE Investigators. Risk factors for ischaemic and intracerebral haemorrhagic stroke in 22 countries (the INTERSTROKE study): a case-control study. Lancet 2010;376:112–23.

50. Bamford J, Sandercock P, Dennis M, et al. Classification and natural history of clinically identifiable subtypes of cerebral infarction. Lancet 1991;337: 1521–6.

51. Adams HP Jr, Bendixen BH, Kappelle LJ, et al. Classification of subtype of acute ischemic stroke. Definitions for use in a multicenter clinical trial. TOAST. Trial of org 10172 in acute stroke treatment. Stroke 1993;24:35–41.

52. Andrew NE, Thrift AG, Cadilhac DA. The prevalence, impact and economic implications of atrial fibrillation in stroke: what progress has been made? Neuroepidemiology 2013;40:227–39.

53. Sposato LA, Cipriano LE, Saposnik G, et al. Diagnosis of atrial fibrillation after stroke and transient ischaemic attack: a systematic review and meta-analysis. Lancet Neurol 2015;14:377–87.

54. Arquizan C, Lamy C, Mas JL. Simultaneous supratentorial multiple cerebral infarctions. Rev Neurol 1997;153:748–53.

55. Bogousslavsky J, Cachin C, Regli F, et al. Cardiac sources of embolism and cerebral infarction–clinical consequences and vascular concomitants: the Lausanne Stroke Registry. Neurology 1991;41:855–9.

56. Palacio S, Hart RG. Neurologic manifestations of cardiogenic embolism: an update. Neurol Clin 2002;20:179–93.

57. Alzamora MT, Sorribes M, Heras A, et al, for the "ISISCOG Study Group". Ischemic stroke incidence in Santa Coloma de Gramenet (ISISCOG), Spain. A community-based study. BMC Neurol 2008;27(8):5.

58. Aquil N, Begum I, Ahmed A, et al. Risk factors in various subtypes of ischemic stroke according to TOAST criteria. J Coll Physicians Surg Pak 2011; 21(5):280–3.

59. Bejot Y, Caillier M, Ben Salem D, et al. Ischaemic stroke subtypes and associated risk factors: a French population based study. J Neurol Neurosurg Psychiatry 2008;79:1344–8.

60. Biswas M, Sen S, Simmons J. Etiology and risk factors of ischemic stroke in Indian-American patients from a hospital-based registry in New Jersey, USA. Neurol Asia 2009;14(2):81–6.

61. Carod-Artal FJ, Casanova Lanchipa JO, Cruz Ramírez LM, et al. Stroke subtypes and comorbidity among ischemic stroke patients in Brasilia and Cuenca: a Brazilian-Spanish cross-cultural study. J Stroke Cerebrovasc Dis 2014;23(1):140–7.

62. Consoli D, Paciaroni M, Galati F, et al, behalf of SI-SIFO Group. Prevalence of patent foramen ovale in ischaemic stroke in Italy: results of SISIFO study. Cerebrovasc Dis 2015;39(3–4):162–9.

63. D'Anna L, Gigli GL, Gregoraci G, et al. Identification of stroke etiology may contribute to improve the outcome in dedicated units. J Stroke Cerebrovasc Dis 2015;24(4):802–10.

64. Feigin V, Carter K, Hackett M, et al, Auckland Regional Community Stroke Study Group. Ethnic disparities in incidence of stroke subtypes: Auckland Regional Community Stroke Study, 2002-2003. Lancet Neurol 2006;5(2):130–9.

65. Goldstein LB, Matchar DB, Hoff-Lindquist J, et al. Veterans Administration Acute Stroke (VASt) Study: lack of race/ethnic-based differences in utilization of stroke-related procedures or services. Stroke 2003;34(4):999–1004.

66. Grau AJ, Weimar C, Buggle F, et al. Risk factors, outcome, and treatment in subtypes of ischemic stroke: the German stroke data bank. Stroke 2001;32(11):2559–66.

67. Gutierrez J, Koch S, Dong C, et al. Racial and ethnic disparities in stroke subtypes: a multiethnic sample of patients with stroke. Neurol Sci 2014; 35(4):577–82.

68. Hajsadeghi S, Kashani Amin L, Bakhshandeh H, et al. The diagnostic value of N-terminal pro-brain natriuretic peptide in differentiating cardioembolic ischemic stroke. J Stroke Cerebrovasc Dis 2013; 22(4):554–60.

69. Jung KH, Lee SH, Kim BJ, et al, Korean Stroke Registry Study Group. Secular trends in ischemic stroke characteristics in a rapidly developed country: results from the Korean Stroke Registry Study (secular trends in Korean stroke). Circ Cardiovasc Qual Outcomes 2012;5(3):327–34.

70. Kaul S, Sunitha P, Suvarna A, et al. Subtypes of ischemic stroke in a metropolitan city of South India (one year data from a hospital based stroke registry). Neurol India 2002;50(1):14–8.

71. Kolominsky-Rabas PL, Weber M, Gefeller O, et al. Epidemiology of ischemic stroke subtypes according to TOAST criteria: incidence, recurrence, and long-term survival in ischemic stroke subtypes: a population-based study. Stroke 2001;32:2735–40.

72. Lang Q, Zhou M, Feng H, et al. Research on the relationship between fibrinogen level and subtypes of the TOAST criteria in the acute ischemic stroke. BMC Neurol 2013;13:207.

73. Lange MC, Cabral NL, Moro CHC, et al. Incidence and mortality of ischemic stroke subtypes in Joinville, Brazil: a population-based study. Arq Neuropsiquiatr 2015;73:648–54.

74. Lavados PM, Sacks C, Prina L, et al. Incidence, case-fatality rate, and prognosis of ischaemic stroke subtypes in a predominantly Hispanic-Mestizo population in Iquique, Chile (PISCIS project): a community-based incidence study. Lancet Neurol 2007;6:140–8.

75. Leyden JM, Kleinig TJ, Newbury J, et al. Adelaide stroke incidence study: declining stroke rates but many preventable cardioembolic strokes. Stroke 2013;44:1226–31.

76. Liu X, Xu G, Wu W, et al. Subtypes and one-year survival of first-ever stroke in Chinese patients: the Nanjing Stroke Registry. Cerebrovasc Dis 2006;22(2–3):130–6.

77. Markus HS, Khan U, Birns J, et al. Differences in stroke subtypes between black and white patients with stroke: the South London ethnicity and stroke study. Circulation 2007;116(19):2157–64.

78. Marnane M, Duggan CA, Sheehan OC, et al. Stroke subtype classification to mechanism-specific and undetermined categories by TOAST, A-S-C-O, and causative classification system: direct comparison in the North Dublin population stroke study. Stroke 2010;41:1579–86.

79. Medic S, Beslac-Bumbasirevic L, Kisic-Tepavcevic D, et al. Short-term and long-term stroke survival: the belgrade prognostic study. J Clin Neurol 2013;9(1):14–20.

80. Nacu A, Fromm A, Sand KM, et al. Age dependency of ischaemic stroke subtypes and vascular risk factors in Western Norway: the Bergen Norwegian stroke Cooperation Study. Acta Neurol Scand 2016;133(3):202–7.

81. Nam HS, Kim HC, Kim YD, et al. Long-term mortality in patients with stroke of undetermined etiology. Stroke 2012;43(11):2948–56.

82. Ntaios G, Papavasileiou V, Makaritsis K, et al. Association of ischaemic stroke subtype with long-term cardiovascular events. Eur J Neurol 2014;21(8): 1108–14.

83. Paciaroni M, Silvestrelli G, Caso V, et al. Neurovascular territory involved in different etiological subtypes of ischemic stroke in the Perugia Stroke Registry. Eur J Neurol 2003;10:361–5.

84. Pikija S, Cvetko D, Malojčić B, et al. A population-based prospective 24-month study of stroke: incidence and 30-day case-fatality rates of first-ever

strokes in Croatia. Neuroepidemiology 2012;38: 164–71.

85. Porcello Marrone LC, Diogo LP, de Oliveira FM, et al. Risk factors among stroke subtypes in Brazil. J Stroke Cerebrovasc Dis 2013;22(1):32–5.

86. Renjen PN, Beg MA, Ahmad K. Epidemiological study of incidence and risk factors of ischemic stroke subtypes according to trial of ORG 10172 in acute stroke treatment criteria: a 3 years, hospital-based study. Int J Med Public Health 2015;5(1):50–4.

87. Saposnik G, Caplan LR, Gonzalez LA, et al. Differences in stroke subtypes among natives and caucasians in Boston and Buenos Aires. Stroke 2000; 31(10):2385–9.

88. Schulz UG, Rothwell PM. Differences in vascular risk factors between etiological subtypes of ischemic stroke: importance of population-based studies. Stroke 2003;34:2050–9.

89. Sciolla R, Ferrari G, Leone M, SINPAC (Società INter-regionale Piemonte e Valle d'Aosta per le Cerebrovasculopatie) Group. Stroke and transient ischaemic attack in 18 neurology departments from two Italian regions: the SINPAC database. Neurol Sci 2005;26(4):208–17.

90. Sen S, Dahlberg K, Case A, et al. Racial-ethnic differences in stroke risk factors and subtypes: results of a prospective hospital-based registry. Int J Neurosci 2013;123(8):568–74.

91. Shibazaki K, Kimura K, Iguchi Y, et al. Plasma brain natriuretic peptide can be a biological marker to distinguish cardioembolic stroke from other stroke types in acute ischemic stroke. Intern Med 2009; 48(5):259–64.

92. Song S, Burgess RE, Kidwell CS. Racial differences by ischemic stroke subtype: a comprehensive diagnostic approach. Stroke Res Treat 2012;2012: 735097.

93. Stead LG, Gilmore RM, Bellolio MF, et al. Cardioembolic but not other stroke subtypes predict mortality independent of stroke severity at presentation. Stroke Res Treat 2011;2011:281496.

94. Syed NA, Khealani BA, Ali S, et al. Ischemic stroke subtypes in Pakistan: the Aga Khan University Stroke Data Bank. J Pak Med Assoc 2003;53(12): 584–8.

95. Toso V, Carolei A, Gensini GF, et al, SIRIO Study Investigators. The stroke in Italy and related impact on outcome (SIRIO) study: design and baseline data. Neurol Sci 2006;27(Suppl 3):S263–7.

96. van den Herik EG, de Lau LM, Mohamad A, et al. Association of two single nucleotide polymorphisms from genomewide association studies with clinical phenotypes of cerebral ischemia. Int J Stroke 2012;7(3):219–23.

97. Zecca B, Mandelli C, Maino A, et al. A bioclinical pattern for the early diagnosis of cardioembolic stroke. Emerg Med Int 2014;2014:242171.

98. Hayden DT, Hannon N, Callaly E, et al. Rates and Determinants of 5-Year Outcomes After Atrial Fibrillation-Related Stroke: a Population Study. Stroke 2015;46(12):3488–93.

99. Sanna T, Diener HC, Passman RS, et al, for the CRYSTAL AF Investigators. Cryptogenic stroke and underlying atrial fibrillation. N Engl J Med 2014;370:2478–86.

100. Gladstone DJ, Spring M, Dorian P, et al, for the EMBRACE Investigators and Coordinators. Atrial fibrillation in patients with cryptogenic stroke. N Engl J Med 2014;370:2467–77.

Radiological Portrait of Embolic Strokes

Gautam Sachdeva, MD, Ali Saeed, MD, Vishal Jani, MD, Anmar Razak, MD*

KEYWORDS

- Cardioembolism • Stroke • Atrial fibrillation • Radiology • Computed tomography

KEY POINTS

- Stroke is the leading cause of adult disability and the fifth leading cause of death in the United States.
- In 2010, the cost of stroke to the health care system in the United States was estimated to be $71.55 billion, and it is projected to double over the next 20 years.
- Cardioembolism is a leading pathophysiologic cause of stroke, with estimates of being implicated in up to 30% of all cases.
- Certain radiological features on neuroimaging may help distinguish between different pathoetiological processes and help guide further work up and treatment strategies.

INTRODUCTION

Stroke affects nearly 800,000 people every year and is the leading cause for adult disability in the United States. It is estimated that 1 in every 4 adults will have a stroke in their lifetime and as such, it is a disease that has been intensely analyzed and is of utmost concern within the health care system. With the recent advances in novel therapeutics (thrombolysis, mechanical intervention, and comprehensive rehabilitation), stroke has recently dropped to the fifth leading cause of death in the United States. Despite this improvement in mortality, it continues to burden the health care system through its cost, estimated in 2010 to be nearly $71.55 billion. With the aging population, the prevalence is expected to increase by nearly 20% in 2030, with the cost projected to more than double.[1]

Stroke is generally divided into ischemic or hemorrhagic type, with the overwhelming majority, nearly 80%, being ischemic. It is important to differentiate between these 2 types, as their subsequent management strategies differ significantly. Ischemic strokes are most commonly classified according to the TOAST classification system, which includes 5 main etiologic categories (**Box 1**). As will be discussed later, certain radiological features can help differentiate between some of these etiologic subtypes, thus aiding in guiding further work up and prevention strategies. For example, large artery atherosclerotic embolic strokes, like cardioembolic strokes, tend to be cortical, multifocal, or result in large vessel occlusion (LVO) strokes. On the other hand, small vessel occlusion strokes tend to be smaller, subcortical, and centered near perforator vessel-rich areas (lacunar) (eg, basal ganglia and thalamus). A further distinct radiological feature is watershed distribution strokes, which imply profound global hypoperfusion if bilateral or if unilateral, may suggest a large vessel atherosclerotic critical stenosis. It is still important to recognize, however, that in a minority of cases (2%–5%), embolic strokes, including cardioembolism, may result in lacunar or watershed infarcts if the clot burden is singular and small (lacunar) or multiple and small (watershed

Disclosure Statement: No disclosures from any of the authors.
Department of Neurology and Opthalmology, Clinical Center, Michigan State University, 804 Service Road, Room: A217, East Lansing, MI 48824, USA
* Corresponding author.
E-mail address: anmar.razak@hc.msu.edu

Cardiol Clin 34 (2016) 269–278
http://dx.doi.org/10.1016/j.ccl.2015.12.008
0733-8651/16/$ – see front matter © 2016 Elsevier Inc. All rights reserved.

shower of emboli).[2–4] Of these categories, cardioembolic is the most common and accounts for up 30% of ischemic strokes etiologies.[5]

One of the most prominent abnormalities that results in cardioembolic stroke is atrial fibrillation. In 2010, the prevalence of atrial fibrillation ranged between 2.7 and 6.1 million, with estimates of this statistic to double by 2050.[6] Atrial fibrillation occurs when the left atrium of the heart beats in an irregular and rapid fashion. The abnormal rhythm can result in stagnant pooling of blood in the heart, leading to clot formation and the potential of embolization to the brain resulting in stroke. It is reported that atrial fibrillation as an independent risk factor increases the risk of stroke fivefold.[7] Furthermore, data suggest that strokes related to atrial fibrillation tend to be more debilitating and transient ischemic attacks related to atrial fibrillation tend to last longer when compared with strokes related to carotid disease.[8,9]

CLINICAL PRESENTATION OF EMBOLIC STROKES

Stroke is defined as brain, spinal cord, or retinal cell death attributable to ischemia, based on neuropathological, neuroimaging, and/or clinical evidence of permanent injury.[10] With cardioembolic stroke predominantly affecting the brain, lateralizing clinical signs are particularly evident. Although many stroke subtypes share clinical features, a careful assessment can often lead an experienced examiner to favor a cardioembolic pathophysiologic origin. Taking an accurate history also provides vital pieces of information which may help determine if a stroke is ultimately cardioembolic in origin. Determining for example, if there is any known history of prior or exiting atrial fibrillation, presence of a prosthetic heart valve, known history of heart failure, or severe valvular disease may raise the index of suspicion that an ischemic stroke may be cardioembolic in origin.

Cardioembolic strokes tend to occur and progress rather abruptly in their presentation as compared with other stroke subtypes. Lacunar strokes and or atherothrombotic strokes may present with stuttering symptoms over time, giving the body a chance to develop alternative blood flow patterns, whereas cardioembolic strokes typically cause an abrupt loss of blood flow in which there has been no chance for vascular remodeling or diversion of flow. As quickly as they develop, cardioembolic strokes may also quickly resolve or decrease in clinical magnitude due to a clot potentially breaking up and traveling to more distal vessels. Additionally, strokes resulting in visual field deficits, aphasias, and neglect are more likely to be cardioembolic in origin as compared to other stroke etiologies. This may be a manifestation of the observation that cardioembolic clots tend to be large, and as such they favor larger diameter vessels such as the middle cerebral artery and its branches.[11] Watershed stroke may also result in weakness and aphasia; however, such strokes typically produce proximal greater than distal weakness patterns and a transcortical aphasia subtype (motor, sensory). Because larger-diameter arteries are implicated in cardioembolic strokes, it stands to reason why other classic stroke presentations such as pure motor syndrome and/or a pure sensory syndrome that often involve smaller penetrating arteries supplying the internal capsule and thalamus should raise more suspicion of a lacunar subtype when such clinical presentations present themselves. It is also important to recognize that because of their cardiac origin, emboli may result in a multifocal stroke pattern that does not obey only 1 particular vascular distribution, resulting in bilateral symptom manifestations. When multifocal or bihemispheric strokes are encountered, cardioembolism as the underlying mechanism of stroke should be a leading suspicion.

EMERGENCY MANAGEMENT OF ACUTE STROKE

The phrase "Time is brain" emphasizes the urgency in management and treatment of acute ischemic stroke. The quantification of this phrase was originally described by Jeffrey L. Saver, who showed that a typical patient loses 1.9 million neurons per minute if the stroke is left untreated.[12] The

National Institute of Neurologic Disorders and Stroke (NINDS) established stroke evaluation and treatment benchmarks that make up the basis of any stroke evaluation in the emergency room. The goal for acute management of stroke patients entails examination, imaging, laboratory tests, and intravenous thrombolytics initiation in a target time of less than 60 minutes. **Table 1** lays out the breakdown of target times for the emergent stroke patient evaluation per the American Heart Association guidelines.[13]

The emergency evaluation and management of acute stroke starts with ensuring stability of the patient with airway, breathing, and circulation assessment. The second step is ruling out any reversible conditions, such as hypoglycemia, clinically mimicking clinical stroke symptoms. After stability is confirmed, the next step is determining the patient's candidacy for treatment with intravenous thrombolysis and/or intra-arterial therapy. This includes obtaining relevant clinical history and ruling out contraindications to treatment, early triaging of the patient to CT/MRI to rule out hemorrhage and other pathologies, and performing a stroke rating scale called the National Institute of Health Stroke Scale (NIHSS).[13]

In the pertinent history, establishing the time of symptom onset and usage of recent anticoagulants is critical for the treatment decision. If the patient has aphasia and is unable to provide the information, it is defined as the time when the patient was last seen normal without any neurologic symptoms. This should be confirmed from reliable sources. A limited number of laboratory tests, including hematological, coagulation, and biochemistry tests are recommended during the initial evaluation, but only the blood glucose assessment and coagulation studies (if the patient is on oral anticoagulants) should precede the initiation of intravenous therapy. Baseline electrocardiogram (EKG) to look for cardiac rhythm irregularities and baseline cardiac

enzymes are recommended but should not delay intravenous tissue plasminogen activator (tPA) administration.[13]

Rapidly acquired imaging of the brain, either with noncontrast head CT, or less commonly MRI, is required before intravenous tPA administration to exclude intracerebral hemorrhage or a mass lesion as the cause of the patient's presentation. Acute ischemic strokes in most cases are not accompanied by any changes on CT scan within the first 3 to 4.5 hours. If present, however, early ischemic changes regardless of extent are not a contraindication to intravenous tPA, although a frank hypodensity especially when occupying more than one-third of middle cerebral artery territory is a valid reason to withhold treatment because of the increased risk of hemorrhage. A noninvasive vascular study, either computed tomography angiography or magnetic resonance angiography (MRA) of the head and neck is strongly recommended if either intra-arterial thrombolysis or mechanical thrombectomy is contemplated, although it should not delay intravenous tPA administration.[13–15]

Physical examination of patients suspected of having an acute stroke is centered on a focused neurologic examination meant to confirm the diagnosis, help localize the affected part of the brain, and stratify the severity of the stroke. The NIHSS (**Table 2**) is the most widely used and validated standardized tool used for this purpose. It helps to objectively quantify the neurologic examination of the patient and monitor improvement or deterioration in the patient's clinical status and facilitates communicating the patient's clinical status to other health team professionals. It also helps in determining the outcome and prognosis. It is composed of 11 items that integrate most components of the neurologic examination, including level of consciousness, select cranial nerves, motor, sensory, cerebellar function, language, and inattention. The score ranges from 0 to 42 with less than 8, 8 to 16 and greater than 17 signifying mild, moderate, and severe impairment, respectively.[16] Within this tool, examination findings of facial paresis, arm weakness/pronator drift, and language impairment (dysarthria or aphasia) are highly suggestive of an acute stroke diagnosis.[17] Certain abnormal findings on NIHSS like visual fields, best gaze, best language, and extinction/inattention are predictors of cortical large vessel stroke. Symptoms pertaining to pure motor, pure sensory, sensory motor deficits, ataxic hemiparesis, and dysarthria on NIHSS evaluation are predictors of subcortical or lacunar strokes secondary to small vessel lipohyalinosis. Posterior circulation strokes have the weakest representation on the NIHSS, with ataxia out of proportion to the weakness being the best predictor.[18–20]

Table 1
Timeline benchmarks for acute stroke management

Benchmarks	Target Time
Door to emergency room doctor evaluation, history, NIHSS, laboratrory tests	<10 min
Stroke team notification	<15 min
Door to CT head	<25 min
CT head and laboratory interpretation	<45 min
Intravenous TPA given if patient is eligible	<60 min

Table 2
National Institutes of Health stroke scale

Category	Scale Definition
1a	Level of consciousness: (eg, alert, drowsy)	0 = Alert 1 = Drowsy 2 = Stuporous 3 = Coma
1b	LOC questions: (month, age)	0 = Answers both correctly 1 = Answers one correctly 2 = Both incorrect
1c	LOC commands: (open and close eyes; make fist and let go)	0 = Obeys both correctly 1 = Obeys one correctly 2 = Both incorrect
2	Best gaze: (eyes follow examiner's finger/face horizontally)	0 = Normal 1 = Partial gaze palsy 2 = Forced deviation
3	Visual: test visual fields upper and lower quadrants on both sides	0 = No visual loss 1 = Cannot see in 1 quadrant 2 = Cannot see in 2 quadrants 3 = Cannot see in any quadrant
4	Facial palsy: (show teeth, raise eyebrows, and squeeze eyes shut)	0 = Normal 1 = Minor paralysis 2 = Partial paralysis 3 = Complete paralysis
5 & 6	Motor arm & leg: arms—extend the arms with palms down 90° (if sitting) or 45° (if supine); drift is scored if the arm falls before 10 s Begin with the nonparetic limb. Legs—with patient in the supine position, extend the legs 30°; drift is scored if the leg falls before 5 s	0 = No drift for elapsed time 1 = Drift (but does not hit bed) 2 = Cannot resist gravity (drifts to bed) 3 = No effort against gravity (falls to bed quickly, but can move limb) 4 = No movement U = Untestable 5a = Left arm 5b = Right arm 6a = Left leg 6b = Right leg
7	Limb ataxia: perform finger-nose-finger and heel–shin tests on both sides	0 = Absent 1 = Present in 1 limb 2 = Present in 2 limbs
8	Sensory: pin-prick to face, arm, leg, trunk; compare side to side.	0 = Normal; no sensory loss 1 = Mild-to-moderate loss 2 = Severe-to-total loss
9	Best language: name items, describe a picture, and read sentences; tests ability to express ideas verbally	0 = Normal; no aphasia 1 = Mild-to-moderate aphasia 2 = Severe aphasia 3 = No usable speech
10	Dysarthria: evaluate speech clarity by patient repeating listed words	0 = Normal articulation 1 = Mild-to-moderate dysarthria 2 = Nearly unintelligible or worse U = Intubated or other physical barrier
11	Extinction and inattention: using touch and visual stimuli, evaluate for extinction or inattention	0 = No neglect 1 = Inattention or extinction in 1 sensory modality 2 = Complete neglect

IMAGING MODALITIES IN ACUTE STROKE

The noncontrast head CT (NCCT) is the imaging modality of choice in the hyperacute phase given the ease of availability, rapidity of acquisition, and cost-effectiveness.[21]

NCCT is highly sensitive for acute hemorrhage with its hyperdense signal changes usually immediately visible. Ischemic infarcts on the other hand are often not documented by CT before 3 hours from onset, but the diagnostic yield of CT increases progressively with time, so that nearly 60% can be detected by 24 hours; by 7 days, virtually 100% of infarcts are demonstrated on CT.[14,22,23] Early signs of acute ischemia that can be visible on the initial NCCT include loss of gray white interface in the lateral margins of the insula (insular ribbon) and focal hypoattenuation of the parenchyma, especially in large vessel occlusion (LVO) strokes.[24] Detection of these early changes is facilitated by the use of a standardized scoring tool called The Alberta Stroke Program Early CT Score (ASPECTS). This is a 10-point quantitative score that was developed to assess early ischemic changes on initial CT in patients with acute stroke in the anterior circulation. In this score, the middle cerebral artery (MCA) territory is divided into 10 regions, and 1 point is subtracted for every region of hypoattenuation. The score is inversely proportional to stroke severity, and a value of 7 or less signifies an increase in the risk of symptomatic intracerebral hemorrhage complication and poor outcome at 3 months.[25]

In addition to possible early ischemic changes or lack thereof, initial NCCT can show images suggestive of intracranial vascular thrombus/embolus, which can be seen as hyperdense cordlike structures in a major intracranial artery, most commonly the MCA stem (but can also be seen in the anterior or posterior cerebral arteries as well as the basilar artery). This is sometimes referred to as the MCA hyperdense sign and can indicate an embolus from a proximal source such as the carotid artery (artery-to-artery embolus) or a more proximal source of embolism (cardiac or systemic) (**Fig. 1**).[26]

Other imaging modalities include advanced CT techniques such as CT angiogram and CT perfusion, which assist in providing a comprehensive study of intracranial and extracranial vasculature, distinguishing infarct core from the ischemic penumbra. This can help in better selection of patients for intra-arterial TPA or thrombolytic therapy.[27]

MRI brain is an alternative imaging modality, which is highly sensitive for the detection of acute stroke. MRI diffusion weighted image (DWI) sequence can detect ischemic changes

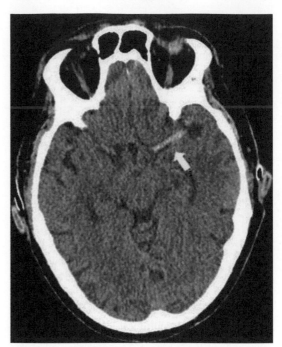

Fig. 1. Hyperdense middle cerebral artery (MCA) sign on the left (*yellow arrow*) indicative of an occlusive embolus within the vessel lumen in a patient with atrial fibrillation.

within 3 to 30 minutes of symptom onset compared with CT, in which changes are often delayed. It is as sensitive as CT scan for the detection of acute or chronic hemorrhage (with susceptibility images).[28,29] MRA can help detect vascular occlusions and can be used as a part of acute stroke work up. Limitations to MRI compared with CT use are cost, availability, decreased resolution of early intracerebral hemorrhage, patient intolerance/claustrophobia, and exclusions in patients with ferromagnetic fragments, aneurysm clips, otic or cochlear implants, old prosthetic heart valves, pacemakers, and neurostimulators.[30]

IMAGING APPEARANCE OF CARDIOEMBOLIC STROKE

Certain findings on imaging modalities can sometimes suggest the underlying source or etiology of the stroke, although this is not always reliable; additionally, further testing is always required for confirmation. For example, patients with cardioembolic source of stroke sometimes exhibit acute multiple territorial infarcts or a single but large cortical infarct. Multiple infarcts are typically multifocal and may involve bilateral hemispheres spanning different vascular territories, (eg, left middle cerebral artery and right posterior cerebral

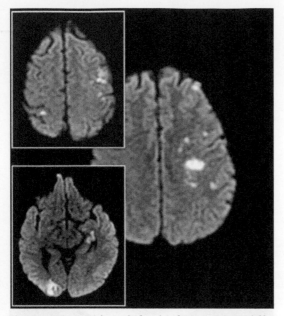

Fig. 2. Patient with multifocal infarcts on MRI diffusion weighted sequence. Hyperintense (*white*) lesions are seen in the left frontal lobe and the right parietal and occipital lobes. The patient in this case had atrial fibrillation.

artery territories) (**Fig. 2**). Cortical infarcts in cardioembolic cases are classically wedge shaped with the base pointing toward the surface and apex inwards (**Fig. 3**). Cardiac emboli are generally large in size, producing large vessel occlusions intracranially, which can be visualized on imaging (hyperdense MCA or basilar artery sign) (see **Fig. 1**; **Fig. 4**). However, they can also be small and multiple, causing distal branch occlusions (shower of emboli) (**Fig. 5**).[30,31]

Cerebral embolism, and in particular cardioembolism, is also associated with early and frequent hemorrhagic transformation (up to 71% of cases), early recanalization of occluded vessels, as well as abrupt occlusion without evidence of atherosclerotic disease. About 95% of hemorrhagic infarcts are caused by cardioembolism (**Fig. 6**).[32–34] It is important to recognize that systemic embolism (hypercoagulable states) and aortic arch atherosclerotic disease strokes can also share similar imaging characteristics to cardioembolism findings described previously.[35]

Compared with cardioembolism and systemic embolism, solitary lesions in a unilateral anterior circulation territory or small, scattered lesions in 1 vascular territory are sometimes related to large artery atherosclerosis (extra or intracranial artery to artery embolism) (**Fig. 7**). Cardioembolism in these cases can still be the culprit and cannot be completely ruled out, especially if vascular imaging fails to identify atherosclerostic large vessel disease.[36]

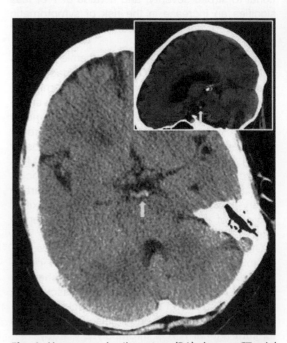

Fig. 4. Hypersense basilar artery (BA) sign on CT axial and sagittal (small subset) images indicative of embolic occlusion of the artery (*yellow arrows*). The axial image shows the thrombus extending into the right posterior cerebral artery.

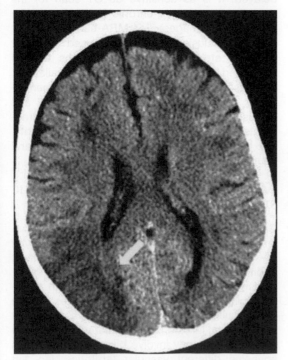

Fig. 3. Right parieto-occipital wedge shaped infarct on CT scan (*yellow arrow*).

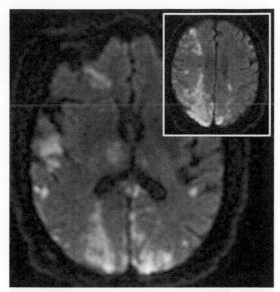

Fig. 5. Extensive multifocal bilateral showering infarcts on MRI diffusion weighted sequence seen as hyperintense lesions in anterior and posterior circulation territories of the both hemispheres. The culprit in this case was an atrial thrombus.

Other image findings of stroke subtypes that point away from cardioembolism include lacunar infarcts, which are small vessel strokes causing infarcts less than 20 mm in size. These classically result from the occlusion of small deep penetrating end vessels, including

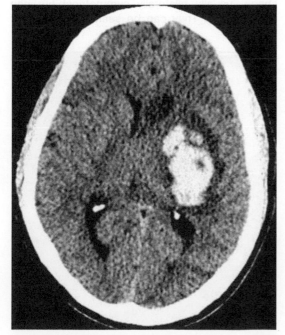

Fig. 6. Early hemorrhagic transformation in a patient with a left middle cerebral artery cardioembolic stroke.

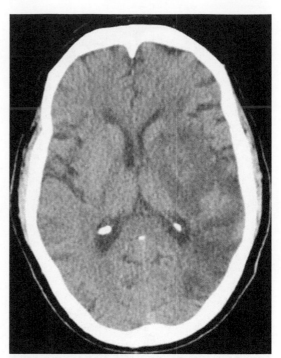

Fig. 7. Subacute infarct in the left middle cerebral artery distribution (left frontal and parietal lobe hypodensities) due to artery-to-artery thromboembolism in a patient with critical left internal carotid artery stenosis.

lenticulostriate, thalamoperforators, recurrent artery of Heubner, and pontine perforators. The location of these strokes is usually in the basal ganglia, thalamus, brain stem, and corona radiata subcortical territories (**Fig. 8**). The mechanism is usually lipohyalinosis of these end arteries, although embolism and intracranial atherosclerotic disease can also be responsible in a small subset of cases.[31,37] Typical radiographic features include small discrete foci of hypodensity on CT and diffusion restriction on MRI. They are usually 3 to 20 mm in diameter, with an average size of about 10 mm. They are usually solitary, although they have a high recurrence rate, and multiple areas of acute and subacute infarct foci may be seen simultaneously (**Fig. 9**).[18,38]

Finally, watershed infarcts (also referred to as border zone infarcts) are ischemic lesions located at junctions of 2 major arterial territories. They constitute approximately 10% of all ischemic cerebral infarcts.[33] They are divided into 2 major types: external (cortical) and internal (subcortical). The external border zone infarcts are large, oval, or wedge-shaped, and are located either at the frontal cortex between anterior cerebral artery (ACA) and MCA territories, at

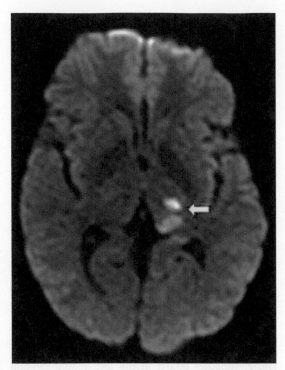

Fig. 8. Acute left thalamic lacunar stroke on MRI (*yellow arrow*).

the occipital cortex between MCA and posterior cerebral artery (PCA) territories, or at the paramedian white matter between ACA and MCA territories (**Fig. 10**). The common etiology of these

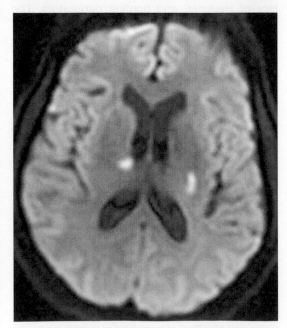

Fig. 9. Bilateral basal ganglia (BG) nonembolic lacunar strokes on MRI. Typically these are seen as early recurrent strokes in patients with highly uncontrolled vascular risk factors.

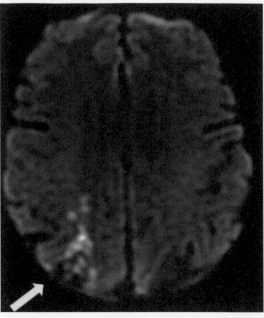

Fig. 10. External (cortical) watershed infarct between the right middle cerebral and right posterior cerebral artery vascular territory (*yellow arrow*).

infarcts is microemboli from cardiac source or atherosclerotic plaques of the major arteries. These microemboli disseminate to the cortical borderzone areas, which have low perfusion pressure with limited ability to wash out emboli. The internal (subcortical) infarcts are linear in shape, usually bilaterally symmetrical but can be unilateral. They can be seen as a string of

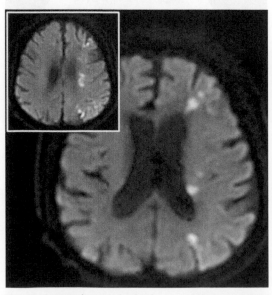

Fig. 11. Internal watershed infarct on MRI in a patient with severe critical left internal carotid artery stenosis.

pearls on MRI parallel to the lateral ventricle, which is the site of border zones between the deep penetrating end vessels (lenticulostriate arteries, recurrent artery of Huebner, anterior choroidal artery) and the major vessels (ACA, MCA and PCA) in the centrum semiovale and coronoa radiata (**Fig. 11**). The causative mechanisms here are usually either profound systemic hypotension causing bilateral lesions, or regional cerebral hypoperfusion secondary to severe intra/extracranial carotid artery stenosis resulting in unilateral internal watershed stroke, although microembolism can still be a cause.[39,40]

SUMMARY

Certain stroke etiologies produce different and characterstic image appearances that can help distinguish the underlying etiology or pathology and assist in guiding further work up and management decisions. Familiarizing oneself with these image characteristics and paring them with history and neurologic examination findings provide an invaluable tool in acute stroke diagnosis and management, the details of which may vary depending on the underlying cause.

REFERENCES

1. Ovbiagele B, Goldstein LB, Higashida RT, et al. Forecasting the future of stroke in the united states: a policy statement from the American Heart Association and American Stroke Association. Stroke 2013; 44:2361–75.
2. Cacciatore A, Russo LS Jr. Lacunar infarction as an embolic complication of cardiac and arch angiography. Stroke 1991;22:1603–5.
3. Lodder J, Bamford JM, Sandercock PA, et al. Are hypertension or cardiac embolism likely causes of lacunar infarction? Stroke 1990;21:375–81.
4. Torvik A. The pathogenesis of watershed infarcts in the brain. Stroke 1984;15:221–3.
5. Kolominsky-Rabas PL, Weber M, Gefeller O, et al. Epidemiology of ischemic stroke subtypes according to toast criteria: Incidence, recurrence, and long-term survival in ischemic stroke subtypes: a population-based study. Stroke 2001;32: 2735–40.
6. Mozaffarian D, Benjamin EJ, Go AS, et al. Heart disease and stroke statistics–2015 update: a report from the american heart association. Circulation 2015;131:e29–322.
7. Wolf PA, Abbott RD, Kannel WB. Atrial fibrillation as an independent risk factor for stroke: the Framingham study. Stroke 1991;22:983–8.
8. Harrison MJ, Marshall J. Atrial fibrillation, TIAs and completed strokes. Stroke 1984;15:441–2.
9. Anderson DC, Kappelle LJ, Eliasziw M, et al. Occurrence of hemispheric and retinal ischemia in atrial fibrillation compared with carotid stenosis. Stroke 2002;33:1963–7.
10. Sacco RL, Kasner SE, Broderick JP, et al. An updated definition of stroke for the 21st century: a statement for healthcare professionals from the American Heart Association/American Stroke Association. Stroke 2013;44:2064–89.
11. Arboix A, Alió J. Cardioembolic stroke: clinical features, specific cardiac disorders and prognosis. Curr Cardiol Rev 2010;6:150–61.
12. Saver JL. Time is brain–quantified. Stroke 2006;37: 263–6.
13. Jauch EC, Saver JL, Adams HP Jr, et al. Guidelines for the early management of patients with acute ischemic stroke: a guideline for healthcare professionals from the American Heart Association/American Stroke Association. Stroke 2013;44(3):870–947.
14. Merino JG, Warach S. Imaging of acute stroke. Nat Rev Neurol 2010;6:560–71.
15. Gilberto gonzález R. Acute ischemic stroke—imaging and intervention. Berlin: Springer-Verlag; 2015.
16. Briggs DE, Felberg RA, Malkoff MD, et al. Should mild or moderate stroke patients be admitted to an intensive care unit? Stroke 2001;32:871–6.
17. Simel LBG, David L. Is this patient having a stroke? JAMA 2015;293:2391–402.
18. Fisher C. Lacunar infarcts: a review cerebrovascular. Cerebrovasc Dis 1991;1:311–20.
19. Martin-Schild S, Albright KC, Tanksley J, et al. Zero on the NIHSS does not equal the absence of stroke. Ann Emerg Med 2011;57:42–5.
20. Sartor EA, Albright K, Boehme AK, et al. The nihss score and its components can predict cortical stroke. J Neurol Disord Stroke 2013;2:1026.
21. Wardlaw JM, Seymour J, Cairns J, et al. Immediate computed tomography scanning of acute stroke is cost-effective and improves quality of life. Stroke 2004;35:2477–83.
22. Bryan RN, Levy LM, Whitlow WD, et al. Diagnosis of acute cerebral infarction: comparison of CT and MR imaging. AJNR Am J Neuroradiol 1991;12(4): 611–20.
23. Sarwar M, Batnitzky S, editors. Imaging of Non-Traumatic Ischemic and Hemorrhagic Disorders of the Central Nervous System. Springer Science & Business Media; 2012. p. 193–220.
24. Norman CLT, Barkovich AJ, Gean-Marton A, et al. Loss of the insular ribbon: another early ct sign of acute middle cerebral artery infarction. Radiology 1990;176:801–6.
25. Barber PA, Demchuk AM, Zhang J, et al. Validity and reliability of a quantitative computed tomography score in predicting outcome of hyperacute stroke before thrombolytic therapy. Lancet 2000;355: 1670–4.

26. Berge E, Nakstad PH, Sandset PM. Large middle cerebral artery infarctions and the hyperdense middle cerebral artery sign in patients with atrial fibrillation. Acta Radiol 2001;42:261–8.

27. Koenig M, Kraus M, Theek C, et al. Quantitative assessment of the ischemic brain by means of perfusion-related parameters derived from perfusion ct. Stroke 2001;32:431–7.

28. Li F, Han S, Tatlisumak T, et al. A new method to improve in-bore middle cerebral artery occlusion in rats: demonstration with diffusion- and perfusion-weighted imaging. Stroke 1998;29: 1715–9 [discussion: 1719–20].

29. Chalela JA, Kidwell CS, Nentwich LM, et al. Magnetic resonance imaging and computed tomography in emergency assessment of patients with suspected acute stroke: a prospective comparison. Lancet 2007;369:293–8.

30. Culebras A, Kase CS, Masdeu JC, et al. Practice guidelines for the use of imaging in transient ischemic attacks and acute stroke. A report of the stroke council, american heart association. Stroke 1997;28:1480–97.

31. Ringelstein EB, Koschorke S, Holling A, et al. Computed tomographic patterns of proven embolic brain infarctions. Ann Neurol 1989;26:759–65.

32. Molina CA, Montaner J, Abilleira S, et al. Timing of spontaneous recanalization and risk of hemorrhagic transformation in acute cardioembolic stroke. Stroke 2001;32:1079–84.

33. Jörgensen L, Torvik A. Ischaemic cerebrovascular diseases in an autopsy series part 2. Prevalence, location, pathogenesis, and clinical course of cerebral infarcts. J Neurol Sci 1969;9:285–320.

34. Fisher M, Adams RD. Observations on brain embolism with special reference to the mechanism of hemorrhagic infarction. J Neuropathol Exp Neurol 1951;10:92–4.

35. Jung JM, Kwon JY, Kim HJ, et al. Ischemic lesion burden and characteristics of aortic atheroma. J Stroke Cerebrovasc Dis 2014;23:278–82.

36. Kang DW, Chalela JA, Ezzeddine MA, et al. Association of ischemic lesion patterns on early diffusion-weighted imaging with toast stroke subtypes. Arch Neurol 2003;60:1730–4.

37. Lee DK, Kim JS, Kwon SU, et al. Lesion patterns and stroke mechanism in atherosclerotic middle cerebral artery disease: early diffusion-weighted imaging study. Stroke 2005;36:2583–8.

38. Arboix A, Marti-Vilalta JL. Lacunar stroke. Expert Rev Neurother 2009;9:179–96.

39. Derdeyn CP, Khosla A, Videen TO, et al. Severe hemodynamic impairment and border zone–region infarction. Radiology 2001;220:195–201.

40. Del Sette M, Eliasziw M, Streifler JY, et al. Internal borderzone infarction: a marker for severe stenosis in patients with symptomatic internal carotid artery disease. For the North American Symptomatic Carotid Endarterectomy (NASCET) group. Stroke 2000;31:631–6.

Atrial Fibrillation and Cognitive Decline
Phenomenon or Epiphenomenon?

 CrossMark

Shadi Kalantarian, MD, MPH[a], Jeremy N. Ruskin, MD[b],*

KEYWORDS

• Atrial fibrillation • Cognitive impairment • Dementia

KEY POINTS

• Atrial fibrillation is associated with cognitive impairment.
• The association is independent of history of clinical stroke.
• Silent cerebral infarction, proinflammatory state, and brain hypoperfusion due to beat-to-beat variability in cardiac cycle length are plausible but unproven mechanisms underlying this association.

INTRODUCTION

Atrial fibrillation (AF), the most prevalent cardiac arrhythmia, is a costly disease that is associated with significant morbidity and mortality.[1] Emerging evidence suggests a link between AF and cognitive impairment (from mild to severe dementia).[2] One school of thought has been that dementia is merely a secondary phenomenon that occurs alongside AF with the aging of the population as a result of shared risk factors; however, there are new data to support other potential mechanisms underlying this association. These data go beyond coincidence and common risk factors. This article, therefore, aims to review current evidence surrounding 3 areas of debate: (1) the characteristics and magnitude of the association between AF and cognitive impairment, (2) plausible mechanisms underlying this association, and (3) potential treatment strategies that might target the proposed mechanistic pathways.

ATRIAL FIBRILLATION AND COGNITIVE IMPAIRMENT

It is well established that AF increases the risk of clinical stroke by fourfold to fivefold,[1] and patients with history of stroke are at higher risk of developing dementia.[3] It is also known that AF and cognitive impairment share several common risk factors, including but not limited to, advanced age, diabetes,[4,5] hypertension,[5,6] and heart failure.[7] Therefore, it is not surprising to observe a significant association between AF and cognitive impairment in patients with first-ever or recurrent stroke (relative risk [RR] 2.70, 95% confidence interval [CI] 1.82–4.00).[2] However, a recent meta-analysis demonstrated a 34% increase in the risk of cognitive impairment in patients with AF (RR 1.40, CI 1.19–1.64) in the *absence of a history of clinical stroke* and after adjustment for several shared risk factors.[2] This observation suggests that there are mechanistic pathways other than clinical stroke and shared risk factors that link AF and cognitive impairment.

Supported in part by the Deane Institute for Integrative Research in Atrial Fibrillation and Stroke at Massachusetts General Hospital.

[a] Internal Medicine Residency Program, Yale New Haven Hospital, 20 York Street, New Haven, CT 06510, USA;
[b] Cardiac Arrhythmia Service, Massachusetts General Hospital, Harvard Medical School, 55 Fruit Street, Boston, MA 02114, USA
* Corresponding author. Cardiac Arrhythmia Service, Massachusetts General Hospital, Harvard Medical School, 55 Fruit Street, Boston, MA 02114, USA
E-mail address: jruskin@partners.org

Cardiol Clin 34 (2016) 279–285
http://dx.doi.org/10.1016/j.ccl.2015.12.011

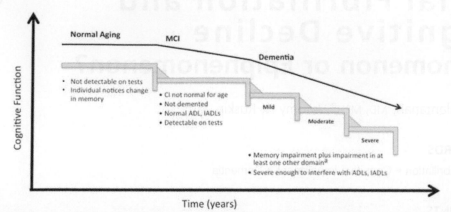

Fig. 1. Spectrum of cognitive decline. [a]Cognitive function has several domains, including memory, language, attention, motor, visuospatial function, executive functioning, and verbal fluency. ADL, activities of daily living (ie, mobility, bathing, dressing, self-feeding, personal hygiene and grooming, independent toileting); CI, cognitive impairment; IADLs, instrumental ADLs (ie, shopping, housekeeping, accounting, food preparation/medications, telephone/transportation); MCI, mild cognitive impairment.

Cognitive impairment has a wide spectrum ranging from mild cognitive impairment to severe dementia (**Fig. 1**). AF is not only associated with the entire spectrum of cognitive impairment, but also appears to be related to a faster decline in cognition and development of dementia at earlier ages.[8] Among the dementia subtypes, Alzheimer disease is the most common, affecting approximately 5.3 million Americans of all ages in 2015, followed by vascular dementia, previously known as multi-infarct dementia, which comprises 10% of dementia cases.[9] However, data suggest that pathologic evidence of Alzheimer and vascular dementia coexist in approximately half of patients with dementia.[9] Given the association of AF with stroke, the association between AF and vascular dementia is likely. Nonetheless, data were previously lacking on the magnitude of the association between AF and subtypes of dementia.

The Intermountain Heart Collaborative Study[10] is the largest prospective study that investigated the association between AF and different types of dementia (Alzheimer disease, and vascular, senile, and nonspecific dementia). In this study, AF was associated with a significant increase in the incidence of all dementia subtypes over a 5-year follow-up. Although this study has been criticized for risk of misclassification of dementia subtypes owing to the use of *International Classification of Diseases, Ninth Revision* (ICD-9) codes as the diagnostic method, their findings are supported by the Rotterdam Study where more sensitive methods, such as neurologic and psychiatric assessment, as well as imaging, were used to distinguish subtypes of dementia (Alzheimer vs vascular dementia).[11]

Finally, cognitive function has several domains that do not seem to be equally affected by AF.

Evidence suggests that AF is associated with poorer performance in global cognitive ability, but people with AF appear to perform disproportionately worse in tasks related to abstract reasoning, immediate and delayed recall, and executive functioning.[12,13]

MECHANISMS UNDERLYING THE ASSOCIATION BETWEEN ATRIAL FIBRILLATION AND COGNITIVE IMPAIRMENT

Fig. 2 summarizes the possible mechanisms underlying the association between AF and cognitive impairment.

Hypercoagulable States and Brain Infarcts

AF is associated with an increased risk of thromboembolism likely through several mechanisms including but not limited to blood stasis and a hypercoagulable state. Several studies show elevated plasma fibrinogen levels in patients with chronic AF, independent of the presence of valvular heart disease, cardiac dysfunction, or coronary artery disease. Warfarin therapy or conversion to sinus rhythm did not normalize the fibrinogen levels in these patients.[14] AF is independently associated with increased plasma levels of prothrombin fragment 1 + 2, and the levels appear to decline after anticoagulation.[15] Additionally, subjects with AF and dementia exhibit increased thrombin generation and fibrin turnover compared with those without dementia. Another contributor to a procoagulant/prothrombotic state is local cardiac platelet activation and endothelial dysfunction in patients with acute-onset AF.[16]

Thromboembolic events in AF can lead to clinically overt stroke or may remain silent without causing any acute neurologic deficits. This

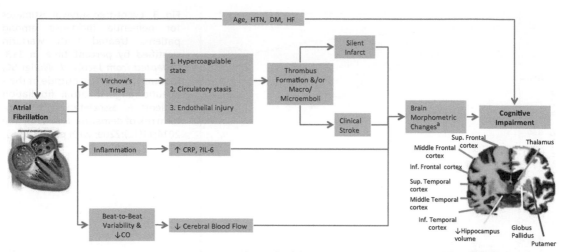

Fig. 2. Putative mechanisms underlying the association between AF and cognitive impairment. [a]Some of reported brain morphometric changes include hippocampus atrophy, white matter hyperintensities, and frontal medial lobe atrophy. CO, cardiac output; DM, diabetes mellitus; HF, heart failure; HTN, hypertension. *Up arrows* indicate increase, *Down arrows* indicate decrease, ? means questionable or possible.

appears to depend on the size and location of brain infarcts. For instance, small infarcts in cortical or subcortical areas of the frontal or parietal lobes may not cause any appreciable acute neurologic deficits, whereas even small infarcts in the speech or motor cortex can lead to acute aphasia or paralysis.[17] Silent cerebral infarcts are identified in more than 40% of MRI images of patients with AF and AF is associated with more than twofold increase in the odds of developing silent infarcts.[18] Although silent infarcts may not cause acute neurologic deficits, new studies suggest a significant association between silent infarcts and the development of cognitive decline.[19] Silent infarcts in patients with AF have a microembolic mechanism and are identified as small, well-demarcated bilateral lesions, often in clusters, most prevalent in the frontal lobes.[19] This pattern of distribution seems to be similar to vascular dementia, in which most silent strokes seem to affect frontal circuit components (frontal cortex, basal ganglia, thalamus) that play an important role in executive functioning.[20] Therefore, the term "silent infarct" is probably a misnomer. Although these injuries do not initially present as focal neurologic deficits, with the accumulation of silent infarcts and repetitive brain injuries over time, they may manifest as cognitive impairment.

There is a paucity of evidence regarding the effect of anticoagulation on silent cerebral infarcts and the risk of cognitive impairment. Several studies did not show a significant reduction in risk of cognitive impairment in patients on warfarin therapy,[21] whereas a few showed a trend toward reduced risk of cognitive impairment associated with anticoagulation.[22] The controversy originates from the lack of assessment of quality of

anticoagulation management and merely focusing on presence or absence of exposure to warfarin. One recent study[23] addressed this shortcoming by evaluating the time in therapeutic range (TTR) to assess the effectiveness of warfarin therapy. The Intermountain Heart Collaborative Study[23] demonstrated a consistent increase in risk of dementia with decreasing percentage of time in therapeutic range (**Fig. 3**). The association between warfarin therapy and dementia was a "U"-shaped curve with increased risks of dementia among patients with overexposure and underexposure to warfarin (ie, supratherapeutic and subtherapeutic international normalized ratios [INRs]). This is likely due to cumulative brain injury from microbleeds and silent infarcts, respectively.

On the other hand, it is known that elderly people with dementia are at higher risk of having poor anticoagulation management with more frequent out-of-range INRs. Data from the Atrial Fibrillation Clopidogrel Trial With Irbesartan for Prevention of Vascular Events (ACTIVE W) trial[24] shows that even mild cognitive impairment at baseline is a predictor of less-effective anticoagulation (measured by a time in therapeutic range of less than 65% over 1.5 year). In addition, mild cognitive impairment (Mini-Mental State Examination [MMSE] <26) was found to be associated with more vascular events (6.7% vs 3.6% per 100 patient-years; $P = .002$) and more bleeding (9.6% vs 7% per 100 patient-years; $P = .04$). Therefore, critics have argued that the result of the Intermountain Heart Collaborative Study is partially biased by lack of exclusion of patients with mild cognitive impairment at baseline. These subjects are at increased risk for both ineffective anticoagulation and dementia in the future.

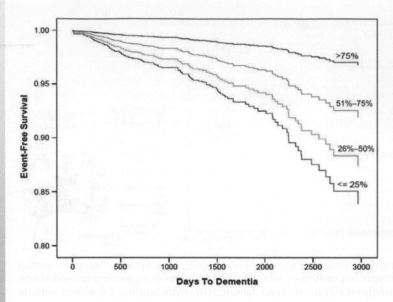

Fig. 3. Event-free survival estimates for dementia incidence among patients treated with warfarin stratified by percent time in TTR. (*Adapted from* Jacobs V, Woller SC, Stevens S, et al. Time outside of therapeutic range in atrial fibrillation patients is associated with long-term risk of dementia. Heart Rhythm 2014;11(12):2209; with permission.)

Proinflammatory State

A proinflammatory state has been reported in patients with AF[25,26] and in patients with dementia[27] independently. C-reactive protein (CRP), a marker of inflammation, is associated with development and persistence of AF,[26] and its levels correlate with AF burden.[28] This association appears to be more significant in the presence of elevated complement components (C3, C4).[29] The association between AF and elevated CRP persists across all levels of CHADS2 scores.[30] This supports the concept that the presence of several comorbidities, including heart failure, hypertension, advanced age, and history of stroke, cannot fully explain the inflammatory state in patients with AF. Additionally, a proinflammatory state measured by CRP or interleukin (IL)-6 levels in patients with AF is associated with worse outcomes, including increased risk of death, stroke,[31] and recurrence of AF after cardioversion.[32] The proinflammatory state in patients with dementia has been described in several studies; elevated CRP levels are associated with significantly increased risk for all dementia subtypes (Alzheimer disease and vascular dementia) independent of cardiovascular risk factors and disease.[27]

The effect of anti-inflammatory agents on the development of cognitive impairment in patients with AF is unknown. It is known from prior studies that statin therapy is associated with reduced inflammatory markers such as CRP.[33] One randomized controlled trial[34] assigned patients with AF on oral warfarin therapy to 1 of 2 treatment groups: atorvastatin40/ezetemibe 10 or placebo. Several endpoints including levels of inflammatory

markers and changes in brain volumes, as well as the risk of cognitive impairment, were assessed. The results of this study demonstrated a significant reduction in brain atrophy (specifically left amygdala) and memory decline associated with statin therapy. Analysis of inflammatory markers revealed significant decrease in CRP levels and several other inflammatory markers in the statin treatment group compared with placebo. Among the inflammatory markers, a reduction in IL-1 receptor antagonist (IL-1RA), IL-9, IL-2, and IL-12, as well as macrophage inflammatory protein-1beta, correlated significantly with improvement in neurocognitive function, memory, and speed.[34,35]

Changes in Brain Perfusion

AF eliminates the contribution of atrial transport to cardiac output and causes beat-to-beat variability in the cardiac cycle. These changes have been shown to be associated with disproportionate reductions in perfusion to different brain regions.[36] A rapid ventricular rate during AF also reduces the diastolic filling time and contributes further to lower cardiac output. In theory, therefore, rate control strategies in patients with a sustained rapid ventricular response during AF should improve brain perfusion. Efimova and colleagues[37] studied a group of patients with medically refractory rapidly conducted AF who were candidates for atrioventricular (AV) junction ablation and ventricular pacing and compared their brain perfusion before and 3 months after the procedure. A control group without AF was also included in the study. Brain perfusion was assessed by brain single-photon emission computed tomography scanning, and regional perfusion was correlated with domains of neurocognitive function as measured by neurocognitive testing. Brain perfusion was globally reduced in patients with AF compared with the control group. Cardiac output and brain perfusion improved significantly after AV junctional ablation and placement of a permanent pacemaker in patients with rapidly conducted AF. There was a significant correlation between reduced brain perfusion in the superior frontal region and attention and immediate memory. Reduced brain perfusion in the inferior frontal region was associated with worse psychomotor speed.

Rhythm control strategies, on the other hand, should improve cardiac output by restoring atrial transport and eliminating beat-to-beat variability in the cardiac cycle length. In an observational study by Bunch and colleagues,[38] patients with AF who underwent a catheter ablation procedure to eliminate AF had a significantly lower risk of developing dementia in the future, comparable to patients without any history of AF. These results are yet to be confirmed by randomized controlled trials such as the Catheter Ablation versus Antiarrhythmic Drug Therapy for Atrial Fibrillation (CABANA) trial that is still ongoing.

Brain Morphometric Changes

Brain morphometric changes are frequently seen in brain imaging of patients with dementia. Total brain volume loss is one of the most common findings in patients with dementia, particularly Alzheimer disease.[39] AF has also been shown to be associated with reduced total brain volume even in the absence of a history of stroke.[40] This association is stronger among patients with persistent/permanent AF compared with paroxysmal AF and among those with increased time from the first diagnosis of the disease.

The hippocampus, a key neurologic center for learning and memory, is affected in Alzheimer disease[41,42] and vascular dementia,[43,44] as well as diabetes[45] and hypertension.[46] Recent evidence also suggests a significant association between hippocampal atrophy and cognitive impairment in patients with AF in the absence of stroke.[47]

Data from the Alzheimer's Disease Neuroimaging Initiative[48] shows evidence of volume loss in the middle temporal lobes and entorhinal cortex in patients with AF. In this study, entorhinal cortex atrophy was correlated with worse performance on the MMSE. This is consistent with data from postmortem[49] and imaging studies[41,42,50] in Alzheimer disease that identify middle temporal lobe structures, and in particular the entorhinal cortex, amygdala, and hippocampus as the sites of earliest change in Alzheimer disease.

White matter hyperintensities on MRI were found to be associated with a more than threefold increase in the risk of stroke (3.3, 95% CI 2.6–4.4) and a twofold increase in risk of dementia (1.9, 1.3–2.8) and death (2.0, 1.6–2.7).[51] Also, studies suggest an association between white matter hyperintensities and a faster decline in global cognitive performance, executive function, and processing speed.[51] The pathophysiology of these lesions is not well described but it appears that reduced cardiac output and brain perfusion, as well as microvacular disease, are correlated with their presence.[51] Controversy exists among studies on the association between AF and evidence of white matter hyperintensities on MRI. The Rotterdam study was among the first studies that investigated the presence of white matter lesions in patients with AF using 1.5-T MRI scanning.[52] Although analysis of this cohort showed a borderline significant association between AF and severe periventricular white matter lesions, later studies failed to reproduce these results.[47,53] One observational study also showed a higher severity of deep and subcortical white matter hyperintensities in patients with AF.[54] These controversial findings are in part due to the lack of a standardized and accurate method for quantifying white matter lesions. In addition, studies that did not show a significant association between AF and white matter lesions were either underpowered to detect an association,[53] or included a younger population with potentially a higher brain reserve capacity.[47]

DISCUSSION/SUMMARY

AF is associated with cognitive impairment ranging from mild to overt dementia and this association is independent of clinical stroke and multiple shared risk factors. Silent cerebral infarction, proinflammatory states, and brain hypoperfusion due to beat-to-beat variability in cardiac cycle length leading to brain morphometric changes are *plausible but unproven mechanisms* underlying this association. To date, no effective preventive measures or treatments have been identified that definitively mitigate the risk of dementia in patients with AF. Anticoagulation with warfarin has not been shown to reduce risk of dementia, most likely owing to poor anticoagulation management with frequent out-of-range INRs. Whether the use of the novel anticoagulants will offer greater protection than warfarin in this population remains to be determined. Rate control strategies may improve brain perfusion and memory but this has not been studied in a randomized controlled trial. More data are required from ongoing trials, such as CABANA, to determine whether rhythm control through AF ablation or antiarrhythmic drugs may reduce the risk of future dementia. Overall, this is a novel field that requires multiple observational studies with long-term follow-up, as well as large-scale randomized controlled trials with accurate neurocognitive testing and brain imaging to better elucidate the mechanisms underlying the association between AF and cognitive impairment and to ultimately define effective preventive strategies and treatment options.

REFERENCES

1. Mozaffarian D, Benjamin EJ, Go AS, et al. Heart disease and stroke statistics–2015 update: a report from the American Heart Association. Circulation 2015;131(4):e29–322.

2. Kalantarian S, Stern TA, Mansour M, et al. Cognitive impairment associated with atrial fibrillation: a meta-analysis. Ann Intern Med 2013;158(5 Pt 1):338–46.

3. Gorelick PB, Scuteri A, Black SE, et al. Vascular contributions to cognitive impairment and dementia: a statement for healthcare professionals from the American Heart Association/American Stroke Association. Stroke 2011;42(9):2672–713.

4. Cheng G, Huang C, Deng H, et al. Diabetes as a risk factor for dementia and mild cognitive impairment: a meta-analysis of longitudinal studies. Intern Med J 2012;42(5):484–91.

5. Knopman D, Boland LL, Mosley T, et al. Cardiovascular risk factors and cognitive decline in middle-aged adults. Neurology 2001;56(1):42–8.

6. Elias MF, Wolf PA, D'Agostino RB, et al. Untreated blood pressure level is inversely related to cognitive functioning: the Framingham Study. Am J Epidemiol 1993;138(6):353–64.

7. Vogels RL, Scheltens P, Schroeder-Tanka JM, et al. Cognitive impairment in heart failure: a systematic review of the literature. Eur J Heart Fail 2007;9(5):440–9.

8. Thacker EL, McKnight B, Psaty BM, et al. Atrial fibrillation and cognitive decline: a longitudinal cohort study. Neurology 2013;81(2):119–25.

9. Alzheimer's Association. 2015 Alzheimer's disease facts and figures. Alzheimers Dement 2015;11(3):332–84.

10. Bunch TJ, Weiss JP, Crandall BG, et al. Atrial fibrillation is independently associated with senile, vascular, and Alzheimer's dementia. Heart Rhythm 2010;7(4):433–7.

11. Breteler MM. Vascular involvement in cognitive decline and dementia. Epidemiologic evidence from the Rotterdam study and the Rotterdam scan study. Ann N Y Acad Sci 2000;903:457–65.

12. Elias MF, Sullivan LM, Elias PK, et al. Atrial fibrillation is associated with lower cognitive performance in the Framingham offspring men. J Stroke Cerebrovasc Dis 2006;15(5):214–22.

13. Farina E, Magni E, Ambrosini F, et al. Neuropsychological deficits in asymptomatic atrial fibrillation. Acta Neurol Scand 1997;96(5):310–6.

14. Lip GY. Fibrinogen and cardiovascular disorders. QJM 1995;88(3):155–65.

15. Roldan V, Marín F, Blann AD, et al. Interleukin-6, endothelial activation and thrombogenesis in chronic atrial fibrillation. Eur Heart J 2003;24(14):1373–80.

16. Akar JG, Jeske W, Wilber DJ. Acute onset human atrial fibrillation is associated with local cardiac platelet activation and endothelial dysfunction. J Am Coll Cardiol 2008;51(18):1790–3.

17. Yatsu FM, Shaltoni HM. Implications of silent strokes. Curr Atheroscler Rep 2004;6(4):307–13.

18. Kalantarian S, Ay H, Gollub RL, et al. Association between atrial fibrillation and silent cerebral infarctions: a systematic review and meta-analysis. Ann Intern Med 2014;161(9):650–8.

19. Gaita F, Corsinovi L, Anselmino M, et al. Prevalence of silent cerebral ischemia in paroxysmal and persistent atrial fibrillation and correlation with cognitive function. J Am Coll Cardiol 2013;62(21):1990–7.

20. Konno S, Meyer JS, Terayama Y, et al. Classification, diagnosis and treatment of vascular dementia. Drugs Aging 1997;11(5):361–73.

21. Mavaddat N, Roalfe A, Fletcher K, et al. Warfarin versus aspirin for prevention of cognitive decline in atrial fibrillation: randomized controlled trial (Birmingham Atrial Fibrillation Treatment of the Aged Study). Stroke 2014;45(5):1381–6.

22. Barber M, Tait RC, Scott J, et al. Dementia in subjects with atrial fibrillation: hemostatic function and the role of anticoagulation. J Thromb Haemost 2004;2(11):1873–8.

23. Jacobs V, Woller SC, Stevens S, et al. Time outside of therapeutic range in atrial fibrillation patients is associated with long-term risk of dementia. Heart Rhythm 2014;11(12):2206–13.

24. Flaker GC, Pogue J, Yusuf S, et al. Cognitive function and anticoagulation control in patients with atrial fibrillation. Circ Cardiovasc Qual Outcomes 2010;3(3):277–83.

25. Asselbergs FW, van den Berg MP, Diercks GF, et al. C-reactive protein and microalbuminuria are associated with atrial fibrillation. Int J Cardiol 2005;98(1):73–7.

26. Aviles RJ, Martin DO, Apperson-Hansen C, et al. Inflammation as a risk factor for atrial fibrillation. Circulation 2003;108(24):3006–10.

27. Schmidt R, Schmidt H, Curb JD, et al. Early inflammation and dementia: a 25-year follow-up of the

Honolulu-Asia Aging Study. Ann Neurol 2002;52(2): 168–74.

28. Chung MK, Martin DO, Sprecher D, et al. C-reactive protein elevation in patients with atrial arrhythmias: inflammatory mechanisms and persistence of atrial fibrillation. Circulation 2001;104(24):2886–91.

29. Dernellis J, Panaretou M. Effects of C-reactive protein and the third and fourth components of complement (C3 and C4) on incidence of atrial fibrillation. Am J Cardiol 2006;97(2):245–8.

30. Crandall MA, Horne BD, Day JD, et al. Atrial fibrillation and CHADS2 risk factors are associated with highly sensitive C-reactive protein incrementally and independently. Pacing Clin Electrophysiol 2009;32(5):648–52.

31. Conway DS, Buggins P, Hughes E, et al. Prognostic significance of raised plasma levels of interleukin-6 and C-reactive protein in atrial fibrillation. Am Heart J 2004;148(3):462–6.

32. Watanabe E, Arakawa T, Uchiyama T, et al. High-sensitivity C-reactive protein is predictive of successful cardioversion for atrial fibrillation and maintenance of sinus rhythm after conversion. Int J Cardiol 2006;108(3):346–53.

33. Mozaffarian D, Minami E, Letterer RA, et al. The effects of atorvastatin (10 mg) on systemic inflammation in heart failure. Am J Cardiol 2005;96(12): 1699–704.

34. Lappegard KT, Pop-Purceleanu M, van Heerde W, et al. Improved neurocognitive functions correlate with reduced inflammatory burden in atrial fibrillation patients treated with intensive cholesterol lowering therapy. J Neuroinflammation 2013;10:78.

35. Tendolkar I, Enajat M, Zwiers MP, et al. One-year cholesterol lowering treatment reduces medial temporal lobe atrophy and memory decline in stroke-free elderly with atrial fibrillation: evidence from a parallel group randomized trial. Int J Geriatr Psychiatry 2012;27(1):49–58.

36. Friedman HS, O'Connor J, Kottmeier S, et al. The effects of atrial fibrillation on regional blood flow in the awake dog. Can J Cardiol 1987;3(5):240–5.

37. Efimova I, Efimova N, Chernov V, et al. Ablation and pacing: improving brain perfusion and cognitive function in patients with atrial fibrillation and uncontrolled ventricular rates. Pacing Clin Electrophysiol 2012;35(3):320–6.

38. Bunch TJ, Crandall BG, Weiss JP, et al. Patients treated with catheter ablation for atrial fibrillation have long-term rates of death, stroke, and dementia similar to patients without atrial fibrillation. J Cardiovasc Electrophysiol 2011; 22(8):839–45.

39. Scahill RI, Schott JM, Stevens JM, et al. Mapping the evolution of regional atrophy in Alzheimer's disease: unbiased analysis of fluid-registered serial MRI. Proc Natl Acad Sci U S A 2002;99(7):4703–7.

40. Stefansdottir H, Arnar DO, Aspelund T, et al. Atrial fibrillation is associated with reduced brain volume and cognitive function independent of cerebral infarcts. Stroke 2013;44(4):1020–5.

41. Lehericy S, Baulac M, Chiras J, et al. Amygdalohippocampal MR volume measurements in the early stages of Alzheimer disease. AJNR Am J Neuroradiol 1994;15(5):929–37.

42. Jack CR Jr, Petersen RC, Xu YC, et al. Medial temporal atrophy on MRI in normal aging and very mild Alzheimer's disease. Neurology 1997;49(3):786–94.

43. Dolek N, Saylisoy S, Ozbabalik D, et al. Comparison of hippocampal volume measured using magnetic resonance imaging in Alzheimer's disease, vascular dementia, mild cognitive impairment and pseudodementia. J Int Med Res 2012;40(2):717–25.

44. Kril JJ, Patel S, Harding AJ, et al. Patients with vascular dementia due to microvascular pathology have significant hippocampal neuronal loss. J Neurol Neurosurg Psychiatry 2002;72(6):747–51.

45. Korf ES, van Straaten EC, de Leeuw FE, et al. Diabetes mellitus, hypertension and medial temporal lobe atrophy: the LADIS study. Diabet Med 2007;24(2):166–71.

46. den Heijer T, Launer LJ, Prins ND, et al. Association between blood pressure, white matter lesions, and atrophy of the medial temporal lobe. Neurology 2005;64(2):263–7.

47. Knecht S, Oelschläger C, Duning T, et al. Atrial fibrillation in stroke-free patients is associated with memory impairment and hippocampal atrophy. Eur Heart J 2008;29(17):2125–32.

48. Qureshi AI, Saed A, Tasneem N, et al. Neuroanatomical correlates of atrial fibrillation: a longitudinal MRI study. J Vasc Interv Neurol 2014;7(5):18–23.

49. Braak H, Braak E. Neuropathological staging of Alzheimer-related changes. Acta Neuropathol 1991;82(4):239–59.

50. Juottonen K, Laakso MP, Partanen K, et al. Comparative MR analysis of the entorhinal cortex and hippocampus in diagnosing Alzheimer disease. AJNR Am J Neuroradiol 1999;20(1):139–44.

51. Debette S, Markus HS. The clinical importance of white matter hyperintensities on brain magnetic resonance imaging: systematic review and meta-analysis. BMJ 2010;341:c3666.

52. de Leeuw FE, de Groot JC, Oudkerk M, et al. Atrial fibrillation and the risk of cerebral white matter lesions. Neurology 2000;54(9):1795–801.

53. Lazarus R, Prettyman R, Cherryman G. White matter lesions on magnetic resonance imaging and their relationship with vascular risk factors in memory clinic attenders. Int J Geriatr Psychiatry 2005;20(3):274–9.

54. Kobayashi A, Iguchi M, Shimizu S, et al. Silent cerebral infarcts and cerebral white matter lesions in patients with nonvalvular atrial fibrillation. J Stroke Cerebrovasc Dis 2012;21(4):310–7.

Cardiac Monitoring for Atrial Fibrillation in Cryptogenic Stroke

Sukit M. Ringwala, MD, MPH[a], Todd T. Tomson, MD[a],
Rod S. Passman, MD, MSCE[b],*

KEYWORDS

- Stroke • Atrial fibrillation • Cardiac monitoring

KEY POINTS

- Despite an extensive initial evaluation, the cause of up to a third of ischemic strokes remains undetermined.
- New atrial fibrillation (AF) detection in patients with cryptogenic stroke is critical because it warrants anticoagulation for the secondary prevention of stroke.
- Observational studies and prospective randomized controlled trials illustrate that a substantial proportion of patients with cryptogenic stroke have AF detected by post-stroke cardiac monitoring.
- Monitoring for more extended periods of time increases the proportion of patients in whom AF is detected. Insertable cardiac monitors provide the highest yields of AF detection.
- Based on the current evidence, prolonged monitoring for AF in patients with cryptogenic stroke beyond the guideline-recommended 30 days may be beneficial.

BACKGROUND

Stroke is among the most feared adverse events in all of medicine. Annually, more than 600,000 cases of ischemic stroke are reported in the United States.[1] For people who experience ischemic stroke, morbidity and mortality have been estimated at 70% to 80%.[2,3] In fact, stroke is the leading cause of long-term disability and is responsible for $36.5 billion per year in health care costs.[4] Accurate determination of stroke cause has a substantial impact on secondary prevention therapies. Therefore, a comprehensive diagnostic evaluation is recommended, which includes but is not limited to brain imaging, vascular imaging, tests of hypercoagulability, and cardiac evaluation to assess for cardiac sources of emboli.[1,5]

Despite a complete diagnostic evaluation, a definitive cause cannot be identified for approximate one-third of ischemic strokes. These strokes are referred to as being cryptogenic in origin, and antiplatelet therapy is the recommended treatment. The most commonly used classification scheme for stroke cause is the TOAST (Trial of ORG 10172 in Acute Stroke Treatment) classification. TOAST defines cryptogenic stroke as brain infarction that is not attributable to a cardiac source of embolism, large artery atherosclerosis, or small artery disease despite extensive vascular, cardiac, and serologic evaluation. Cryptogenic stroke is, therefore, a diagnosis of exclusion.[6]

Thromboembolism due to atrial fibrillation (AF) is an established cause of both ischemic stroke and

Financial Disclosures: Dr R.S. Passman receives research support and honoraria from Medtronic.
[a] Department of Clinical Cardiac Electrophysiology, Northwestern Memorial Hospital, 676 North Saint Claire Street, Suite 600, Chicago, IL 60657, USA; [b] Department of Clinical Cardiac Electrophysiology, The Bluhm Cardiovascular Institute, Northwestern Memorial Hospital, Northwestern University Feinberg School of Medicine, 676 North Saint Claire Street, Suite 600, Chicago, IL 60657, USA
* Corresponding author.
E-mail address: r-passman@northwestern.edu

Cardiol Clin 34 (2016) 287–297
http://dx.doi.org/10.1016/j.ccl.2015.12.010

transient ischemic attack (TIA). Although first described in patients with mitral stenosis, the Framingham study conclusively demonstrated a 5-fold increased risk of stroke even in patients with nonvalvular AF.[7] Even though the association between AF and stroke is clear, the often paroxysmal and asymptomatic nature of AF has made the diagnosis challenging. Overall, about 40% of patients with AF are entirely asymptomatic; studies of patients with a known history of paroxysmal AF (PAF) demonstrate that 79% to 94% of AF episodes are asymptomatic.[8–11] Furthermore, the clustering and rarity of episodes over a short time frame has further complicated efforts at detection.[9–12] Despite these challenges, diagnosing AF in a survivor of ischemic stroke or TIA is of paramount importance as it potentially changes treatment from antiplatelet therapy to anticoagulation and by doing so may further reduce the risk of recurrent stroke.[13–15]

Anticoagulation following ischemic stroke is indicated only for those patients diagnosed with AF outside of some rare circumstances. Thus, an emerging component in managing patients after ischemic stroke has been the use of cardiac monitoring to assess for atrial arrhythmias after a comprehensive stroke workup has been negative and the event has been categorized as cryptogenic. Current guidelines recommend prolonged rhythm monitoring for approximately 30 days within 6 months of the index event in order to detect atrial fibrillation. This recommendation is a class IIA recommendation.[16] Importantly, data suggest that detection rates are likely to underestimate the total prevalence of AF with this strategy.[5] To date, the optimum duration of monitoring is unknown. This review discusses the various methods of monitoring for AF in patients with cryptogenic stroke with a focus on observational studies and prospective randomized controlled trials that have evaluated the use of external monitors and insertable cardiac monitors (ICMs) in this population.

OBSERVATIONAL STUDIES OF EXTERNAL MONITORS: INPATIENT MONITORING

Although the label of cryptogenic stroke is usually applied after a full workup of the stroke mechanism has been completed, observational studies that assessed cardiac monitoring in the inpatient setting laid the initial groundwork for continuous monitoring after discharge (**Table 1**).[17–35] Sulter and colleagues[17] evaluated the utility of stroke care monitoring units in the first 48 hours after a stroke. These units performed at least 48 hours of continuous inpatient heart rhythm monitoring

as opposed to serial heart rate monitoring in the conventional monitoring group. The AF detection rate was 18.5% in the continuous monitoring group compared with 3.5% in the conventional monitoring group. Bansil and Karim[18] assessed 48 hours of cardiac monitoring in 150 consecutive patients who presented with stroke. The detection rate for new AF in the first 48 hours after stroke was 8%. More recently, Kallmünzer and colleagues[19] showed that among patients without AF on presenting electrocardiogram (ECG), new AF detection rates were 9.2% using telemetry monitoring. The median time to AF detection was 22 hours. Notably, in two-thirds of the 37 patients with a history of AF and no evidence of AF on presentation, AF was not detected during the inpatient monitoring period (median monitoring time of 75.5 hours). There is a concern that AF episodes on inpatient telemetry monitoring may go undetected or unnoticed. In a study of 133 consecutive patients admitted to a stroke unit for stroke or TIA, no AF episodes were detected on continuous telemetry over a mean observation time of 73.4 hours. However, simultaneous Holter monitors were placed on the same patients and demonstrated an actual AF incidence of 6% with a mean recording time of 29.8 hours.[36]

OBSERVATIONAL STUDIES OF EXTERNAL MONITORS: HOLTER MONITORING

In recognition that AF may go undetected or may not have occurred during continuous inpatient monitoring, observational studies have evaluated the utility of ambulatory monitoring after hospitalization for stroke. Holter monitoring for 24 hours after stroke has been shown to detect more AF compared with serial ECGs.[21] An observational study by Thakkar and Bagarhatta[25] reported an AF detection rate with 24-hour Holter monitoring of 5.8%. Studies on ambulatory monitoring have also suggested that AF detection rates were up to 6% after 72 hours of continuous ECG monitoring.[20] A multicenter trial was performed in 2013 and further supported the idea that 72-hour Holter monitoring was superior in detecting AF compared with 24-hour monitoring, with a 4.3% detection rate after 72 hours compared with a 2.6% with only 24 hours of monitoring.[24] The number needed to screen with 72 hours to make a new diagnoses of AF was 55 patients. Holter monitoring for a duration of 7 days was evaluated in 281 patients in the FIND-AF trial.[22] From the total cohort of patients, 224 patients had no history of AF on presentation and 12.5% of these patients had newly detected AF at 7 days. This detection rate was significantly higher than the 4.8%

Table 1
Observational studies for external cardiac monitors

		AF Duration (s)	N	New AF Detection Rate
Inpatient continuous monitoring	Sulter et al,[17] 2003	NR	54	Intervention arm (telemetry), 18.5%; conventional arm (heart rate checks), 3.5%
	Bansil & Karim,[18] 2004	NR	150	4%
	Kallmünzer et al,[19] 2012	>30	346	16%
Holter	Schuchert et al,[20] 1999	60	82	6%
	Gunalp et al,[21] 2006	Any AF	26	42%
	Stahrenberg et al,[22] 2010 (FIND-AF)	>30	224	7-d, 12.5% 24-h, 4.8%
	Doliwa Sobocinski et al,[23] 2012	10	249	30-d intermittent, 6%; 24-h Holter, 0.8%
	Grond et al,[24] 2013	>30	1135	24-h, 2.6%; 72-h, 4.3%
	Thakkar & Bagarhatta,[25] 2014	>30	52	24-h Holter, 5.8%
Holter and inpatient continuous monitoring	Rizos et al,[26] 2010	>30	136	CEM, 21.3%
	Rizos et al,[27] 2012	>30	496	Overall detection rate, 8.3%; Holter, 2.8%; CEM 5.4%
	Gumbinger et al,[28] 2012	≥30	192	Holter, 1%; CEM, 6.8%
	Suissa et al,[29] 2013	>30	946	Holter, 2.26%; CEM, 12.5%
Event monitors	Barthélémy et al,[30] 2003	≥30	28	Automatic event recorder, 14.3%
	Flint et al,[31] 2012	>30	239	Automatic event recorder: >30 s, 6.7%; >5 s, 11.0%
Holter and event monitor	Jabaudon et al,[32] 2004	Variable	149	Holter (N = 139), 5.0%; event monitor (N = 88), 5.7%
MCOT	Tayal et al,[33] 2008	Variable	56	MCOT: >30 s, 3%; < or >30 s, 13%
	Miller et al,[34] 2013	Variable	156	MCOT: <30 s, 11.5%; ≥30 s, 4.5%
	Kalani et al,[35] 2015	>30	85	MCOT: 4.7%

Abbreviations: CEM, continuous ECG monitoring; MCOT, mobile cardiac outpatient telemetry; N, number of patients that met inclusion criteria and did not have a history of AF.

detection rate with 24-hour monitoring. Moreover, the data showed that the cumulative detection rate continued to increase from day 1 to day 7, suggesting that even longer monitoring would continue to provide additional yield. Further analysis of the FIND-AF trial also illustrated that the prevalence of AF increased with age and that the number needed to screen with a 7-day Holter monitor to detect new AF was inversely proportional to age.[37] Holter monitoring over even longer periods of time has also been reviewed. Doliwa Sobocinski and colleagues[23] found that intermittent monitoring 10 seconds, twice per day, for 30 days had higher AF detection rates than continuous 24-hour Holter monitoring. Collectively, the data on Holter monitoring affirm that longer monitoring after cryptogenic stroke is more likely to result in higher rates of AF detection.

OBSERVATIONAL STUDIES OF EXTERNAL MONITORS: OUTPATIENT EVENT MONITORING

Ambulatory cardiac monitoring with event recorders has allowed for extended periods of monitoring for up to 30 days after a cryptogenic stroke with the benefit of detecting asymptomatic arrhythmia with automatic triggering. Barthélémy and colleagues[30] studied the effectiveness of long-term automatically triggered event recorders in detecting AF. Among 28 patients without an underlying cause of stroke, AF was detected in 14.3% of the patients using automatically triggered event recorders. With the Stroke and Monitoring for PAF in Real Time (SMART) registry, Flint and colleagues[31] extended the use of event monitors to 30 days. Of the 239 patients who completed the monitor study, AF was detected in 29 patients (12.1%). Only 6.1% of the AF events were patient triggered, which means almost 94% of the AF events would have been missed without automatically triggered monitoring. More than half of the first AF events were detected after 10 days, emphasizing the need for prolonged monitoring in the patient population. Jabaudon and colleagues[32] examined AF detection rates initially using 24-hour Holter monitors followed by a 7-day event monitor in those patients in whom AF was still not detected. Among the 139 patients who underwent Holter monitoring, AF was detected in 5% of the patients. Compliance for ambulatory event monitoring was 73.3%. Among the 88 patients who completed the ambulatory monitor, AF was detected in an additional 5.7% of the patients. This study further underscores that additional monitoring beyond a 24-hour Holter with an automatically triggered ambulatory monitoring device increased the yield of AF detection.

OBSERVATIONAL STUDIES OF EXTERNAL MONITORS: OUTPATIENT MOBILE CARDIAC TELEMETRY MONITORING

Mobile cardiac outpatient telemetry (MCOT) has allowed for continuous telemetry monitoring for extended durations in the ambulatory setting. Three retrospective studies have been performed evaluating its efficacy in finding unrecognized AF after cryptogenic stroke. Among 56 patients with cryptogenic stroke who underwent MCOT monitoring for 21 days, 23% of patients were found to have new AF.[33] However, most of these episodes were brief in duration; the AF detection rate was approximately 5% for events greater than 30 seconds. Similarly, findings by Miller and colleagues[34] illustrated an AF detection rate of 19.5% at 21 days in a cohort of 156 patients. The detection rate was 3.9% for 48 hours of monitoring, 9.2% for 7 days, and 15.1% for 14 days. The rate of MCOT compliance was 80% for at least 14 days and 62% for at least 21 days. Kalani and colleagues[35] retrospectively evaluated MCOT use after ischemic stroke with a monitoring duration of 14 to 30 days. Of the 85 patients who met the study criteria, 64.7% completed 30 days of MCOT, 21.2% completed only 21 days of MCOT, and 8.2% completed only 7 days of MCOT. The AF detection rate was 4.7%, which was lower than previous studies. The yield in those patients who completed the full 30 days of monitoring was 1.8%. The investigators surmised that an extensive evaluation of patients with cryptogenic stroke with multiple modalities of cardiac imaging, including transthoracic echocardiography, transesophageal echocardiography, and cardiac MRI, as was done in their cohort may lower the yield of AF detection in patients who remain categorized as cryptogenic.

RANDOMIZED CONTROLLED TRIALS COMPARING EXTERNAL MONITORING STRATEGIES

Several randomized controlled trials comparing external monitoring strategies have been conducted. In the first randomized trial of cardiac monitoring after cryptogenic stroke by Kamel and colleagues,[38] the rate of AF detection was lower than expected. In this relatively small study, 40 patients with cryptogenic stroke or TIA were randomized in a 1:1 fashion to either 21 days of MCOT or to routine follow-up. No patients in either study arm were diagnosed with AF. However, 25% of the patients in the monitoring arm never wore the monitor; the patients who did wear the monitor were only compliant with it 64% of the assigned days. These results primarily highlight the difficulties inherent in the use of external monitors that may be uncomfortable or unwieldy to wear, particularly in patients who may have neurologic impairment.

A somewhat larger randomized trial performed in the United Kingdom by Higgins and colleagues[39] was more in line with observational data. In this study, 100 patients with cryptogenic stroke were randomized to either standard practice to detect AF or to standard practice plus 7 days of cardiac event monitoring within the first 14 days after stroke. Standard practice in this study consisted of additional 12-lead ECGs (after the admission ECG showing sinus rhythm), echocardiograms, and 24-hour Holter monitoring. The primary end point of the study was the detection of AF greater than 20 seconds within 14 days of presentation. Significantly more AF was detected in the group of patients who received event monitors, with AF detected in 18% of monitored patients versus only 2% of standard practice patients. This significant improvement in AF detection with event monitoring persisted at 90 days. In addition to showing an increased detection of AF, the study also showed that anticoagulation use in the monitored patients was significantly higher than in the standard-practice patients (16% vs 0% at 14 days and 22% vs 6% at 90 days), although the study was not powered to show a reduction in recurrent strokes related to anticoagulation. As opposed to the previously mentioned randomized trial, compliance with ambulatory monitoring was better in this study, with greater than 80% of patients successfully completing transmission of recorded data at 7 days.

The EMBRACE (Event Monitor Belt for Recording Atrial Fibrillation after a Cerebral Ischemic Event) trial is the largest randomized controlled trial to date of external monitoring strategies in cryptogenic stroke.[2] In this study, 572 patients, 55 years old or older, with no known history of AF, and cryptogenic stroke or TIA within the previous 6 months were randomized either to monitoring with a 30-day event monitor (intervention group) or to conventional 24-hour Holter monitoring (control group). All patients had an initial workup, including a 24-hour Holter monitor, which failed to uncover the cause of stroke or TIA. The primary outcome was detection of AF lasting 30 seconds or longer within 90 days after randomization. Significantly more AF was detected in the intervention group than the control group, with AF detected in 16.1% of patients monitored with a 30-day event monitor versus 3.2% of patients monitored with a 24-hour Holter monitor. The number of patients needed to screen with a 30-day event monitor to detect one additional case of AF was only 8 patients. Interestingly, AF was detected clinically by means other than monitoring in only 0.5% of enrollees, suggesting that monitoring is the only method of detecting AF in most of these patients given the paroxysmal and often asymptomatic nature of the disease. In addition, when AF detection was analyzed as a function of the number of weeks of monitoring, there was an incremental increase in the yield of AF detection with each additional week of monitoring. Similar to the randomized trial by Higgins and colleagues,[39] the EMBRACE investigators found that oral anticoagulation use was significantly increased in the intervention group, 18.6% of whom were prescribed anticoagulation at 90 days, compared with the control group, 11.1% of whom were prescribed anticoagulation at 90 days. Adherence to monitoring was also similar in this study, with 82% of patients in the intervention group completing more than 3 weeks of monitoring.

A fourth randomized controlled trial of external monitoring strategies, the Find-AFRANDOMISED trial, has completed enrollment.[40] An estimated 400 patients with a history of acute ischemic stroke and no prior history of AF were enrolled. Patients were randomized in a 1:1 fashion either to prolonged monitoring with 10 days of Holter monitoring at baseline and at 3 and 6 months after randomization or to standard of care with at least 24 hours of continuous ECG monitoring at baseline. The primary outcome of this study is newly detected AF lasting at least 30 seconds within 6 months.

Overall, these randomized trials confirm the general trend seen in observational studies that more prolonged monitoring for AF in patients with cryptogenic stroke results in a higher detection rate of AF. They also highlight the fact that compliance with external monitors is suboptimal, with only 4 of 5 patients compliant with the monitor in the best of situations.

OBSERVATIONAL STUDIES OF INSERTABLE CARDIAC MONITORS

Insertable cardiac monitors (ICMs) with AF-sensing algorithms have been available since 2009. The most commonly used devices in the United States use Lorenz plots to evaluate beat-to-beat variability of the RR intervals in 2-minute time sequences. The sensitivity and negative predictive value for AF detection is 96.1% and 97.4%, respectively, with an overall accuracy for AF duration of 98.5%.[41] The most recent iteration of these devices (Reveal LINQ, Medtronic Inc, Dublin, Ireland) transfers data wirelessly via nightly automatic submissions.[42] The device, about 1 mL in volume, is injected subcutaneously in the left parasternal region using local anesthetic and allows for continuous monitoring throughout the 3-year battery life of the device. In addition, the device requires minimal patient compliance and may allow for early detection of AF and prompt intervention before the next event. Adverse events are uncommon and generally limited to pocket infection and device erosion. Given many of the logistic benefits for patients as well as the ease of device implantation, ICMs are becoming more readily adopted for arrhythmia detection. Single-arm studies of ICMs have been carried out over the last several years (**Table 2**). The first attempt by Dion and colleagues[43] included 24 patients and found a 0% incidence of AF, but the device used in the study (Medtronic Reveal Plus ILR 9526) contained no specific AF-sensing algorithm and instead considered AF any tachycardia greater than 165 beats per minute that lasted greater than 30 seconds. Using a device with specific AF sensing algorithms (Medtronic RevealXT), Cotter and colleagues[44] found a 25.5% incidence of AF over a follow-up period of 229 days. As in the general population, univariate predictors of AF were found to include increasing age, interatrial conduction block, left atrial volume, and the occurrence of atrial premature contractions on preceding external monitoring. Similarly, Etgen and colleagues[45] used the same model device in 22 patients with cryptogenic stroke and found a similar incidence of AF detection, though in this case no differences in clinical characteristics were found between those patients

Table 2
Observational studies of ICM use following cryptogenic stroke

Author	N	Time from Event to Implant	Definition of AF	Device	Mean Age (y)	Duration of Monitoring (mo)	Median Time to AF Detection (d)	Yield (%)
Cotter et al,[44] 2013	51	174 d	2 min	Reveal XT	51.5	7.5	48	25.5
Etgen et al,[45] 2013	22	152.8 d	≥6 min	Reveal XT	61.6	120.0	153	27.3
Ritter et al,[46] 2013	60	13 d	≥2 min	Reveal XT	63.0	12.6	64	17.0

with and without AF. Of those found to have AF, 67% were asymptomatic. The largest of these uncontrolled studies enrolled 60 patients and, in addition to implanting the ICM, patients also simultaneously wore a 7-day Holter monitor.[46] AF was detected by the ICM in 10 patients (17%), but only 1 patient (1.7%) had AF detected on the 7-day Holter. As in the previous study, there were no clinical features, either on baseline demographics or brain imaging, that were useful in distinguishing those with and without device-detected AF. There were no complications from device implantation reported in any of these trials.[43–46]

RANDOMIZED CONTROLLED TRIALS OF INSERTABLE CARDIAC MONITORS VERSUS EXTERNAL MONITORS

The CRYSTAL AF (Cryptogenic Stroke and underlying Atrial Fibrillation) is the only randomized controlled trial thus far to compare the utility of ICMs to routine care.[5] Patients were 40 years of age or older with no previous history of AF or atrial flutter and had a negative comprehensive workup for the cause of an ischemic stroke or TIA including vascular imaging, MRI, transesophageal echocardiogram, a hypercoagulable workup for those less than 55 years of age, and at least 24 hours of continuous cardiac monitoring for all patients. The presence of a pacemaker or implantable cardioverter-defibrillator was an exclusion criterion. A total of 441 patients were enrolled and followed for up to 345 days. The primary end point was an AF event lasting greater than 30 seconds in the first 6 months. Key secondary end points included the time to first detection within the first 12 months, stroke recurrence, and utilization of oral anticoagulation between the two groups. The time from index event to randomization was approximately 38 days, and the time between

randomization to device implantation was approximately 9 days. An intention-to-treat analysis revealed an AF detection rate of 8.9% in the ICM group and 1.4% in the control group (hazard ratio 6.4). At 12 months, the difference in detection rates remained statistically significant at 12.4% in the intervention arm compared with 2% in the conventional monitoring arm (hazard ratio 7.3). At 36 months of follow-up, the rate of detection of AF was 30.0% in the ICM group versus 3.0% in the control group (hazard ratio 8.8) (**Fig. 1**). The median time from randomization to detection of AF at 36 months was 84 days in the ICM arm and 52 days in the control arm, which is notably longer than the current guideline-recommended duration for monitoring of 30 days and is beyond the reach of most external monitors. The median value for maximum time in AF was 11.2 hours, with more than 90% of those patients with AF having at least one episode greater than 6 minutes in duration and nearly half (46%) the patients having at least one AF episode greater than 12 hours in duration. Among the first ICM-detected AF episodes, 79% were asymptomatic. The number needed to screen with an ICM to detect an AF episode at 6 months was 14, at 12 months was 10, and at 36 months was 4. Although the study was not powered to assess a reduction in recurrent stroke risk, there was a favorable trend in those randomized to the ICM arm of the study (7.1% vs 9.1%). In order to find 5 additional patients with AF in those randomized to routine care, an additional 202 ECGs, 52 Holters, and 1 event monitor were performed. Although age and baseline PR interval were week predictors of AF, it is interesting to note that there was no evidence for an association between brain infarction pattern and AF detection.[47] The results of CRYSTAL AF convey that ECG monitoring with an ICM is superior to conventional follow-up for detection of AF

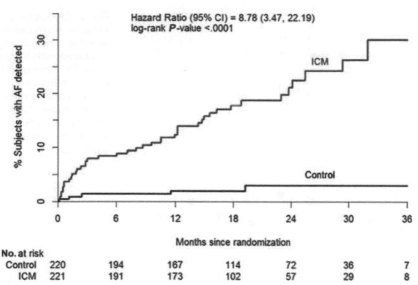

Fig. 1. Three-year follow-up for CRYSTAL AF. (*Adapted from* Sanna T, Diener HC, Morillo CA, et al. Cryptogenic stroke and underlying atrial fibrillation. N Engl J Med 2014;370(26):2484.)

after cryptogenic stroke and that monitoring may be necessary for greater than 30 days in order to detect the first episode of AF. The major limitations of these devices are their invasive nature and cost.

The sensitivity of long-term ICM monitoring was compared with various forms of short-term external monitoring by Choe and colleagues[48] with data from the CRYSTAL AF cohort. This analysis simulated several intermittent monitoring strategies and compared them with ICM continuous monitoring. The intermittent monitoring included short-term monitoring that simulated 24-hour and 48-hour Holter monitoring and external event recorders lasting between 7 and 30 days. The lowest sensitivity for AF was 1.3% with a single 24-hour Holter. The highest sensitivity was with a 30-day monitor (22.8%), assuming 100% compliance with monitoring. All of the intermittent monitoring strategies had a lower sensitivity than that of continuous monitoring with negative predictive values ranging from 82% to 85% (**Fig. 2**). These findings reaffirmed that long-term continuous monitoring was more effective at detecting AF than any short-term or intermittent monitoring strategy and emphasize the need for continuous long-term monitoring even if a short-term external monitor does not detect AF.

Although CRYSTAL AF explored the use of ICM in the setting of a highly controlled clinical trial, the rate of AF detection has also been assessed in a real-world setting. In the cohort of 1247 patients implanted with an ICM for cryptogenic stroke indications, the AF detection rate was 4.6% at 30 days and 12.2% at 182 days.[1] At 6 months, this was a 37% relative increase in AF detection at 6 months

compared with the detection rate in CRYSTAL AF. The median time to detection was 58 days, which was also congruent with optimal AF monitoring of greater than that recommended in the guidelines. The increased AF-detection rates seen on ICMs in routine clinical practice are likely because, unlike in CRYSTAL AF, routine practice may not always include an extensive evaluation including assessments such as transesophageal echocardiography and greater than 24 hours of cardiac monitoring. In turn, the detection rates for AF after ICM implant are higher.[1,5]

META-ANALYSES OF MONITORING TECHNIQUES

Several recent meta-analyses have looked at the available data related to monitoring for AF in patients with stroke. A meta-analysis by Dussault and colleagues[49] investigated the effects of the duration of monitoring on AF detection rates in patients after the diagnosis of stroke. A total of 8715 patients with recent stroke or TIA, not necessarily cryptogenic in nature, from 31 studies were included. Overall, new AF was diagnosed in 7.4% of patients. Although there was significant heterogeneity between studies, longer durations of monitoring were associated with a significant increase in AF detection when duration of monitoring was analyzed as both a continuous variable or as a dichotomous variable. When analyzed as a continuous variable, AF detection increased from 4.4% at 24 hours to 15.2% at 30 days to 29.2% at 180 days (**Fig. 3**). When analyzed as a dichotomous variable, long-term monitoring for 7 or more

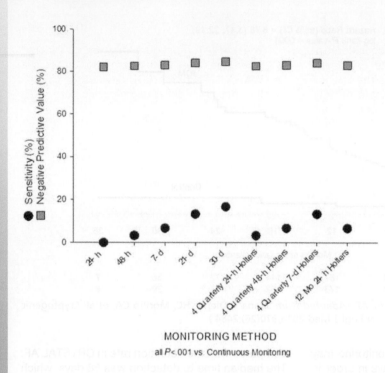

Fig. 2. Simulation of sensitivity and negative predictive value of various external monitoring techniques compared with ICM. (*Adapted from* Choe WC, Passman RS, Brachmann J, et al. A comparison of atrial fibrillation monitoring strategies after cryptogenic stroke (from the Cryptogenic Stroke and Underlying AF Trial). Am J Cardiol 2015;116(6):891; with permission.)

days resulted in detection of AF in 15% of patients versus only 5.1% of patients monitored for 3 days or less. When only randomized controlled trials were analyzed, long-term monitoring was associated with a 7.3 odds of detecting AF compared with traditional short-term monitoring.

The results of a similar meta-analysis by Kishore and colleagues[50] are consistent with the finding of

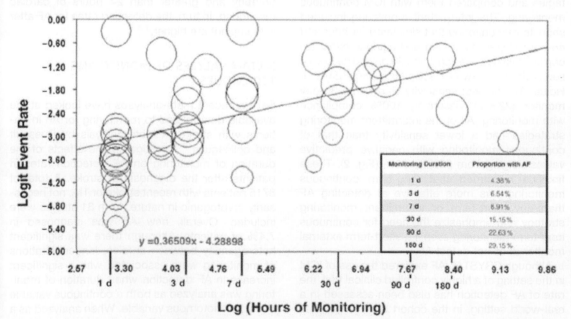

Fig. 3. AF detection increases with increasing duration of monitoring after stroke. (*Adapted from* Dussault C, Toeg H, Nathan M, et al. Electrocardiographic monitoring for detecting atrial fibrillation after ischemic stroke or transient ischemic attack: systematic review and meta-analysis. Circ Arrhythm Electrophysiol 2015;8(2):266; with permission.)

the previous study. A total of 32 studies, including 5038 patients, were analyzed. Like the previously discussed study, this meta-analysis included unselected patients with stroke, not just patients with cryptogenic stroke. The overall detection rate of AF was 11.5%, and prolonged monitoring was associated with an increased yield of newly diagnosed AF. When AF monitoring was extended from 24 hours to 72 hours, AF detection increased by 2% to 4% for each additional 24 hours of monitoring. When external loop recorders were repeated at 3 or 6 months after an initial monitor, AF detection increased from 6% to 8% with the initial monitor to 14% with repeat monitoring. The investigators acknowledge that their findings were limited by the heterogeneity of the included studies, including heterogeneity in study design, sample size, monitoring techniques, AF definition, and patient populations.

Afzal and colleagues[51] performed a meta-analysis looking specifically at patients with cryptogenic stroke. This analysis compared the effectiveness of ICMs with wearable external monitors for detection of AF in patients with cryptogenic stroke. Overall, AF was detected in 17.6% of patients. Patients with ICMs were monitored for a median of 365 days, whereas patients with external monitors were monitored for a median of 21 days. Significantly higher AF detection was achieved with ICM monitoring (23.3% of patients) compared with wearable devices (13.6% of patients). No significant difference was present in AF detection between studies whereby monitoring was started at less than 29 days from the event compared with the studies whereby monitoring was started after 29 days. The median duration between index event and ICM implantation was 72 days compared with wearable monitors, which had a mean duration of 25 days.

COST-EFFECTIVENESS OF MONITORING

The cost-effectiveness of long-term cardiac monitoring in the setting of cryptogenic stroke is an important issue as it adds perspective to the financial burden of the disease process on the patients and the health care system. Almost half of the total cost attributed to stroke management is from inpatient and emergency department costs. Given this cost burden, secondary prevention of stroke with a cost-conscious management strategy in diagnosis and therapy is critical. Kamel and colleagues[52] performed a cost-utility analysis for extended outpatient cardiac monitoring after ischemic stroke. Their model predicted a new AF detection rate of 44 cases for every 1000 monitored patients, which would result in a projected

cost-utility ratio of $13,000 per quality-adjusted life-years with an estimated net cost of $440,000 per patient. The cost-effectiveness of using an ICM for AF detection after a cryptogenic stroke has also been assessed. A cost-effectiveness Markov-model analysis of the CRYSTAL-AF findings shows that the incremental cost-effectiveness ratio for ICM use in a cryptogenic stroke population is $28,308, an amount lower than that of cholesterol therapy and antihypertensive treatment.[53]

FUTURE IMPLICATIONS

A review of the data shows that monitoring for longer durations after cryptogenic stroke leads to higher yields in AF detection. The optimal monitoring period has yet to be determined but is likely beyond the up to 30 days recommended in stroke prevention guidelines. Detection of new AF after ischemic stroke cannot be directly translated to a cause-and-effect relationship, especially when the AF is first detected months to years from the initial event. However, the morbidity and mortality associated with the failure to diagnose and treat AF in a survivor of ischemic stroke may be enough justification to change management based on any AF detection, regardless of timing or duration. It must be acknowledged that fundamental questions remain. First, we do not know whether short, subclinical episodes of AF detected on monitoring of any nature confer the same risk as longer, clinically evident episodes. Second, it is not known whether anticoagulating patients in response to relatively brief, device-detected subclinical AF episodes confer the same reduction in stroke risk seen in trials of patients with clinically evident AF.

Although ICMs provide the highest yields of AF detection, there is still a likely role for external monitors in patients who are expected to be compliant with monitoring and follow-up visits. If external monitoring is chosen as the first-line assessment, it is imperative that the search for AF continues even if extended external monitoring is negative given the low sensitivity of even a 30-day monitor. The development of smartphone ECG technologies, other wearable long-term cardiac monitors with AF detection algorithms, and insertable monitors with longer-term batteries capable of measuring physiologic parameters beyond heart rhythm may provide further opportunities for elucidating the causes of cryptogenic stroke. Although the sum of the data supports the concept that AF is prevalent in a cryptogenic stroke population, it must be emphasized that the mechanism of stroke in most of these patients remains elusive.

REFERENCES

1. Ziegler PD, Rogers JD, Ferreira SW, et al. Real-world experience with insertable cardiac monitors to find atrial fibrillation in cryptogenic stroke. Cerebrovasc Dis 2015;40(3–4):175–81.

2. Gladstone DJ, Spring M, Dorian P, et al. Atrial fibrillation in patients with cryptogenic stroke. N Engl J Med 2014;370(26):2467–77.

3. Gladstone DJ, Bui E, Fang J, et al. Potentially preventable strokes in high-risk patients with atrial fibrillation who are not adequately anticoagulated. Stroke 2009;40(1):235–40.

4. Mozaffarian D, Benjamin EJ, Go AS, et al. Heart disease and stroke statistics–2015 update: a report from the American Heart Association. Circulation 2015;131(4):e29–322.

5. Sanna T, Diener HC, Morillo CA, et al. Cryptogenic stroke and underlying atrial fibrillation. N Engl J Med 2014;370(26):2478–86.

6. Adams HP Jr, Bendixen BH, Kappelle LJ, et al. Classification of subtype of acute ischemic stroke. Definitions for use in a multicenter clinical trial. TOAST. Trial of Org 10172 in Acute Stroke Treatment. Stroke 1993;24(1):35–41.

7. Wolf PA, Abbott RD, Kannel WB. Atrial fibrillation as an independent risk factor for stroke: the Framingham Study. Stroke 1991;22(8):983–8.

8. Page RL, Wilkinson WE, Clair WK, et al. Asymptomatic arrhythmias in patients with symptomatic paroxysmal atrial fibrillation and paroxysmal supraventricular tachycardia. Circulation 1994;89(1):224–7.

9. Strickberger SA, Ip J, Saksena S, et al. Relationship between atrial tachyarrhythmias and symptoms. Heart Rhythm 2005;2(2):125–31.

10. Quirino G, Giammaria M, Corbucci G, et al. Diagnosis of paroxysmal atrial fibrillation in patients with implanted pacemakers: relationship to symptoms and other variables. Pacing Clin Electrophysiol 2009;32(1):91–8.

11. Verma A, Champagne J, Sapp J, et al. Discerning the incidence of symptomatic and asymptomatic episodes of atrial fibrillation before and after catheter ablation (DISCERN AF): a prospective, multicenter study. JAMA Intern Med 2013;173(2):149–56.

12. Ziegler PD, Glotzer TV, Daoud EG, et al. Incidence of newly detected atrial arrhythmias via implantable devices in patients with a history of thromboembolic events. Stroke 2010;41(2):256–60.

13. Albers GW, Hart RG, Lutsep HL, et al. AHA scientific statement. Supplement to the guidelines for the management of transient ischemic attacks: a statement from the Ad Hoc Committee on Guidelines for the Management of Transient Ischemic Attacks, Stroke Council, American Heart Association. Stroke 1999;30(11):2502–11.

14. van Walraven C, Hart RG, Singer DE, et al. Oral anticoagulants vs aspirin in nonvalvular atrial fibrillation: an individual patient meta-analysis. JAMA 2002;288(19):2441–8.

15. Hart RG, Halperin JL, Pearce LA, et al. Lessons from the stroke prevention in atrial fibrillation trials. Ann Intern Med 2003;138(10):831–8.

16. Kernan WN, Ovbiagele B, Black HR, et al. Guidelines for the prevention of stroke in patients with stroke and transient ischemic attack: a guideline for healthcare professionals from the American Heart Association/American Stroke Association. Stroke 2014;45(7):2160–236.

17. Sulter G, Elting JW, Langedijk M, et al. Admitting acute ischemic stroke patients to a stroke care monitoring unit versus a conventional stroke unit: a randomized pilot study. Stroke 2003;34(1):101–4.

18. Bansil S, Karim H. Detection of atrial fibrillation in patients with acute stroke. J Stroke Cerebrovasc Dis 2004;13(1):12–5.

19. Kallmunzer B, Breuer L, Hering C, et al. A structured reading algorithm improves telemetric detection of atrial fibrillation after acute ischemic stroke. Stroke 2012;43(4):994–9.

20. Schuchert A, Behrens G, Meinertz T. Impact of long-term ECG recording on the detection of paroxysmal atrial fibrillation in patients after an acute ischemic stroke. Pacing Clin Electrophysiol 1999;22(7):1082–4.

21. Gunalp M, Atalar E, Coskun F, et al. Holter monitoring for 24 hours in patients with thromboembolic stroke and sinus rhythm diagnosed in the emergency department. Adv Ther 2006;23(6):854–60.

22. Stahrenberg R, Weber-Krüger M, Seegers J, et al. Enhanced detection of paroxysmal atrial fibrillation by early and prolonged continuous Holter monitoring in patients with cerebral ischemia presenting in sinus rhythm. Stroke 2010;41(12):2884–8.

23. Doliwa Sobocinski P, Anggårdh Rooth E, Frykman Kull V, et al. Improved screening for silent atrial fibrillation after ischaemic stroke. Europace 2012;14(8):1112–6.

24. Grond M, Jauss M, Hamann G, et al. Improved detection of silent atrial fibrillation using 72-hour Holter ECG in patients with ischemic stroke: a prospective multicenter cohort study. Stroke 2013;44(12):3357–64.

25. Thakkar S, Bagarhatta R. Detection of paroxysmal atrial fibrillation or flutter in patients with acute ischemic stroke or transient ischemic attack by Holter monitoring. Indian Heart J 2014;66(2):188–92.

26. Rizos T, Rasch C, Jenetzky E, et al. Detection of paroxysmal atrial fibrillation in acute stroke patients. Cerebrovasc Dis 2010;30(4):410–7.

27. Rizos T, Güntner J, Jenetzky E, et al. Continuous stroke unit electrocardiographic monitoring versus 24-hour Holter electrocardiography for detection of

paroxysmal atrial fibrillation after stroke. Stroke 2012;43(10):2689–94.

28. Gumbinger C, Krumsdorf U, Veltkamp R, et al. Continuous monitoring versus HOLTER ECG for detection of atrial fibrillation in patients with stroke. Eur J Neurol 2012;19(2):253–7.

29. Suissa L, Lachaud S, Mahagne MH. Optimal timing and duration of continuous electrocardiographic monitoring for detecting atrial fibrillation in stroke patients. J Stroke Cerebrovasc Dis 2013;22(7):991–5.

30. Barthélémy JC, Féasson-Gérard S, Garnier P, et al. Automatic cardiac event recorders reveal paroxysmal atrial fibrillation after unexplained strokes or transient ischemic attacks. Ann Noninvasive Electrocardiol 2003;8(3):194–9.

31. Flint AC, Banki NM, Ren X, et al. Detection of paroxysmal atrial fibrillation by 30-day event monitoring in cryptogenic ischemic stroke: the Stroke and Monitoring for PAF in Real Time (SMART) Registry. Stroke 2012;43(10):2788–90.

32. Jabaudon D, Sztajzel J, Sievert K, et al. Usefulness of ambulatory 7-day ECG monitoring for the detection of atrial fibrillation and flutter after acute stroke and transient ischemic attack. Stroke 2004;35(7):1647–51.

33. Tayal AH, Tian M, Kelly KM, et al. Atrial fibrillation detected by mobile cardiac outpatient telemetry in cryptogenic TIA or stroke. Neurology 2008;71(21):1696–701.

34. Miller DJ, Khan MA, Schultz LR, et al. Outpatient cardiac telemetry detects a high rate of atrial fibrillation in cryptogenic stroke. J Neurol Sci 2013;324(1–2):57–61.

35. Kalani R, Bernstein R, Passman R, et al. Low yield of mobile cardiac outpatient telemetry after cryptogenic stroke in patients with extensive cardiac imaging. J Stroke Cerebrovasc Dis 2015;24(9):2069–73.

36. Lazzaro MA, Krishnan K, Prabhakaran S. Detection of atrial fibrillation with concurrent Holter monitoring and continuous cardiac telemetry following ischemic stroke and transient ischemic attack. J Stroke Cerebrovasc Dis 2012;21(2):89–93.

37. Wachter R, Weber-Krüger M, Seegers J, et al. Age-dependent yield of screening for undetected atrial fibrillation in stroke patients: the Find-AF study. J Neurol 2013;260(8):2042–5.

38. Kamel H, Navi BB, Elijovich L, et al. Pilot randomized trial of outpatient cardiac monitoring after cryptogenic stroke. Stroke 2013;44(2):528–30.

39. Higgins P, MacFarlane PW, Dawson J, et al. Noninvasive cardiac event monitoring to detect atrial fibrillation after ischemic stroke: a randomized, controlled trial. Stroke 2013;44(9):2525–31.

40. Weber-Kruger M, Gelbrich G, Stahrenberg R, et al. Finding atrial fibrillation in stroke patients: randomized evaluation of enhanced and prolonged Holter monitoring–Find-AF(RANDOMISED) –rationale and design. Am Heart J 2014;168(4):438–45.e1.

41. Hindricks G, Pokushalov E, Urban L, et al. Performance of a new leadless implantable cardiac monitor in detecting and quantifying atrial fibrillation: results of the XPECT trial. Circ Arrhythm Electrophysiol 2010;3(2):141–7.

42. Tomson TT, Passman R. The reveal LINQ insertable cardiac monitor. Expert Rev Med Devices 2015;12(1):7–18.

43. Dion F, Saudeau D, Bonnaud I, et al. Unexpected low prevalence of atrial fibrillation in cryptogenic ischemic stroke: a prospective study. J Interv Card Electrophysiol 2010;28(2):101–7.

44. Cotter PE, Martin PJ, Ring L, et al. Incidence of atrial fibrillation detected by implantable loop recorders in unexplained stroke. Neurology 2013;80(17):1546–50.

45. Etgen T, Hochreiter M, Mundel M, et al. Insertable cardiac event recorder in detection of atrial fibrillation after cryptogenic stroke: an audit report. Stroke 2013;44(7):2007–9.

46. Ritter MA, Kochhäuser S, Duning T, et al. Occult atrial fibrillation in cryptogenic stroke: detection by 7-day electrocardiogram versus implantable cardiac monitors. Stroke 2013;44(5):1449–52.

47. Bernstein RA, Di Lazzaro V, Rymer MM, et al. Infarct topography and detection of atrial fibrillation in cryptogenic stroke: results from CRYSTAL AF. Cerebrovasc Dis 2015;40(1–2):91–6.

48. Choe WC, Passman RS, Brachmann J, et al. A comparison of atrial fibrillation monitoring strategies after cryptogenic stroke (from the cryptogenic stroke and underlying AF trial). Am J Cardiol 2015;116(6):889–93.

49. Dussault C, Toeg H, Nathan M, et al. Electrocardiographic monitoring for detecting atrial fibrillation after ischemic stroke or transient ischemic attack: systematic review and meta-analysis. Circ Arrhythm Electrophysiol 2015;8(2):263–9.

50. Kishore A, Vail A, Majid A, et al. Detection of atrial fibrillation after ischemic stroke or transient ischemic attack: a systematic review and meta-analysis. Stroke 2014;45(2):520–6.

51. Afzal MR, Gunda S, Waheed S, et al. Role of outpatient cardiac rhythm monitoring in cryptogenic stroke: a systematic review and meta-analysis. Pacing Clin Electrophysiol 2015;38(10):1236–45.

52. Kamel H, Hegde M, Johnson DR, et al. Cost-effectiveness of outpatient cardiac monitoring to detect atrial fibrillation after ischemic stroke. Stroke 2010;41(7):1514–20.

53. Diamantopoulos A, Sawyer LM, Lip GY, et al. Cost-effectiveness of an insertable cardiac monitor to detect atrial fibrillation in patients with cryptogenic stroke. Int J Stroke 2016. [Epub ahead of print].

Device-Detected Atrial Fibrillation—Perils and Pitfalls: An Update

 CrossMark

Phani Surapaneni, MD[a], Abdul Safadi, MD[a],
Tahmeed Contractor, MD[b], Mehul B. Patel, MD[c],
Ranjan K. Thakur, MD, MPH, MBA[a],*

KEYWORDS

- Stroke • Atrial fibrillation • Cardioembolism • Anticoagulation

KEY POINTS

- Cardiac implantable electronic devices (CIED) with an atrial lead can reliably detect atrial high-rate events (AHRE), which are supposedly tantamount to having atrial fibrillation (AF) or flutter because several studies have documented a correlation between AHRE and electrocardiogram-documented episodes of AF with a high degree of sensitivity and specificity.
- Atrial rate and duration are two parameters that characterize an AHRE. The definition of AHRE and AHRE burden used to examine stroke rates differs among different trials. The optimal definition of AHRE and burden level that portend a higher risk of stroke, therefore, warranting anticoagulation remains unclear.
- CIED atrial sensitivity settings may affect AHRE detection and burden due to oversensing or undersensing of signals as well as spurious arrhythmias, such as nonsustained atrial tachycardias, detected as AF. Therefore, AHREs should be carefully adjudicated on a case-by-case basis; the presence of AF should be confirmed before considering anticoagulation.
- The AHRE threshold burden beyond which thromboembolic risk is increased remains undefined. It is likely that stroke risk is related to both the longest duration of AHRE as well as total AHRE burden and patient characteristics, such as the CHA_2DS_2VASc score.

INTRODUCTION

Atrial fibrillation (AF) is the most common sustained arrhythmia encountered in clinical practice and has an estimated prevalence as high as 9% in the elderly.[1] The risk of stroke is increased 5-fold in patients with nonrheumatic AF and 17-fold in patients with rheumatic AF.[2,3] One of the foremost goals of managing AF is the reduction of thromboembolic strokes and systemic embolism. Implantable heart rhythm devices, such as implantable cardioverter-defibrillators (ICDs), cardiac resynchronization therapy (CRT) devices (pacemakers [CRT-P] and defibrillators [CRT-D]) and permanent pacemakers (PPMs), are increasingly being used worldwide. These devices are capable of sensing intrinsic atrial activity, and they often detect spontaneous atrial high-rate events (AHRE) in asymptomatic patients. Barring any spurious causes, AHRE seen by these

---

A version of this article was originally published as "Device-Detected Atrial Fibrillation: Perils and Pitfalls" in *Cardiac Electrophysiology Clinics*, Volume 3, Issue 4, December 2011.
Conflict of interest: none.
[a] Sparrow Thoracic and Cardiovascular Institute, Michigan State University, Lansing, MI, USA; [b] Department of Cardiology, Lehigh Valley Health Network, 1240 South Cedar Crest Boulevard, Allentown, PA 18103, USA; [c] Department of Clinical Cardiac Electrophysiology, The Bay Pines Veterans Affairs Health Care System, University of South Florida, Tampa, 10000 Bay Pines Boulevard, Bay Pines, FL 33744, USA
* Corresponding author. Thoracic and Cardiovascular Institute, 405 West Greenlawn, Suite 400, Lansing, MI 48910.
E-mail address: thakur@msu.edu

devices is supposedly tantamount to having AF or atrial flutter (AFL) because several studies have documented a correlation between AHRE and electrocardiogram (ECG)-documented episodes of AF/AFL with a high degree of sensitivity and specificity. However, the critical duration, frequency, or overall burden of AHRE that increases stroke risk is still unknown; thus, the threshold level of AHRE that warrants anticoagulation is still unclear. This article reviews the current literature on the risk of stroke with device-detected AHRE and raises questions that need further clarification.

ATRIAL FIBRILLATION AS A RISK FACTOR FOR STROKE

AF is a major independent risk factor for stroke and accounts for 10% of all ischemic strokes.[4] Almost 25% of strokes in patients aged 80 to 89 years are secondary to AF, and its propensity to cause strokes increases with age.[2] In the United States alone, AF causes approximately 75,000 strokes per year.[5] Because of the large size of emboli compared with other sources, AF-related strokes tend to be more severe and consequently have a greater impact on morbidity as well as mortality.[6,7] Over the last few decades, warfarin has remained the only anticoagulant that has significantly reduced stroke burden in AF.[8] Perceived bleeding risks, need for monitoring international normalized ratio, narrow therapeutic window, and drug as well as dietary interactions are some of the reasons why warfarin is not prescribed in many high-risk patients with AF, especially the elderly.[9,10] However, new treatment alternatives are emerging. Newer oral anticoagulants, such as dabigatran and rivaroxaban, are equally efficacious, with a lower risk of intracranial hemorrhage, and obviate anticoagulation monitoring.[11,12] Left atrial appendage occlusion devices, such as the WATCHMAN (Boston Scientific, Marlborough, MA) device, are also being evaluated for stroke reduction in nonvalvular AF and may replace the need for long-term anticoagulation, at least in some patients.[13] Availability of these alternative options may make thromboembolic prophylaxis possible in more patients.

Alongside better treatment methods, advanced diagnostic modalities, such as transtelephonic ECG monitoring, mobile cardiac outpatient telemetry, and implantable loop recorders, are more effective in diagnosing AF, especially paroxysmal AF.[14,15] These advanced techniques have detected paroxysmal AF in up to 25% of patients with cryptogenic stroke.[15] It is known that the risk of ischemic stroke with paroxysmal AF is similar to that with permanent AF, and it can be significantly reduced with anticoagulation.[16,17] However,

the degree or duration of paroxysmal AF that increases the risk of stroke is still unknown.

ATRIAL HIGH-RATE EVENTS AND ATRIAL FIBRILLATION

Devices, such as ICDs, CRT devices, and dual-chamber PPMs, provide a wealth of information on atrial as well as ventricular sensed and paced events. The critical atrial rate that has to be exceeded in order to trigger labeling it AHRE can be programmed, allowing these devices to accurately report their frequency, duration, and overall burden compared with sensed or paced atrial rhythm. Several studies have documented positive correlation between PPM-identified AHRE and ECG-documented episodes of AF or AFL with a high degree of sensitivity and specificity.[18,19] However, the correlation is imperfect because oversensing (far-field sensing, double counting, T-wave oversensing in sinus tachycardia, and so forth) can lead to false-positive reporting of AF (**Fig. 1**) and undersensing (eg, P-wave sensitivity set too low or too high) can lead to underdetection of AF (**Fig. 2**).

AHREs have been found in nearly 50% of dual-chamber PPM recipients with or without known AF.[20,21] Subsequent studies that excluded patients with known AF reported AHREs in approximately 30% of PPM recipients.[18,22] A similar incidence (~25%) has been found in CRT device recipients, and patients with these events showed less echocardiograph response to CRT as well as a greater number of adverse cardiac outcomes, such as appropriate/inappropriate ICD shocks and hospitalizations for heart failure.[23,24] Risk factors for developing AHREs include a previous history of AF,[25] underlying sinus node dysfunction,[21] and right ventricular (RV) pacing.[22,26] In the Mode Selection Trial (MOST), AF increased by 1% for every 1% increase in RV pacing.[26] Similarly Cheung and colleagues[22] found that in PPM recipients with a cumulative RV pacing 50% or greater, the risk of AF was doubled (hazard ratio [HR] = 2.2; 95% confidence intervals [CI] = 1.0–4.7; P = .04).

The duration of AHREs vary considerably. For example, Cheung and colleagues[22] found that 60% of the population had an AHRE duration of more than 1 hour and in 16% AHRE episode lasted more than 1 week. Brief episodes may precede longer episodes, as almost 50% of patients with an AHRE less than 1 hour had subsequent episodes lasting 1 hour or greater. However, some of the early onset, brief episodes in the immediate postimplant phase, may be secondary to the temporary proarrhythmic state due to the inflammatory effect of atrial lead implantation. An analysis of the Silent

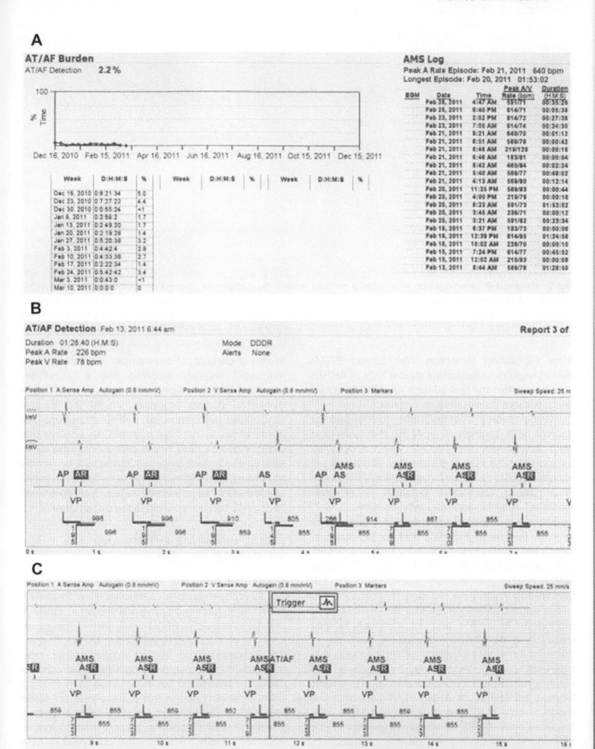

Fig. 1. Pacemaker interrogation strips from a patient with a dual-chamber pacemaker demonstrates far-field sensing of R waves leading to inappropriate detection of AT/AF. Panel (A) shows an overall AF burden of 2.2% and weekly burden from 0% to 5%. A typical episode of automatic mode switch (AMS) occurred on February 13, 2011 at 6:44 AM, lasting 1 hour 28 minutes and 50 seconds (*bottom, right column*). Panel (B) shows atrial and ventricular pacing for the first 3 cycles. V-pacing is followed by far-field R-wave sensing falling in the refractory period (AR). After an AS-VP event, AP-VP is again far-field sensed in the atrium and leads to AMS and VVI pacing. This pacing leads to double counting of atrial activity (far-field paced R waves and intrinsic atrial activity), leading to detection of AT/AF in panel (C). bpm, beats per minute; AR, atrial refractory; V, ventricular.

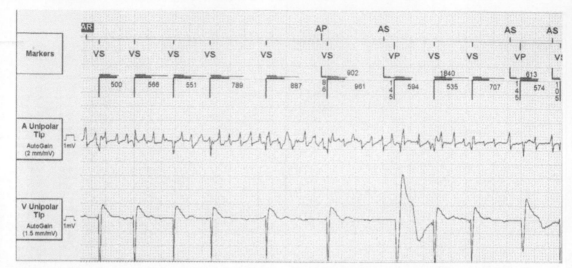

Fig. 2. Pacemaker interrogation strip from a patient with a dual-chamber pacemaker demonstrates AF undersensing. AF is present in the atrial channel, whereas the ventricular channel shows a well-controlled, irregular rhythm. The marker channel at the top clearly shows appropriate sensing of ventricular activity, whereas atrial activity is undersensed. A, atrium; V, AS, atrial sensed; V, ventricle; VP, ventricular paced; VS, ventricular sensed.

Atrial Fibrillation Detection With Stored EGMs (SAFE) registry revealed that almost 25% of AHREs occurred within the first 30 days after PPM implantation without subsequent recurrence.[27]

Several studies have attempted to estimate the approximate duration of an AHRE that correlates with clinician-documented AF. When a cutoff of 5 minutes and a rate of greater than 250 beats per minute (bpm) are chosen for significant AHRE, there is a strong correlation between pacemaker-identified AHREs and clinically confirmed AF.[19] Similarly, a subanalysis of the MOST population, which used greater than 220 bpm for 5 minutes as significant AHRE, found a high correlation with clinically detected AF (HR = 5.93, $P = .0001$).[28] Shorter cutoffs lead to overdetection, commonly due to far-field R- and T-wave oversensing.[29]

It is critical to adjudicate that the AHRE events are indeed AF or AFL and not spuriously labeled because of its clinical implications. Because of the limited memory allocated for intracardiac electrograms, pacing devices may store only limited electrogram data to corroborate that the events labeled as AHRE, or AHRE-triggered automatic mode switch (AMS) events are indeed AF or AFL. Because most AHRE episodes are asymptomatic and found incidentally on device interrogation, symptom correlation is usually absent.[19] Atrial undersensing can lead to nondetection of low amplitude atrial signals and, thus, underestimate AF burden, whereas oversensing issues can lead to erroneous overestimation of AF burden. In the absence of correlate-stored electrograms, the diagnosis may be impossible to confirm; one has to make decisions about therapeutic interventions

in this uncertainty. For example, Kohno and colleagues[30] recently reported that a cumulative increase in atrial pacing and the use of an atrial overdrive pacing algorithm might be closely associated with spurious AHRE detection. The admonition, as best as possible, to confirm that the device-detected AHRE represents true AF or AFL is even more pertinent in the era of remote monitoring, when potentially every AHRE (meeting predefined atrial rate and duration criteria) leading to an AMS can be reported to the pacemaker clinic.

ATRIAL HIGH-RATE EVENTS AND THROMBOEMBOLISM

Recent studies that have assessed the risk of thromboembolism associated with AHRE detected in pacing devices are shown in **Table 1**. Initial evidence of increased risk came from a subanalysis of 312 patients enrolled in MOST,[28] which was a randomized trial of dual-chamber rate-modulated pacing versus single-chamber ventricular rate–modulated pacing in patients with sinus node dysfunction.[26] In this subanalysis, an AHRE was defined as an atrial rate 220 bpm or greater lasting at least 5 minutes. Over a median follow-up of 27 months, AHREs were observed in 51% of the population and were an independent predictor of mortality (HR = 2.48, $P = .009$) and nonfatal stroke (HR = 2.79; $P = .001$). The MOST study subanalysis concluded that AHRE detected by pacemakers in patients with sinus node dysfunction can identify patients that are more than twice as likely to die or have a stroke and 6 times as likely to develop AF as similar patients without AHRE.

Table 1
Clinical studies evaluating risk of thromboembolism with device-detected AHRE

No.	Study and Year	No. of Subjects	Design	Population	Significant AHRE Definition	Results
1.	Glotzer et al,[28] 2003	312	RCT subanalysis	Dual-chamber pacemaker recipients	Atrial rate ≥220 bpm lasting ≥5 min	Increased risk of death and nonfatal stroke with AHRE
2.	Capucci et al,[31] 2005	725	Prospective, observational	Dual-chamber pacemaker recipients	AF for 5 min or 1 d	Increased risk of TE in patients with AHRE >1 d duration
3.	TRENDS study,[32] 2009	2486	Prospective, observational	Pacemaker/ defibrillator recipients with ≥stroke risk factor	Atrial rate ≥175 bpm lasting ≥20 s	Increased risk of TE in patients with AHRE ≥5.5 h
4.	ASSERT study,[33,34] 2010	2580	Randomized trial	Pacemaker/ defibrillator recipients with hypertension and aged ≥65 y	Atrial rate ≥190 bpm lasting ≥6 min	Increased ischemic stroke and TE in AHRE group

Abbreviations: ASSERT, Asymptomatic Atrial Fibrillation and Stroke Evaluation in Pacemaker Patients and the Atrial Fibrillation Reduction Atrial Pacing Trial; RCT, randomized controlled trial; TE, thromboembolism.

However, this study was conducted in patients with early generation pacemakers that had limited device memory and diagnostic capability to accurately assess duration/rate of the AHRE.

Following this, Capucci and colleagues[31] conducted a larger, prospective, multicenter observational study in patients who received PPMs for bradycardia. A total of 725 patients were monitored for arterial embolic events (including stroke, transient ischemic attack, and peripheral arterial embolism) over a median follow-up of 22 months. An AHRE duration of greater than 5 minutes was considered significant in this study. Using a Cox proportional hazard model, the association between 2 different AHRE durations (more than 5 minutes and 1 day) and thromboembolism was assessed. Although a higher incidence of arterial embolism was found in patients with an AHRE duration greater than 1 day ($P = .03$), a similar increase was not found in patients with an AHRE duration greater than 5 minutes. The exact AHRE duration associated with stroke risk could not be estimated from this study, as patients with an AHRE duration ranging from 5 minutes to 24 hours were included in the same group and these patients were not further stratified. Thus, the risk of thromboembolism and the need for anticoagulation in patients with an AHRE greater than 5 minutes remained unclear.

The TRENDS study was a prospective observational study conducted in ICD, CRT, or PPM recipients with a $CHADS_2$ score of 1 or greater.[32] A total of 2486 patients with at least 30 days of device data were followed for a mean of 1.4 years. An atrial rate of greater than 175 bpm lasting 20 seconds or longer was used to define AHRE. AHRE burden, defined as the longest AHRE duration in a 30-day period, was divided into 3 subsets: zero, low (<5.5 hours), and high (≥5.5 hours). The annual risk of thromboembolism or transient ischemic events was significantly greater in the high-burden subset when compared with the zero/low-burden subsets (2.4% vs 1.1%). After adjusting for stroke risk factors and antithrombotic treatment, the HR for thromboembolic events in the high-AHRE-burden group compared with the zero-burden group did not achieve statistical significance ($HR = 2.20$; $CI = 0.96$–3.8; $P = .06$). A significant limitation of this study was the low-event rate (1.3%) in the study population when compared with the observed rate (4%) in patients with a similar $CHADS_2$ score (ie, >2). This finding precluded further stratification of the population into increasing AHRE burden levels. Although this study provided some indication suggesting an increased risk of thromboembolism in patients with high AHRE burden, further clarification was required.

The Asymptomatic AF and Stroke Evaluation in Pacemaker Patients and the AF Reduction Atrial Pacing Trial (ASSERT) assessed dual-chamber PPM or ICD recipients with hypertension and aged at least 65 years.[33] Unlike prior studies, patients with known AF or on warfarin or other anticoagulant therapy were excluded. A total of 2580 patients from 136 centers were followed for approximately 3 years. In this study, AHRE was defined as an episode of device-detected atrial rate greater than 190 bpm, lasting greater than 6 minutes, which was found in a third of the population. The risk of ischemic stroke and systemic embolism was significantly higher in the AHRE group than the non-AHRE group (relative risk = 2.49; CI = 1.28–4.84; P = .007).[34] This risk remained significantly higher in the AHRE group in subsequent analyses after excluding those with surface ECG-detected AF (thus isolating device-detected AF), controlling for stroke risk factors, and limiting comparison with the high-risk group (ie, CHADS$_2$ $\geq$2). Although this study did not substratify groups based on AHRE burden to define a specific AHRE threshold value that increases stroke risk, it removed confounding from other clinical factors and, thus, gave a better assessment of risk of ischemic stroke due to device-detected AHRE.

UNANSWERED QUESTIONS

Although cardiac implantable electronic device [CIED]–detected AHRE implies underlying AF/AFL and potentially increased risk of thromboembolism, many questions remain unanswered:

1. How should we define CIED-detected AF? The definition of AHRE, which is a surrogate marker of paroxysmal AF, differs among different trials; the best definition for this remains unclear. Atrial rate and duration are 2 parameters that characterize an AHRE. Initial studies indicate that a rate of greater than 250 bpm and a duration of more than 5 minutes correlates best with clinician-confirmed AF. The ASSERT trial used a slightly lower rate (190 bpm) for AHRE, and it is possible that results of ASSERT would have differed had investigators used a different definition of AHRE. Requiring a longer duration of high atrial rate for a cutoff may lead to underestimating the AF burden, whereas the converse may lead to overestimation. So, what is the optimal atrial rate and duration to define an AHRE?

2. What is the best atrial sensitivity setting to prevent undersensing or oversensing? The interplay between atrial-sensitivity setting and atrial and far-field signal size measured by the device may lead to oversensing or undersensing of AHREs and can significantly change the recorded AHRE burden in a given patient. Sometimes, increasing atrial sensitivity (lower threshold value) can lead to a paradoxic undersensing of AF because of inappropriate atrial noise reversion.[35]

3. What is the critical AHRE burden that warrants therapeutic intervention? The threshold burden beyond which thromboembolic risk is increased remains undefined. It is likely that stroke risk is related to both the longest duration of AHRE as well as total AHRE burden; these issues need further study.

4. Should we routinely anticoagulate patients with CIED-detected AHREs? Based on the result of the ASSERT trial, it seems appropriate to anticoagulate high-risk patients with significant AHREs (as defined by an atrial rate of >190 bpm and duration >6 minutes). Ghali and colleagues[36] have observed that clinicians initiate anticoagulation in device-detected AHRE if they had a prior history of AF or a significant burden. There are no studies that have looked at outcomes after anticoagulation in device-detected AHRE.

5. Should we actively monitor device recipients for AHREs via continuous remote monitoring systems? The Clinical Evaluation of Remote Notification to Reduce Time to Clinical Decision (CONNECT) trial demonstrated that wireless remote monitoring with predefined automatic alerts significantly reduced the time to a clinical decision in response to the alert, compared with standard in-office follow-up.[37] Other studies of remote monitoring also demonstrated beneficial outcomes.[38,39] The IMPACT study was a randomized single-blinded control study that included ICD and CRT-D device recipients.[40] It compared the benefit of using Biotronik (Biotronik, Berlin, Germany) home monitoring technology to detect AF/AFL to initiate anticoagulation as soon as possible with a predefined anticoagulation plan compared with conventional device follow-up in the clinic every 3 months and physician-initiated anticoagulation, as per the discretion of the treating physician. As in ASSERT, this study also excluded patients with known AF and patients already on anticoagulation. Unfortunately, the study was terminated prematurely because of meeting the futility end point. The question of anticoagulation is still very important in this population, but the study design of the IMPACT trial did not answer the question.

SUMMARY

AF is an important risk factor for stroke and thromboembolism, and AF-related stroke has a high morbidity and mortality. CIED-detected AHRE is usually tantamount to having clinical AF, but there are many exceptions. Although the risk of stroke with clinical AF is relatively well known, the thromboembolic risk of CIED-detected AHRE is unclear because studies have used differing criteria of atrial high rate and duration for defining AHRE. Recently, the ASSERT study demonstrated an increased risk of stroke in patients with CIED-detected AHRE, even in the absence of a previous history of clinical AF. However, some areas that need further study are an accurate definition of what constitutes a significant CIED-detected AHRE; a threshold AHRE burden level that confers a stroke risk and, thus, the need for anticoagulation; as well as the ideal monitoring strategy, namely, continuous remote monitoring versus periodic surveillance in the device clinic.

REFERENCES

1. Go AS, Hylek EM, Phillips KA, et al. Prevalence of diagnosed atrial fibrillation in adults: national implications for rhythm management and stroke prevention: the Anticoagulation and Risk Factors in Atrial Fibrillation (ATRIA) study. JAMA 2001;285:2370–5.

2. Wolf PA, Abbott RD, Kannel WB. Atrial fibrillation as an independent risk factor for stroke: the Framingham study. Stroke 1991;22:983–8.

3. Wolf PA, Dawber TR, Thomas HE Jr, et al. Epidemiologic assessment of chronic atrial fibrillation and risk of stroke: the Framingham study. Neurology 1978;28:973–7.

4. Hart RG, Pearce LA, Rothbart RM, et al. Stroke with intermittent atrial fibrillation: incidence and predictors during aspirin therapy. Stroke Prevention in Atrial Fibrillation Investigators. J Am Coll Cardiol 2000;35:183–7.

5. Chugh SS, Blackshear JL, Shen WK, et al. Epidemiology and natural history of atrial fibrillation: clinical implications. J Am Coll Cardiol 2001;37:371–8.

6. Harrison MJ, Marshall J. Atrial fibrillation, TIAs and completed strokes. Stroke 1984;15:441–2.

7. Anderson DC, Kappelle LJ, Eliasziw M, et al. Occurrence of hemispheric and retinal ischemia in atrial fibrillation compared with carotid stenosis. Stroke 2002;33:1963–7.

8. Morley J, Marinchak R, Rials SJ, et al. Atrial fibrillation, anticoagulation, and stroke. Am J Card 1996; 77:38A–44A.

9. Beyth RJ, Antani MR, Covinsky KE, et al. Why isn't warfarin prescribed to patients with nonrheumatic atrial fibrillation? J Gen Intern Med 1996;11:721–8.

10. O'Hare JA, Ul-Iman N, Geoghegan M. Non-anticoagulation in atrial fibrillation. Ir J Med Sci 1994;163: 448–50.

11. Connolly SJ, Ezekowitz MD, Yusuf S, et al. Dabigatran versus warfarin in patients with atrial fibrillation. N Engl J Med 2009;361:1139–51.

12. Ehrens I, Lip GYH, Peters K. What do the RE-LY, AVERROES and ROCKET-AF trials tell us for stroke prevention in atrial fibrillation. Thromb Haemost 2011;105(4):574–8.

13. Holmes DR, Reddy VY, Turi ZG, et al. Percutaneous closure of the left atrial appendage versus warfarin therapy for prevention of stroke in patients with atrial fibrillation: a randomized non-inferiority trial. Lancet 2009;374:534–42.

14. Gaillard N, Deltour S, Vilotijevic B, et al. Detection of paroxysmal atrial fibrillation with transtelephonic EKG in TIA or stroke patients. Neurology 2010;74: 1666–70.

15. Tayal AH, Tian M, Kelly KM, et al. Atrial fibrillation detected by mobile cardiac outpatient telemetry in cryptogenic TIA or stroke. Neurology 2008;71: 1696–701.

16. Hohnloser SH, Pajitnev D, Pogue J, et al. Incidence of stroke in paroxysmal versus sustained atrial fibrillation in patients taking oral anticoagulation or combined antiplatelet therapy: an ACTIVE W substudy. J Am Coll Cardiol 2007;50:2156–61.

17. Friberg L, Hammar N, Rosenqvist M. Stroke in paroxysmal atrial fibrillation: report from the Stockholm Cohort of Atrial Fibrillation. Eur Heart J 2010; 31:967–75.

18. Schuchert A, Lepage S, Ostrander JJ, et al. Automatic analysis of pacemaker diagnostic data in the identification of atrial tachyarrhythmias in patients with no prior history of them. Europace 2005;7: 242–7.

19. Pollak WM, Simmons JD, Interian A Jr, et al. Clinical utility of intra-atrial pacemaker stored electrograms to diagnose atrial fibrillation and flutter. Pacing Clin Electrophysiol 2001;24:424–9.

20. Defaye P, Dournaux F, Mouton E. Prevalence of supraventricular arrhythmias from the automated analysis of data stored in the DDD pacemakers of 617 patients: the AIDA study. The AIDA Multicenter Study Group. Automatic Interpretation for Diagnosis Assistance. Pacing Clin Electrophysiol 1998;21:250–5.

21. Gillis AM, Morck M. Atrial fibrillation after DDDR pacemaker implantation. J Cardiovasc Electrophysiol 2002;13:542–7.

22. Cheung JW, Keating RJ, Stein KM, et al. Newly detected atrial fibrillation following dual chamber pacemaker implantation. J Cardiovasc Electrophysiol 2006;17:1323–8.

23. Borleffs CJ, Ypenburg C, van Bommel RJ, et al. Clinical importance of new-onset atrial fibrillation

after cardiac resynchronization therapy. Heart Rhythm 2009;6:305–10.

24. Leclercq C, Padeletti L, Cihák R, et al. Incidence of paroxysmal atrial tachycardias in patients treated with cardiac resynchronization therapy and continuously monitored by device diagnostics. Europace 2010;12:71–7.

25. Orlov MV, Ghali JK, Araghi-Niknam M, et al. Asymptomatic atrial fibrillation in pacemaker recipients: incidence, progression, and determinants based on the atrial high rate trial. Pacing Clin Electrophysiol 2007;30:404–11.

26. Sweeney MO, Hellkamp AS, Ellenbogen KA, et al. Adverse effect of ventricular pacing on heart failure and atrial fibrillation among patients with normal baseline QRS duration in a clinical trial of pacemaker therapy for sinus node dysfunction. Circulation 2003;107:2932–7.

27. Mittal S, Stein K, Gilliam FR 3rd, et al. Frequency, duration, and predictors of newly-diagnosed atrial fibrillation following dual-chamber pacemaker implantation in patients without a previous history of atrial fibrillation. Am J Cardiol 2008;102:450–3.

28. Glotzer TV, Hellkamp AS, Zimmerman J, et al. Atrial high rate episodes detected by pacemaker diagnostics predict death and stroke: report of the Atrial Diagnostics Ancillary Study of the Mode Selection Trial (MOST). Circulation 2003;107:1614–9.

29. Seidl K, Meisel E, VanAgt E, et al. Is the atrial high rate episode diagnostic feature reliable in detecting paroxysmal episodes of atrial tachyarrhythmias? Pacing Clin Electrophysiol 1998;21:694–700.

30. Kohno R, Abe H, Oginosawa Y, et al. Reliability and characteristics of atrial tachyarrhythmias detection in dual chamber pacemakers. Circ J 2011;75(5): 1090–7.

31. Capucci A, Santini M, Padeletti L, et al. Monitored atrial fibrillation duration predicts arterial embolic events in patients suffering from bradycardia and atrial fibrillation implanted with antitachycardia pacemakers. J Am Coll Cardiol 2005;46:1913–20.

32. Glotzer TV, Daoud EG, Wyse DG, et al. The relationship between daily atrial tachyarrhythmia burden from implantable device diagnostics and stroke risk: the TRENDS study. Circ Arrhythm Electrophysiol 2009;2:474–80.

33. Hohnloser SH, Capucci A, Fain E, et al. Asymptomatic Atrial Fibrillation and Stroke Evaluation in Pacemaker Patients and the Atrial Fibrillation Reduction Atrial Pacing Trial (ASSERT). Am Heart J 2006; 152:442–7.

34. Available at: www.theheart.org. Accessed March 24, 2011.

35. Kolb C, Halbfass P, Zrenner B, et al. Paradoxical atrial undersensing due to inappropriate atrial noise reversion of atrial fibrillation in dual-chamber pacemakers. J Cardiovasc Electrophysiol 2005;16: 696–700.

36. Ghali JK, Orlov MV, Araghi-Niknam M, et al. The influence of symptoms and device detected atrial tachyarrhythmias on medical management: insights from A-HIRATE. Pacing Clin Electrophysiol 2007;30: 850–7.

37. Crossley GH, Boyle A, Vitense H, et al. The CONNECT (Clinical Evaluation of Remote Notification to Reduce Time to Clinical Decision) trial: the value of wireless remote monitoring with automatic clinician alerts. J Am Coll Cardiol 2011;57: 1181–9.

38. Varma N, Epstein AE, Irimpen A, et al, for the TRUST Investigators. Efficacy and safety of automatic remote monitoring for implantable cardioverter-defibrillator follow-up: the Lumos-T Safety Reduces Routine Office Device Follow-Up (TRUST) trial. Circulation 2010;122:325–32.

39. Crossley GH, Chen J, Choucair W, et al. Clinical benefits of remote versus transtelephonic monitoring of implanted pacemakers. J Am Coll Cardiol 2009; 54:2012–9.

40. Ip J, Waldo AL, Lip GY, et al. Multicenter randomized study of anticoagulation guided by remote rhythm monitoring in patients with implantable cardioverter-defibrillator and CRT-D devices: rationale, design, and clinical characteristics of the initially enrolled cohort the IMPACT study. Am Heart J 2009;158:364–70.

Atrial Fibrillation Ablation and Stroke

Philip Aagaard, MD, PhD[a], David Briceno, MD, PhD[a], Zoltan Csanadi, MD, PhD[b],
Sanghamitra Mohanty, MD[c], Carola Gianni, MD[c], Chintan Trivedi, MD, MPH[c],
Edina Nagy-Baló, MD, PhD[b], Stephan Danik, MD[d], Conor Barrett, MD[d],
Francesco Santoro, MD[e], J. David Burkhardt, MD, PhD[c], Javier Sanchez, MD[c],
Andrea Natale, MD, PhD, FESC, FHRS[c,f,g,h,i,j],*, Luigi Di Biase, MD, PhD, FHRS[c,e,k],*

KEYWORDS

• Anticoagulation • Atrial fibrillation • Silent cerebral ischemia • Stroke

KEY POINTS

- Catheter ablation has become a widely available and accepted treatment to restore sinus rhythm (SR) in patients with atrial fibrillation (AF) who fail antiarrhythmic drug therapy.
- Although generally safe, the procedure carries a non-negligible risk of complications, including a small risk of periprocedural stroke and transient ischemic attack (TIA) as well as risk of silent cerebral ischemia (SCI).
- Embolic events cluster in the first 24 hours after ablation, although the high-risk period extends to at least 2 weeks postablation.
- Large thromboembolic events mainly relate to dislodgement of pre-formed thrombus. The mechanisms of SCI, on the other hand, are less well understood and may include small thrombotic, tissue, char, and/or air emboli.
- Uninterrupted anticoagulation, maintenance of an adequate ACT during the procedure, and measures to avoid and detect thrombus build-up on sheaths and catheters during the procedure appears useful to reduce the risk of embolic events.
- Although a majority of acute SCI lesions regress at medium-term follow-up, it appears prudent to use techniques that minimize SCI until conclusive data are available.

INTRODUCTION

Catheter ablation offers the opportunity to restore SR without the adverse effects of antiarrhythmic drugs. In the past decade, catheter ablation has become a widely available and accepted treatment modality to restore SR in patients with AF who have failed antiarrhythmic drug therapy. Although generally safe, the procedure involves hardware introduction into the systemic circulation

Disclosures: Dr P. Aagaard reports that he has no conflicts of interest. Dr L. Di Biase is a consultant for Biosense Webster, Stereotaxis, and St Jude Medical and has received speaker honoraria/travel from Pfizer, Janssen, EpiEP, Biotronik, and Boston Scintific. Dr A. Natale is a consultant for Biosense Webster and St Jude Medical and has received speaker honoraria/travel from Medtronic, Boston Scientific, Biotronik, and Janssen.

[a] Department of Medicine, Albert Einstein College of Medicine, Montefiore Hospital, Bronx, NY, USA; [b] Department of Cardiology, University of Debrecen, 22 Móricz Zs, Debrecen H4032, Hungary; [c] Department of Cardiology, Texas Cardiac Arrhythmia Institute, St David's Medical Center, Austin, TX, USA; [d] The Al-Sabah Arrhythmia Institute at Mount Sinai St. Luke, New York, NY, USA; [e] Department of Cardiology, University of Foggia, Foggia, Italy; [f] Division of Cardiology, Stanford University, Stanford, CA, USA; [g] CaseWestern Reserve University, Cleveland, OH, USA; [h] EP Services, California Pacific Medical Center, San Francisco, CA, USA; [i] Interventional Electrophysiology, Scripps Clinic, San Diego, CA, USA; [j] Dell Medical School, University of Texas, Austin, TX, USA; [k] Department of Biomedical Engineering, University of Texas, Austin, TX, USA
* Corresponding authors. Texas Cardiac Arrhythmia Institute, St David's Medical Center, Austin, TX
E-mail addresses: dr.natale@gmail.com; dibbia@gmail.com

Cardiol Clin 34 (2016) 307–316
http://dx.doi.org/10.1016/j.ccl.2015.12.012
0733-8651/16/$ – see front matter © 2016 Elsevier Inc. All rights reserved.

and left atrium as well as energy application to the myocardial tissues. Consequently, the procedure carries a non-negligible risk of complications, including a risk of periprocedural stroke and TIA, as well as SCI. This is a review of the mechanisms, incidence, and impact as well as methods to reduce catheter ablation–related cerebral insults.

CEREBROVASCULAR COMPLICATIONS OF CATHETER ABLATION
Stroke and Transient Ischemic Attack

Periprocedural thromboembolic events cluster during the first 24 hours after catheter ablation, although the high-risk period extends to at least 2 weeks after the procedure.[1] The reported incidence of periprocedural events varies largely between studies. In single-center studies, the reported incidence of stroke is as low as 0%[2] and as high as 5%.[3] A meta-analysis, including 6936 patients, reported incidences of TIA and stroke of 0.2% and 0.3%, respectively.[4]

The incidence of periprocedural thromboembolic events does not seem to vary according to center experience. For example, in a high-volume center study, the overall complication rate decreased from 11.1% to 1.6% during a 10-year period, whereas the incidence of stroke and TIA remained stable.[5] Potential explanations include changes over time in procedure (more extensive lesion sets) and patient selection (indication for ablation expanded to higher risk patients), which are both factors that may have an impact on periprocedural embolic risk.

In a large international survey reporting on periprocedural complications, including 162 centers and 32,569 patients, 5 of 32 deaths were due to stroke.[6] Therefore, although the long-term prognosis seems favorable in most patients who survive a periprocedural stroke, with complete neurologic recovery in most cases,[7] stroke and TIA remain a significant and feared complications of AF ablation.

Silent Cerebral Ischemia

Although clinically overt stroke and TIA are among the most feared catheter ablation complications, SCI may also have adverse effects. It is well known that brain MRI–detected SCI is associated with dementia and cognitive decline in the general population.[8,9] For example, the presence of SCI was associated with a 2-fold risk of dementia in a population-based study (n = 15,000).[8] Factors that seem to affect the onset and severity of dementia include patient age and lesion size.[10] Elderly patients might be at particularly high risk of cognitive decline even from minor lesions due to their smaller reserve (eg, less cortical volume).

It is well established that AF patients have a high burden of MRI-detected SCI, with a prevalence between 6% and 28%.[8,9,11] It is plausible that such silent brain infarcts, accumulated over time, may be responsible for the adverse impacts of AF on neurocognitive function.[12] In a large population study, AF was associated with a 2-fold increase in cognitive dysfunction and dementia, even in patients without overt clinical strokes or TIAs.[12]

Brain MRI has identified a high incidence of new ischemic embolic lesions after catheter ablation of AF (**Table 1**).[13–17] To date, however, no clear link has been established between post-ablation SCI and long-term cognitive decline, and the histopathological significance of MRI-detected brain lesions remains largely unknown. In 1 study, AF ablation was associated with mild dysfunction in some domains on cognitive function testing, which persisted at 90 days postprocedure in up to 20% of patients.[18] The clinical significance of these changes remain unclear. Another study compared neurocognitive function testing in 21 patients undergoing AF ablation with 23 non-AF controls.[19] Overall, 57% of patients who underwent ablation deteriorated from baseline on the verbal memory tests compared with 17% of controls. The study found no association, however, between cognitive decline and SCI, raising the possibility that post-ablation cognitive decline may be multifactorial rather than related to microembolic events per se. This concept is further supported by several other studies that also failed to establish a correlation between SCI and cognitive decline.[6,7,17,20] One study found that postprocedural cognitive decline only occurred in patients who suffered additional non–procedure-related SCI during follow-up.[8]

A majority of acute MRI lesions observed after AF ablation regress without evidence of chronic glial scar when reassessed at short-term follow-up.[20,21] Therefore, it is possible that successful ablation and restoration of SR, although acutely associated with an increase in SCI, may actually decrease the SCI burden in these patients over time, by reducing the risk of subsequent insults. This concept is supported by findings from a large database (n = 24,244) of patients undergoing catheter ablation and cardioversion.[22] In a propensity-matched analysis, ablation was associated with a significantly higher risk of stroke/TIA within the first 30 days postprocedure (relative risk [RR] 1.53; P = .05). Ablation was also associated, however, with a lower risk of non-TIA stroke during long-term follow-up (RR 0.78; P = .03). Furthermore, several other

Table 1
Incidence of MRI-detected silent cerebral ischemia according to ablation technique

Author, Year	N	Activated Clotting Time (s)	Ablation Technique	Silent Cerebral Ischemia (%)
Lickfett et al,[62] 2006	10	>250	Irrigated-tip RFA	10
Schwarz et al,[19] 2010	21	>300	Irrigated-tip RFA	14
Gaita et al,[13] 2010	232	250–300	Irrigated-tip RFA[c,d]	14
Schrickel et al,[14] 2010	53	>250	Irrigated-tip RFA	11
Herrera Siklody et al,[16] 2011	27	>300	RFA	33
	23	—	Irrigated-tip RFA	7.4
	24	—	Cryoablation	4.3
Neumann et al,[55] 2011	44	>300	Irrigated-tip RFA[d]	6.8
	45	—	Cryoablation	8.9
Deneke et al,[20] 2011	86	>300	Irrigated-tip RFA	38
Gaita et al,[15] 2011	36	>300	RFA	39
	36	—	Irrigated-tip RFA	8.3
	36	—	Cryoablation	5.6
Scaglione et al,[63] 2012	80	>300	Irrigated-tip RFA	6.0
Ichiki et al,[54] 2012	100	>250[a]	Irrigated-tip RFA[c]	7.0
Martinek et al,[21] 2013	131	>300[a]	Irrigated-tip RFA	12
Schmidt et al,[57] 2013	99	>250[a]	Irrigated-tip RFA	22
Ichiki et al,[54] 2012	210	>250[a]	Irrigated-tip RFA[c]	12
Haeusler et al,[17] 2013	37	>300	Irrigated-tip RFA	41
Wieczorek et al,[64] 2013	37	>300[a]	Irrigated-tip RFA	27
Verma et al,[58] 2013	60	>350[a]	Irrigated-tip RFA	1.7
Di Biase et al,[61] 2014	146	>300[b]	Irrigated-tip RFA	2.0

Abbreviations: PVI, pulmonary vein isolation; RFA, radiofrequency ablation.
[a] Uninterrupted anticoagulation.
[b] Uninterrupted anticoagulation and heparin bolus prior to transseptal puncture. All studies aimed for PVI only unless otherwise indicated.
[c] Complex fractionated atrial electrocardiogram ablation in addition to PVI.
[d] Lines in addition to PVI.

studies have reported an apparent reduction in the incidence of new SCI on long-term MRI follow-up after AF ablation.[17,20,23] It has, therefore, been speculated that AF ablation may actually protect against neurocognitive decline and early onset dementia.[23] Future prospective studies investigating the long-term impact of AF ablation on cognitive function are warranted to answer this question.

Mechanisms of Silent Cerebral Ischemia

The mechanism of large thromboembolic events in patients with AF is well established and mainly relates to dislodgement of preformed thrombus, particularly from the left atrial appendage. The mechanisms of periprocedural AF ablation-induced SCI, however, are less well understood and may be multifactorial. SCI on postablation MRI may represent thrombotic emboli, air emboli, char, and/or tissue emboli.

Thrombus may form during and after AF ablation through several pathways. Energy application during ablation injures myocardial epithelial cells, with subsequent loss of their anticoagulation properties. Furthermore, interruption of endothelial integrity exposes the subendothelium, which may promote platelet adhesion, activation, and thrombin production.[24] Thrombi formed during this process may later dislodge due to catheter movement, electrical cardioversion, or improved cardiac contractility from restoration of sinus rhythm.[13] Thrombus may also form directly on introduced sheaths and catheters.[25] Furthermore, blood stasis may promote thrombus formation inside sheaths and in blood columns trapped behind ablation balloons.[13] Finally, turbulence occurring during catheter movement and/or contrast injection may also activate the coagulation cascade through platelet activation.[26]

Gas bubble formation is another potential source of emboli during AF ablation procedures.

Transseptal puncture and left atrial sheath insertion both involve a potential risk of air embolization. This risk seems to increase with the use of more complex catheters.[27] Gas emboli may also form during energy application to the myocardial tissue.[28] Studies performed using intracardiac echocardiography (ICE) have demonstrated that gas bubble formation increases sharply when the tissue temperature rises above 60°C.[29]

Tissue emboli can form when transseptal needles are advanced to gain left atrial access. In addition, the application of energy to the myocardium during lesion formation may cause dislodgement and embolization of myocardial tissue fragments or char, particularly during tissue overheating and steam-pops.[30]

Finally, a residual iatrogenic atrial septal defect after transseptal puncture might increase the risk of paradoxic embolism. Recent evidence suggests, however, a high sealing rate of the defect (66%) immediately after the procedure and a very low incidence of persisting interatrial shunt (4%–7%), predominantly left-to-right, at 12 months of follow-up (16–17) that is not associated with an increased risk of symptomatic cerebral/systemic embolism.

It is possible that the long-term impact of embolization may differ between these mechanisms, that is, air emboli may have less long-term impact than thrombotic and tissue emboli. One study performed serial MRI after AF ablation and initially identified 50 new lesions in 14 patients. Follow-up imaging at 3 months revealed that 47 lesions (94%) were no longer detectable.[20] The 3 residual lesions were larger (>10 mm) on initial imaging compared with lesions that resolved. It can be speculated that larger lesions represent thrombotic emboli, whereas smaller lesions mainly largely represent air emboli. Brain biopsy results from animal model studies have demonstrated, however, that even lesions that resolve on MRI leave behind evidence of cerebral ischemic injury, including endothelial proliferation, glia cell activation, and lymphocytic perivascular infiltrates.[27] There is currently no clinical role, however, for routine follow-up MRI imaging postablation and its use should, therefore, be limited to investigational studies.

PERIPROCEDURAL ANTICOAGULATION

The optimal anticoagulation strategy during AF ablation to reduce the incidence of neurologic sequelae remains an area of active investigation. Current guidelines recommend at least 3 weeks of effective anticoagulation (eg, therapeutic international normalized ratio [INR] and novel oral anticoagulant [NOAC] compliance) prior to ablation.[31] If these criteria are not met, transesophageal echocardiography (TEE) is recommended to rule out left atrial thrombus, although many centers routinely perform TEE prior to ablation regardless of anticoagulation status.

Previously, the most common practice was to stop oral anticoagulation and to bridge the patient to low-molecular-weight heparin a few days before the procedure.[32] The COMPARE trial, however, demonstrated that uninterrupted anticoagulation was superior to bridging, both in terms of preventing periprocedural stroke and TIA and reducing bleeding events, in a population at high risk of embolic events.[33] Stroke or TIA occurred in 4.9% (n = 39) of patients when anticoagulation (Coumadin) was discontinued but only in 0.25% (n = 2) when full anticoagulation was continued (INR goal 2–3.5). Therefore, uninterrupted anticoagulation is considered the current best clinical practice.

Many early studies, where MRI-detected SCI was the endpoint, used anticoagulation strategies (ie, anticoagulation discontinuation) that do not reflect the current best clinical practice. Recent studies have shown that performing AF ablation on uninterrupted anticoagulation as well as maintaining an activated clotting time (ACT) of at least greater than 300 seconds at the time of transseptal puncture reduces the incidence of postprocedural MRI-detected SCI to less than 2%.[34,35] The importance of adequate periprocedural anticoagulation is further supported by a study that demonstrated a reduction in the number of embolic signals on transcranial Doppler during ablation when ACT was maintained greater than 320 seconds compared with an ACT greater than 250 seconds.[28] Using advanced Doppler signal analysis, this study also demonstrated that most Doppler signals were due to gas or particulate debris, rather than thrombus, when using an uninterrupted anticoagulation strategy, suggesting that strategies beyond uninterrupted anticoagulation should be considered to further reduce the risk of SCI.

Although vitamin K antagonists (eg, Coumadin) have been the standard of care for stroke prevention in AF patients for decades, recent years have witnessed the rise of NOACs. Although NOACs have demonstrated noninferiority to Coumadin for stroke prevention in AF,[36] the feasibility and safety of NOACs to prevent AF ablation periprocedural thromboembolic events remain a topic of controversy.[37–39] Recently, the VENTURE-AF trial demonstrated the use of uninterrupted oral rivaroxaban was feasible in patients undergoing AF ablation and that event rates were similar to those for uninterrupted vitamin K antagonist therapy.[40] Similar results have been demonstrated with periprocedural anticoagulation using apixaban.[41,42] There is some concern, however, regarding the use of dabigatran for periprocedural anticoagulation. A multicenter prospective registry showed a significantly higher rate of major bleeding as well as a higher rate of the composite endpoint of bleeding and thromboembolic complications (6% and 16%, respectively) with dabigatran compared with warfarin (1% and 6%, respectively).[37] On the other hand, 1 study found no difference in the incidence of symptomatic and asymptomatic cerebral thromboembolism after AF ablation in patients treated with dabigatran and Coumadin, respectively.[43] A higher risk of thromboembolic complications using dabigatran was reported, however, in a meta-analysis.[44] Furthermore, in a study of 210 patients, the incidence of SCI was 26.7% in patients on periprocedural dabigatran compared with 10% in patients on uninterrupted Coumadin ($P<.05$).[35] Therefore, although NOACs are showing great promise as an alternative agent to Coumadin for uninterrupted periprocedural anticoagulation, more data are needed.[45] Currently, periprocedural anticoagulation with dabigatran cannot be advised.

Intraprocedural considerations to reduce the risk of thromboembolic events also involves administration of unfractionated heparin (UFH) and monitoring for thrombus formation on sheaths and catheters using ICE. UFH should be administered as an intravenous bolus, followed by a continuous infusion to maintain target ACT. To prevent thrombus formation on the transseptal sheath, the bolus is usually given before or immediately after the transseptal puncture.[46] The currently recommended ACT target is 300 seconds to 400 seconds, with some centers aiming for a level greater than 350 seconds. The target ACT should be achieved prior to the first energy delivery and rechecked every 20 minutes to 30 minutes to ensure an adequate level throughout the procedure. Additional UFH boluses can be administered as needed. Importantly, when performing ablations on NOACs, it is often necessary to use larger doses of UFH to maintain an adequate ACT level.[43] UFH is discontinued once all catheters and sheaths have exited the left atrium (LA). Removal of sheaths from the groin can be safely performed when the ACT is less than 200 seconds. Some centers use protamine at the end of the procedure to reverse UFH.

Observational data suggest that a majority of cerebral insults occur within 2 weeks after the procedure,[1] and postablation anticoagulation is recommended in all patients for at least 2 months.[31]

There is a variable degree of atrial stunning after AF ablation, which may promote thrombus formation. Furthermore, there is concern that the endothelial damage incurred during the energy application to the LA is thrombogenic.

There is currently no evidence from large randomized trials to guide long-term anticoagulation strategies after AF ablation. Therefore, at present, patients should be risk-stratified according to the same principles (CHADS$_2$ or CHA$_2$DS$_2$-VASc score) used in patients who have not undergone ablation, even if SR is initially restored.[47–49] These scores have recently been shown to provide prognostic value in patients after ablation.[50] Emerging data suggest, however, that successful AF ablation does reduce the stroke risk and that long-term anticoagulation may not be necessary in all patients. A nonrandomized study followed 755 patients for 25 months after ablation.[1] In a subgroup of 180 patients with greater than or equal to 1 stroke risk factor but who remained in sinus rhythm, anticoagulation was stopped at a median of 5 months postablation, without any cardioembolic events. Furthermore, in a recent observational study including 3344 AF ablation patients, anticoagulation was discontinued in patients without significant left atrial mechanical dysfunction who remained in sinus rhythm, regardless of CHADS$_2$.[51] All patients were transitioned to aspirin and in patients with a CHADS$_2$ score with greater than or equal to 1, anticoagulation was restarted only in the event of AF recurrence. Using this strategy, no cardioembolic events occurred during a mean follow-up of 28 months in 347 patients with a mean CHADS$_2$ score with greater than or equal to 2. Although these data are promising, large randomized trials to evaluate the best postprocedural long-term anticoagulation strategy are needed to help guide the best postablation anticoagulation approach.

OTHER FACTORS HAVING AN IMPACT ON THE RISK OF PERIPROCEDURAL EMBOLIC EVENTS
Patient Characteristics

The risk of clinically overt thromboembolic events and SCI is nonuniform across different patient populations. Patients with persistent AF seem at a higher risk than patients with paroxysmal AF.[52] Furthermore, risk seems to increase in the presence of a high CHADS$_2$ score.[52,53] There are conflicting data, however, regarding clinical predictors of MRI-detected SCI. In the largest study to date, no independent clinical predictors could be identified,[13] whereas other studies have identified age, coronary artery disease, left atrial size, septal wall thickness, and number of failed antiarrhythmic drugs as significant predictors of SCI risk.[14,54,55]

Ablation Energy Source

The source of ablation energy also seems to play a role in the genesis of periprocedural brain lesions. Previously, most ablation procedures were performed with closed-tip catheters. Today, however, open-irrigation radiofrequency energy catheters are becoming the standard of care. The thrombogenic potential seems lower with open-irrigated catheters.[56] This may relate to less risk of tissue overheating with tip-irrigation. Alternative energy sources, including cryoenergy, laser, and microwaves, have also been introduced. The risk of embolism seems lowest with cryoablation, perhaps owing to the sharper edges and less endothelial trauma when using this technique compared with more uneven borders and more endothelial damage when closed-tip radiofrequency ablation catheters are used. Other ablation technologies that rely on heating, including microwave and laser, share similar risk of thrombus formation with radiofrequency ablation.[24] To date, however, here are no clear data showing the advantage of either technology, as measured by the more clinically relevant endpoints of stroke and TIA. The lack of difference in harder endpoints (stroke and TIA), however, could be a power problem, because event rates are low. Therefore, MRI-detected SCI has often been studied as a surrogate marker of ablation related embolic risk. In a randomized comparison of 108 patients, radiofrequency ablation with closed-tip catheters, irrigated-tip catheters, and cryoablation had incidences of MRI-detected SCI of 39%, 8.3%, and 5.6%, respectively ($P<.05$). In another study of 74 patients, MRI-detected SCI incidence was 38%, 7%, and 4% in the groups, respectively ($P<.05$).[16] Other studies, however, have found no difference in MRI-detected SCI between tip-irrigated radiofrequency and cryoballoon ablation.[55,57] Important measures to reduce the incidence of brain-detected SCI seems to be uninterrupted anticoagulation, maintaining an adequate intraprocedural ACT, underwater loading, and optimized electrode settings. In 1 study, these measures decreased the incidence of MRI-detected SCI to less than 2%.[58]

Appropriate titration of radiofrequency energy to avoid tissue overheating also seems important to prevent embolic events. In 1 study that used ICE detection of gas bubbles to titrate radiofrequency energy during ablation, there was no thromboembolic complication in the ICE group, compared with a 3% incidence of periprocedural stroke and/or TIA in the patients where ICE titration was not used.[59] Today, such ICE titration is standard at many centers. Irrigated tip catheters and contact force sensing hold the promise to reduce gas emboli formation and tissue and/or char emboli even further, by allowing adequate lesion formation without unnecessarily high temperatures and steam-pops. The recent adoption of these technologies should be considered when interpreting results from studies on AF ablation associated embolic risk that predate these developments.

Sheaths and Catheters

The introduction of sheaths and catheters can also be a source of thrombotic emboli, through activation of the coagulation cascade,[34] and air emboli, by connecting the cardiac chambers with room air. The risk of air emboli pertains particularly to injections or intermittent flushing through of long sheaths, including left atrial access sheaths. Continuous flushing and other measures to eliminate air bubbles are important to reduce this risk.[31] All sheaths and catheters, however, are potential sources of thrombus formation, particularly in the absence of appropriate and timely anticoagulation. As discussed previously, ICE can play an important role during the ablation procedure to detect catheter-related sources of emboli.[25] At many centers, sheaths are retracted to the right atrium once the diagnostic and ablation catheters have been placed in the left atrium, to reduce systemic embolic risk further.

Ablation Protocol and Periprocedural Cardioversion

Other factors that can potentially affect embolic risk include more extensive ablation protocols, total time spent in the left atrium, and periprocedural cardioversion. Although, there are conflicting data regarding the role of additional ablation and time spent in the left atrium in embolic risk,[13,21,54] procedural cardioversion (both pharmacologic and electrical) during AF ablation seems to increase the risk of clinically evident, and silent, embolism. A recent study has reported a 2.75-times increase in the risk of subclinical cerebral embolism related to periprocedural cardioversion.[13] Analogously, cardioversion during the procedure was the most important predictor of cerebral thromboembolism after AF ablation (odds ratio 3.31) in 1 study.[35] Furthermore, the incidence of silent cerebral lesions also seems lower in patients remaining in stable SR throughout ablation compared with patients who undergo periprocedural cardioversion. It has, therefore, been suggested that cardioversion should be deferred until after the procedure once atrial lesions are healed.[13] There are conflicting data, however, regarding periprocedural cardioversion, with some studies showing no association with cerebral embolization.[17,60,61]

SUMMARY

Catheter ablation has become a widely available and accepted treatment modality to restore SR in patients with AF. Although generally safe, the procedure carries a non-negligible risk of complications, including a risk of periprocedural stroke and TIA as well as SCI. Embolic events cluster in the first 24 hours after ablation, although the high-risk period extends to at least 2 weeks post-ablation. The mechanism of large thromboembolic events in patients with AF is well established and mainly relates to dislodgement of preformed thrombus. The mechanisms of SCI are less well understood and may include small thrombotic, tissue, char, and/or air emboli. Uninterrupted anticoagulation, maintenance of an adequate ACT during the procedure, and measures to avoid and detect thrombus build-up on sheaths and catheters during the procedure, seem useful to reduce the risk of embolic events. Stroke and TIA, although rare, are often catastrophic events. The clinical impact of SCI, on the other hand, is not clear but has been associated with cognitive deterioration in some studies. Therefore, although a majority of acute SCI lesions regress at medium-term follow-up, it seems prudent to use techniques to minimize SCI until conclusive data are available.

REFERENCES

1. Oral H, Chugh A, Ozaydin M, et al. Risk of thromboembolic events after percutaneous left atrial radiofrequency ablation of atrial fibrillation. Circulation 2006;114(8):759–65.
2. Lee G, Sparks PB, Morton JB, et al. Low risk of major complications associated with pulmonary vein antral isolation for atrial fibrillation: results of 500 consecutive ablation procedures in patients with low prevalence of structural heart disease from a single center. J Cardiovasc Electrophysiol 2011;22(2):163–8.
3. Kok LC, Mangrum JM, Haines DE, et al. Cerebrovascular complication associated with pulmonary vein ablation. J Cardiovasc Electrophysiol 2002;13(8):764–7.
4. Calkins H, Reynolds MR, Spector P, et al. Treatment of atrial fibrillation with antiarrhythmic drugs or radiofrequency ablation: two systematic literature reviews and meta-analyses. Circ Arrhythm Electrophysiol 2009;2(4):349–61.
5. Hoyt H, Bhonsale A, Chilukuri K, et al. Complications arising from catheter ablation of atrial fibrillation: temporal trends and predictors. Heart Rhythm 2011;8(12):1869–74.
6. Cappato R, Calkins H, Chen SA, et al. Prevalence and causes of fatal outcome in catheter ablation of atrial fibrillation. J Am Coll Cardiol 2009;53(19):1798–803.
7. Patel D, Bailey SM, Furlan AJ, et al. Long-term functional and neurocognitive recovery in patients who had an acute cerebrovascular event secondary to catheter ablation for atrial fibrillation. J Cardiovasc Electrophysiol 2010;21(4):412–7.
8. Vermeer SE, Prins ND, den Heijer T, et al. Silent brain infarcts and the risk of dementia and cognitive decline. N Engl J Med 2003;348(13):1215–22.
9. Vermeer SE, Hollander M, van Dijk EJ, et al. Silent brain infarcts and white matter lesions increase stroke risk in the general population: the rotterdam scan study. Stroke 2003;34(5):1126–9.
10. Gorelick PB, Scuteri A, Black SE, et al. Vascular contributions to cognitive impairment and dementia: a statement for healthcare professionals from the american heart association/american stroke association. Stroke 2011;42(9):2672–713.
11. Vermeer SE, Longstreth WT Jr, Koudstaal PJ. Silent brain infarcts: a systematic review. Lancet Neurol 2007;6(7):611–9.
12. Ott A, Breteler MM, de Bruyne MC, et al. Atrial fibrillation and dementia in a population-based study. The Rotterdam Study. Stroke 1997;28(2):316–21.
13. Gaita F, Caponi D, Pianelli M, et al. Radiofrequency catheter ablation of atrial fibrillation: a cause of silent thromboembolism? magnetic resonance imaging assessment of cerebral thromboembolism in patients undergoing ablation of atrial fibrillation. Circulation 2010;122(17):1667–73.
14. Schrickel JW, Lickfett L, Lewalter T, et al. Incidence and predictors of silent cerebral embolism during pulmonary vein catheter ablation for atrial fibrillation. Europace 2010;12(1):52–7.
15. Gaita F, Leclercq JF, Schumacher B, et al. Incidence of silent cerebral thromboembolic lesions after atrial fibrillation ablation may change according to technology used: comparison of irrigated radiofrequency, multipolar nonirrigated catheter and cryoballoon. J Cardiovasc Electrophysiol 2011;22(9):961–8.
16. Herrera Siklody C, Deneke T, Hocini M, et al. Incidence of asymptomatic intracranial embolic events after pulmonary vein isolation: comparison of different atrial fibrillation ablation technologies in a multicenter study. J Am Coll Cardiol 2011;58(7):681–8.
17. Haeusler KG, Koch L, Herm J, et al. 3 Tesla MRI-detected brain lesions after pulmonary vein isolation for atrial fibrillation: results of the MACPAF study. J Cardiovasc Electrophysiol 2013;24(1):14–21.

18. Medi C, Evered L, Silbert B, et al. Subtle post-procedural cognitive dysfunction after atrial fibrillation ablation. J Am Coll Cardiol 2013;62(6):531–9.

19. Schwarz N, Kuniss M, Nedelmann M, et al. Neuropsychological decline after catheter ablation of atrial fibrillation. Heart Rhythm 2010;7(12):1761–7.

20. Deneke T, Shin DI, Balta O, et al. Postablation asymptomatic cerebral lesions: long-term follow-up using magnetic resonance imaging. Heart Rhythm 2011;8(11):1705–11.

21. Martinek M, Sigmund E, Lemes C, et al. Asymptomatic cerebral lesions during pulmonary vein isolation under uninterrupted oral anticoagulation. Europace 2013;15(3):325–31.

22. Noseworthy PA, Kapa S, Deshmukh AJ, et al. Risk of stroke after catheter ablation versus cardioversion for atrial fibrillation: a propensity-matched study of 24,244 patients. Heart Rhythm 2015; 12(6):1154–61.

23. Deneke T, Jais P, Scaglione M, et al. Silent cerebral events/lesions related to atrial fibrillation ablation: a clinical review. J Cardiovasc Electrophysiol 2015; 26(4):455–63.

24. Zhou L, Keane D, Reed G, et al. Thromboembolic complications of cardiac radiofrequency catheter ablation: a review of the reported incidence, pathogenesis and current research directions. J Cardiovasc Electrophysiol 1999;10(4):611–20.

25. Ren JF, Marchlinski FE, Callans DJ. Left atrial thrombus associated with ablation for atrial fibrillation: identification with intracardiac echocardiography. J Am Coll Cardiol 2004;43(10):1861–7.

26. Nesbitt WS, Mangin P, Salem HH, et al. The impact of blood rheology on the molecular and cellular events underlying arterial thrombosis. J Mol Med (Berl) 2006;84(12):989–95.

27. Haines DE, Stewart MT, Barka ND, et al. Microembolism and catheter ablation II: effects of cerebral microemboli injection in a canine model. Circ Arrhythm Electrophysiol 2013;6(1):23–30.

28. Nagy-Balo E, Tint D, Clemens M, et al. Transcranial measurement of cerebral microembolic signals during pulmonary vein isolation: a comparison of two ablation techniques. Circ Arrhythm Electrophysiol 2013;6(3):473–80.

29. Kalman JM, Fitzpatrick AP, Olgin JE, et al. Biophysical characteristics of radiofrequency lesion formation in vivo: dynamics of catheter tip-tissue contact evaluated by intracardiac echocardiography. Am Heart J 1997;133(1):8–18.

30. Di Biase L, Natale A, Barrett C, et al. Relationship between catheter forces, lesion characteristics, "popping," and char formation: experience with robotic navigation system. J Cardiovasc Electrophysiol 2009;20(4):436–40.

31. Calkins H, Kuck KH, Cappato R, et al. 2012 HRS/EHRA/ECAS expert consensus statement on catheter and surgical ablation of atrial fibrillation: recommendations for patient selection, procedural techniques, patient management and follow-up, definitions, endpoints, and research trial design: a report of the Heart Rhythm Society (HRS) Task Force on Catheter and Surgical Ablation of Atrial Fibrillation. Developed in partnership with the European Heart Rhythm Association (EHRA), a registered branch of the European Society of Cardiology (ESC) and the European Cardiac Arrhythmia Society (ECAS); and in collaboration with the American College of Cardiology (ACC), American Heart Association (AHA), the Asia Pacific Heart Rhythm Society (APHRS), and the Society of Thoracic Surgeons (STS). Endorsed by the governing bodies of the American College of Cardiology Foundation, the American Heart Association, the European Cardiac Arrhythmia Society, the European Heart Rhythm Association, the Society of Thoracic Surgeons, the Asia Pacific Heart Rhythm Society, and the Heart Rhythm Society. Heart Rhythm 2012;9(4): 632–96.e21.

32. Briceno DF, Natale A, Di Biase L. Heparin kinetics: the "Holy Grail" of periprocedural anticoagulation for ablation of atrial fibrillation. Pacing Clin Electrophysiol 2015;38(10):1137–41.

33. Di Biase L, Burkhardt JD, Santangeli P, et al. Periprocedural stroke and bleeding complications in patients undergoing catheter ablation of atrial fibrillation with different anticoagulation management: results from the role of coumadin in preventing thromboembolism in Atrial Fibrillation (AF) patients undergoing catheter ablation (COMPARE) randomized trial. Circulation 2014; 129(25):2638–44.

34. Dorbala S, Cohen AJ, Hutchinson LA, et al. Does radiofrequency ablation induce a prethrombotic state? analysis of coagulation system activation and comparison to electrophysiologic study. J Cardiovasc Electrophysiol 1998;9(11):1152–60.

35. Ichiki H, Oketani N, Ishida S, et al. The incidence of asymptomatic cerebral microthromboembolism after atrial fibrillation ablation: comparison of warfarin and dabigatran. Pacing Clin Electrophysiol 2013;36(11): 1328–35.

36. Ruff CT, Giugliano RP, Braunwald E, et al. Comparison of the efficacy and safety of new oral anticoagulants with warfarin in patients with atrial fibrillation: a meta-analysis of randomised trials. Lancet 2014; 383(9921):955–62.

37. Lakkireddy D, Reddy YM, Di Biase L, et al. Feasibility and safety of dabigatran versus warfarin for periprocedural anticoagulation in patients undergoing radiofrequency ablation for atrial fibrillation: results from a multicenter prospective registry. J Am Coll Cardiol 2012;59(13): 1168–74.

38. Di Biase L, Natale A. Apixaban is dear to me, but dearer still is warfarin. Pacing Clin Electrophysiol 2015;38(2):153–4.

39. Kim JS, She F, Jongnarangsin K, et al. Dabigatran vs warfarin for radiofrequency catheter ablation of atrial fibrillation. Heart Rhythm 2013;10(4):483–9.

40. Cappato R, Marchlinski FE, Hohnloser SH, et al. Uninterrupted rivaroxaban vs. uninterrupted vitamin K antagonists for catheter ablation in non-valvular atrial fibrillation. Eur Heart J 2015;36(28):1805–11.

41. Di Biase L, Lakkireddy D, Trivedi C, et al. Feasibility and safety of uninterrupted periprocedural apixaban administration in patients undergoing radiofrequency catheter ablation for atrial fibrillation: results from a multicenter study. Heart Rhythm 2015;12(6):1162–8.

42. Nagao T, Inden Y, Shimano M, et al. Efficacy and safety of apixaban in the patients undergoing the ablation of atrial fibrillation. Pacing Clin Electrophysiol 2015;38(2):155–63.

43. Kaseno K, Naito S, Nakamura K, et al. Efficacy and safety of periprocedural dabigatran in patients undergoing catheter ablation of atrial fibrillation. Circ J 2012;76(10):2337–42.

44. Dentali F, Riva N, Crowther M, et al. Efficacy and safety of the novel oral anticoagulants in atrial fibrillation: a systematic review and meta-analysis of the literature. Circulation 2012;126(20):2381–91.

45. Di Biase L. Safety and efficacy of novel oral anticoagulants in the setting of atrial fibrillation ablation: is it time to celebrate the "funeral" of warfarin? J Interv Card Electrophysiol 2014;41(2):103–5.

46. Bruce CJ, Friedman PA, Narayan O, et al. Early heparinization decreases the incidence of left atrial thrombi detected by intracardiac echocardiography during radiofrequency ablation for atrial fibrillation. J Interv Card Electrophysiol 2008;22(3):211–9.

47. American College of Cardiology Foundation, American Heart Association, European Society of Cardiology, et al. Management of patients with atrial fibrillation (compilation of 2006 ACCF/AHA/ESC and 2011 ACCF/AHA/HRS recommendations): a report of the American College of Cardiology/American Heart Association Task Force on practice guidelines. Circulation 2013;127(18):1916–26.

48. European Heart Rhythm Association, European Association for Cardio-Thoracic Surgery, Camm AJ, et al. Guidelines for the management of atrial fibrillation: the task force for the management of atrial fibrillation of the European Society of Cardiology (ESC). Eur Heart J 2010;31(19):2369–429.

49. Camm AJ, Lip GY, De Caterina R, et al. 2012 focused update of the ESC Guidelines for the management of atrial fibrillation: an update of the 2010 ESC Guidelines for the management of atrial fibrillation. Developed with the special contribution of the European Heart Rhythm Association. Eur Heart J 2012;33(21):2719–47.

50. Chao TF, Lin YJ, Tsao HM, et al. CHADS(2) and CHA(2)DS(2)-VASc scores in the prediction of clinical outcomes in patients with atrial fibrillation after catheter ablation. J Am Coll Cardiol 2011;58(23):2380–5.

51. Themistoclakis S, Corrado A, Marchlinski FE, et al. The risk of thromboembolism and need for oral anticoagulation after successful atrial fibrillation ablation. J Am Coll Cardiol 2010;55(8):735–43.

52. Scherr D, Sharma K, Dalal D, et al. Incidence and predictors of periprocedural cerebrovascular accident in patients undergoing catheter ablation of atrial fibrillation. J Cardiovasc Electrophysiol 2009;20(12):1357–63.

53. Di Biase L, Burkhardt JD, Mohanty P, et al. Periprocedural stroke and management of major bleeding complications in patients undergoing catheter ablation of atrial fibrillation: the impact of periprocedural therapeutic international normalized ratio. Circulation 2010;121(23):2550–6.

54. Ichiki H, Oketani N, Ishida S, et al. Incidence of asymptomatic cerebral microthromboembolism after atrial fibrillation ablation guided by complex fractionated atrial electrogram. J Cardiovasc Electrophysiol 2012;23(6):567–73.

55. Neumann T, Kuniss M, Conradi G, et al. MEDAFI-Trial (Micro-embolization during ablation of atrial fibrillation): comparison of pulmonary vein isolation using cryoballoon technique vs. radiofrequency energy. Europace 2011;13(1):37–44.

56. Khairy P, Chauvet P, Lehmann J, et al. Lower incidence of thrombus formation with cryoenergy versus radiofrequency catheter ablation. Circulation 2003;107(15):2045–50.

57. Schmidt B, Gunawardene M, Krieg D, et al. A prospective randomized single-center study on the risk of asymptomatic cerebral lesions comparing irrigated radiofrequency current ablation with the cryoballoon and the laser balloon. J Cardiovasc Electrophysiol 2013;24(8):869–74.

58. Verma A, Debruyne P, Nardi S, et al. Evaluation and reduction of asymptomatic cerebral embolism in ablation of atrial fibrillation, but high prevalence of chronic silent infarction: results of the evaluation of reduction of asymptomatic cerebral embolism trial. Circ Arrhythm Electrophysiol 2013;6(5):835–42.

59. Marrouche NF, Martin DO, Wazni O, et al. Phased-array intracardiac echocardiography monitoring during pulmonary vein isolation in patients with atrial fibrillation: impact on outcome and complications. Circulation 2003;107(21):2710–6.

60. Wissner E, Metzner A, Neuzil P, et al. Asymptomatic brain lesions following laserballoon-based pulmonary vein isolation. Europace 2014;16(2):214–9.

61. Di Biase L, Gaita F, Toso E, et al. Does periprocedural anticoagulation management of atrial fibrillation affect the prevalence of silent thromboembolic

lesion detected by diffusion cerebral magnetic resonance imaging in patients undergoing radiofrequency atrial fibrillation ablation with open irrigated catheters? results from a prospective multicenter study. Heart Rhythm 2014;11(5):791–8.

62. Lickfett L, Hackenbroch M, Lewalter T, et al. Cerebral diffusion-weighted magnetic resonance imaging: a tool to monitor the thrombogenicity of left atrial catheter ablation. J Cardiovasc Electrophysiol 2006;17(1):1–7.

63. Scaglione M, Blandino A, Raimondo C, et al. Impact of ablation catheter irrigation design on silent cerebral embolism after radiofrequency catheter ablation of atrial fibrillation: results from a pilot study. J Cardiovasc Electrophysiol 2012;23(8):801–5.

64. Wieczorek M, Lukat M, Hoeltgen R, et al. Investigation into causes of abnormal cerebral MRI findings following PVAC duty-cycled, phased RF ablation of atrial fibrillation. J Cardiovasc Electrophysiol 2013; 24(2):121–8.

Atrial Fibrillation and Stroke
Making Sense of Recent Observations on Anticoagulation

Marco Proietti, MD[a,b], Gregory Y.H. Lip, MD[a,c],*

KEYWORDS

- Oral anticoagulant therapy • Thromboembolic risk • Vitamin K antagonist
- Non-vitamin K antagonist oral anticoagulants • Clinical characteristics

KEY POINTS

- Atrial fibrillation (AF) is associated with an increased stoke and thromboembolic risk, as well as mortality.
- Use of oral anticoagulant (OAC) therapy significantly reduces stroke and all-cause mortality.
- OAC use for stroke prevention in AF means well-managed vitamin K antagonists (VKA) with a time in therapeutic range greater than 70% or a non-VKA OAC (NOACs).
- Different characteristics of the various NOACs allow us to fit the right NOAC drug to particular patient characteristics.

INTRODUCTION

Atrial fibrillation (AF) is the most prevalent heart rhythm disorder, with recent epidemiologic data showing that the worldwide prevalence of AF increased to 33.5 million patients in 2010.[1] In European countries, the estimated prevalence of AF is about 9 million patients, projected to increase to 17.9 million.[1] Among patients age older than 65 years there was an increase in AF diagnosis from 41 to 85 per 1000 patients from 1993 to 2007.[1] AF also accounts for a great proportion of deaths in the general population, because AF independently increases all-cause mortality and cardiovascular mortality risks both in men and women.[1]

Ischemic stroke is the most common cardiovascular adverse event in AF patients, with an overall 5-fold increase in stroke risk[2] and reported incidence of 19.5 per 1000 patient-years in 2002.[3]

Additionally, stroke severity and recurrence risks are higher with AF.[1]

Oral anticoagulation (OAC) therapy with the vitamin K antagonists (VKA; eg, warfarin), has been central for stroke prevention in the management AF.[4] More recently, several drugs with a direct inhibitory effects on thrombin and factor Xa have been developed.[5] These non-VKA oral anticoagulants (NOACs),[5] namely, dabigatran etexilate, rivaroxaban, apixaban, and edoxaban, are proved to be as effective as warfarin for the prevention of stroke and systemic thromboembolism events in patients with AF[6–10] (Table 1). Details of the clinical trials and study outcomes have been discussed in detail.[11,12]

The aim of this review is to provide an overview of current guidelines and summarize current evidence for the prevention of stroke in AF patients.

[a] Institute of Cardiovascular Sciences, University of Birmingham, City Hospital, Birmingham, UK; [b] Department of Internal Medicine and Medical Specialties, Sapienza-University of Rome, Rome, Italy; [c] Aalborg Thrombosis Research Unit, Department of Clinical Medicine, Aalborg University, Aalborg, Denmark
* Corresponding author. University of Birmingham, Institute of Cardiovascular Sciences, City Hospital, Birmingham B18 7QH, UK.
E-mail address: g.y.h.lip@bham.ac.uk

Cardiol Clin 34 (2016) 317–328
http://dx.doi.org/10.1016/j.ccl.2015.12.006
0733-8651/16/$ – see front matter © 2016 Elsevier Inc. All rights reserved.

Table 1
NOAC clinical trials in NVAF patients

Trial	Year	NOAC	Events Rate	Comparator	Events Rate	p for Noninferiority
RE-LY[6]	2009	Dabigatran 110 mg BD	1.53%/y	Adjusted dose warfarin (INR = 2–3)	1.69%/y	<.001
		Dabigatran 150 mg BD	1.11%/y			<.001
ROCKET AF[7]	2011	Rivaroxaban 20 mg OD	1.7% pts-yrs	Adjusted dose warfarin (INR = 2–3)	2.2% pts-yrs	<.001
ARISTOTLE[8]	2011	Apixaban 5 mg BD	1.27%/y	Adjusted dose warfarin (INR = 2–3)	1.60%/y	<.001
ENGAGE AF-TIMI 38[9]	2013	Edoxaban 30 mg OD	1.61% pts-yrs	Adjusted dose warfarin (INR = 2–3)	1.50% pts-yrs	.005
		Edoxaban 60 mg OD	1.18% pts-yrs			<.001

Abbreviations: ARISTOTLE, Apixaban for Reduction in Stroke and Other Thromboembolic Events in Atrial Fibrillation; BD, twice daily; ENGAGE AF-TIMI, Effective Anticoagulation with Factor Xa Next Generation in Atrial Fibrillation–Thrombolysis in Myocardial Infarction; INR, International Normalized Ratio; NOAC, non-vitamin K antagonist oral anticoagulant; NVAF, nonvalvular atrial fibrillation; OD, once daily; pts-yrs, patient-years; RE-LY, Risk of bleeding with 2 doses of dabigatran compared with warfarin in older and younger patients with atrial fibrillation: an analysis of the randomized evaluation of long-term anticoagulant therapy; ROCKET AF, Rivaroxaban Once Daily Oral Direct Factor Xa Inhibition Compared with Vitamin K Antagonism for Prevention of Stroke and Embolism Trial in Atrial Fibrillation.

A BRIEF OVERVIEW OF CURRENT CLINICAL GUIDELINES

For many years, the VKAs were the only available option to treat nonvalvular AF patients with a high risk of developing an ischemic stroke.[13,14] After the introduction of NOACs, the guidelines have evolved accordingly.

In 2006, the American College of Cardiology, American Heart Association, and European Society of Cardiology (ESC) guidelines recommended thromboembolic risk stratification for patients with AF according to $CHADS_2$ (congestive heart failure, hypertension, age, diabetes, prior stroke) risk score[15] (class IIa, level A). Consideration of less validated risk factors such as coronary artery disease, age 65 to 75, female sex, and thyroid disease was mentioned. Accordingly, patients with at least $CHADS_2$ equal to 1 should be treated with VKAs (class I, level A) Antithrombotic therapy with aspirin was still considered acceptable as an alternative to VKA (class I, level A) or to treat patients at lower risk (class I, level A).

In 2010, the ESC published new guidelines[16] on AF management that recommended a risk factor–based approach using the CHA_2DS_2-VASc (congestive heart failure, hypertension, age ≥75 years, diabetes mellitus, stroke/transient ischemic attack, vascular disease, age 65–74 years, sex category) score,[17] considering both 'major' and 'clinically relevant nonmajor' risk factors (class I, level A). Treatment with VKAs was recommended for patients with 1 major or 2 or more clinically relevant nonmajor risk factors (class I, level A). Patients with only 1 'clinically relevant nonmajor' risk factor were recommended to be treated either with VKAs (class I, level A) or aspirin (class I, level B), with a preference for OAC. Patients with low risk could still be recommended treatment with aspirin or no antithrombotic therapy, with a preference for the latter (class I, level B).

In 2012, the American College of Chest Physicians released the ninth version of their Antithrombotic Therapy and Prevention of Thrombosis Evidence-Based Clinical Practice Guidelines.[18] The $CHADS_2$ score was still recommended to stratify thromboembolic risk, but consideration of non-$CHADS_2$ stroke risk factors, such as age 65 to 74, vascular disease, and female sex, may favor OAC therapy. OAC therapy was recommended for with a $CHADS_2$ score of 1 rather than antiplatelet therapy (grade 2B). In patients with nonvalvular AF, the use of dabigatran 150 mg twice daily rather than adjusted-dose VKAs was recommended.[18]

In 2012, the ESC published a focused update of their previous guidelines. The CHA_2DS_2-VASc score was the risk score recommended for the stratification of thromboembolic risk in all patients with nonvalvular AF. Rather than the approach to identify high-risk patients, the guideline recommended a practice shift to identify initially patients with low risk (ie, CHA_2DS_2-VASc 0 in males, or 1 in females), and no antithrombotic treatment is recommended (class I, level B). OAC should be started in all patients with a CHA_2DS_2-VASc score of 2 or greater, choosing between VKA and NOACs, with the highest possible level of evidence (class I, level A).[19] In (male) patients with a CHA_2DS_2-VASc score of 1, OAC could be considered for OAC therapy after assessing the bleeding risk. NOACs were indicated as broadly preferable, in particular considering the better safety profile and the net clinical benefit demonstrated by these drugs, even if with a lower level of evidence (class IIa, level A).[19]

In 2014, three new guidelines were released. First, the American Heart Association/American College of Cardiology/Heart Rhythm Society published their new comprehensive guidelines for the management of patients with AF. The CHA_2DS_2-VASc score was the recommended tool for stratifying thromboembolic risk. In patients with a CHA_2DS_2-VASc score of 2 or greater, OAC therapy was recommended. Patients with a CHA_2DS_2-VASc of 1 could be treated with either OAC, antiplatelet therapy, or nothing.[2] When OAC is prescribed, both warfarin and the 3 NOACs (dabigatran, rivaroxaban, and apixaban) are all indicated, but reiterating an higher level of evidence for warfarin (class I, level A) than for the NOACs, which were indicated with a class I, level B level of evidence.[2]

The 2014 Focused Update of the Canadian Cardiovascular Society Guidelines for the Management of Atrial Fibrillation[20] was released in late 2014. These guidelines still used the $CHADS_2$ score for risk stratification. All patients with a $CHADS_2$ score of 1 or greater are recommended to be prescribed with OAC (strong recommendation, moderate quality evidence), but also recommended OAC for those age 65 to 74. The Canadian Cardiovascular Society recommended NOACs rather than warfarin for OAC therapy (strong recommendation, high quality evidence), adding also edoxaban to the treatment options available.[20]

In the UK, the National Institute for Health and Care Excellence published a new version of their clinical guidelines for AF management.[21] According to these guidelines, based on the CHA_2DS_2-VASc score, patients with a CHA_2DS_2-VASc of 2 or greater were recommended for OAC therapy, clearly stating that all possible options for anticoagulation should be discussed with the patient. In male patients with a score of 1 (ie, a single stroke risk factor), OAC should be considered. Apixaban, dabigatran, and rivaroxaban are indicated as possible alternatives to warfarin, and the choice should be largely discussed with patient, illustrating all potential risks and benefits of NOACs compared with warfarin.[21,22]

In summary, all major guidelines (**Table 2**) recommend use of NOACs as well as well-managed VKA for the prevention of stroke and thromboembolic risk in nonvalvular atrial fibrillation (NVAF) patients. Every guideline emphasizes that the available evidence is insufficient to establish whether one NOAC is more effective and safe than others in the treatment of NVAF patients. Prospective comparative studies, with all difficulties implied, would be needed to establish whether one NOAC could be more effective than another.

Table 2
Recommendations in current guidelines for NOAC use in NVAF patients

Guidelines	ESC/EHRA	ACCP	AHA/ACCF/HRS	CCS	NICE
Year	2012[19]	2012[18]	2014[2]	2014[20]	2014[21]
Recommendations	NOACs preferred to VKA	Dabigatran 150 mg BD preferred to VKA	Dabigatran, rivaroxaban and apixaban as well as VKA	All NOACs preferred to VKA	Dabigatran, rivaroxaban, apixaban as possible alternatives to VKA
Class of recommendation	IIa	II	I	Strong	NA
Level of evidence	A	B	B	High-Quality	NA

Abbreviations: ACCF, American College of Cardiology Foundation; ACCP, American College of Chest Physicians; AHA, American Heart Association; BD, twice daily; CCS, Canadian Cardiovascular Society; EHRA, European Heart Rhythm Society; ESC, European Society of Cardiology; HRS, Heart Rhythm Society; NA, not applicable; NICE, National Institute for Health and Care Excellence; NOACs, non-vitamin K antagonist oral anticoagulants; VKA, vitamin K antagonist.

MAKING SENSE OF RECENT OBSERVATIONS ON AN ORAL ANTICOAGULANT FOR STROKE PREVENTION

Stroke risk is influenced by several factors and concomitant conditions, which are to be taken into account when considering the risk–benefit balance when prescribing OAC therapy.

Gender

Women affected by AF are at greater risk for stroke compared with men,[23] despite adjustment for comorbidities and antithrombotic therapy.[24–27] When female sex is in association with another stroke risk factor, the risk is accentuated, so that female sex may be a stroke risk modifier, rather than a stroke risk factor per se. Hence, gender is incorporated in the stroke risk stratification scheme recommended by most guidelines, the CHA_2DS_2-VASc score.[17]

Recently, a sex-stratified analysis of OAC use in nonvalvular AF patients enrolled in the Global Anticoagulant Registry in the FIELD-Atrial Fibrillation (GARFIELD-AF) study[28] reported no difference in the overall use of OAC therapy for stroke prevention between men and women. Among truly low-risk patients (defined as a CHA_2DS_2-VASc score of 0 in men and 1 in women) who are not candidates for OAC therapy, the percentage of inappropriate treatment (ie, anticoagulant and/or antiplatelet drugs) was 75.6% in women and 71.7% in men. Among high-risk patients, there was no gender difference in anticoagulants use (66% female vs 65.7% male). The overall use of NOACs in the GARFIELD-AF cohort was similar among genders with factor Xa inhibitors used in around 6.5% and direct thrombin inhibitor use around 5.5%. When patients were stratified according to HAS-BLED (hypertension< abnormal renal or liver function, stroke, bleeding, labile International Normalized Ratio [INR], elderly [>65 years old], drugs or alcohol) score,[29] NOACs were prescribed to 8.7% men with low bleeding risk versus 9.9% women with low bleeding risk; in high-risk patients, the percentage decreased, at 3.3% in both groups.[28]

When compared with VKAs, the risk of intracranial hemorrhage (ICH) on NOACs is lower, ranging from 0.23% to 0.50%.[30] Data on gender difference in ICH incidence and clinical outcomes are controversial and not well-studied. ICH was reported to be influenced by interaction between gender, age, and other comorbidities.[31]

Conversely, data from the EURObservation Research Programme Pilot Survey on Atrial Fibrillation (EORP-AF) on gender differences showed that high risk (CHA_2DS_2-VASc $\geq$2), female AF patients were more likely to be treated with OAC compared with their male counterparts (P < .001).[32] Multivariable analysis for OAC use predictors according to genders demonstrated that if a low HAS-BLED score was a determinant for OAC use in both male and female patients (P = .0337 and P = .0284, respectively), whereas CHA_2DS_2-VASc score was a determinant only for female patients (P = .007).

Ethnicity

The impact of ethnicity on risk stroke among AF patients treated with OAC is a matter of debate.[33,34] Data coming from the Kaiser Permanente Southern California show no difference in stroke rates between white and nonwhite patients among patients hospitalized for AF.[35] An analysis on Medicare patients from 2010 to 2011 and age greater than 65 years old showed that even if risk of stroke seems to be higher for both Afro-Caribbean and Hispanic patients, this risk is significantly decreased when adjusted for previous comorbidities.[36]

Asian AF patients have a higher stroke risk compared with non-Asian patient.[34] A post hoc analysis on the NOACs trials cohorts comparing Asians and non-Asian patients found that, despite similar $CHADS_2$ score, Asian patients had higher stroke risk.[34] Thromboembolic risk management in Asians AF patients is hampered by the perception that Asians patients should be treated with a different INR range (1.6–2.6) than non-Asian patients,[37] which could contribute to the reported higher rate of stroke events.[34] Asians patients also report lower time in therapeutic range and higher percentages of time with INR less than 2 compared with non-Asians.[34] Recent evidence reported that Asians patients reported higher stroke rates even at younger age, with an ischemic stroke rate of 1.78% per year in patients aged 50 to 64 years old,[38] which is above the 0.9% treatment threshold for prescribing OAC treatment.[39]

Therefore, the incidence of thromboembolic stroke can vary across ethnic groups, but whether the therapeutic response with NOACs will lead to outcome differences across differing ethnic groups is less clear. The multinational clinical trials of NOACs give an opportunity to explore this issue because they enrolled AF patients worldwide under the same eligibility criteria, and all the risk factors for stroke were available. However, the randomized, controlled trials on NOACs predominantly enrolled Caucasian individuals (75%); Blacks represent less than 2.0% of trial participants, Asians 14%, and Hispanics approximately

4%.[33] Few studies of NOACs have reported outcomes as a function of race and ethnicity, but the available data suggest some racial differences in morbidity and demonstrate the potential efficacy and safety benefits of NOACs.[40]

In general, warfarin use may be more complex in Asians owing to higher risk for bleeding and higher stroke rate comparing with non-Asians. However, excess of bleeding compared with warfarin was not found in Asians when NOACs were used.[34] Superiority in both efficacy and safety has also been observed in the Asian subgroup analysis of the RE-LY (Risk of bleeding with 2 doses of dabigatran compared with warfarin in older and younger patients with atrial fibrillation: an analysis of the randomized evaluation of long-term anticoagulant therapy) trial[41] and the ARISTOTLE (Apixaban for Reduction in Stroke and Other Thromboembolic Events in Atrial Fibrillation) trial.[42] On the contrary, the impact on safety and efficacy in Asian patients were similar to warfarin in ROCKET AF (Rivaroxaban Once Daily Oral Direct Factor Xa Inhibition Compared with Vitamin K Antagonism for Prevention of Stroke and Embolism Trial in Atrial Fibrillation) trial, perhaps suggesting a different impact of rivaroxaban.[43]

Age

Several factors must be considered regarding the influence of age in the decision-making process. A higher likelihood of drug–drug interactions, more frequent adverse effects, and more comorbidities play a pivotal role in making decisions about anticoagulation. Currently, physicians' decisions seem to be guided more by their concerns over bleeding than an evaluation of the patient's risk for stroke in old patients.

Elderly patients are at risk of falls[44] and the risk of falling is perceived as a contraindication for to OAC therapy, frequently leading to therapy discontinuation.[45,46] However, prospective data did not find an association between risk of falls and major bleeding.[47] Thus, large proportions of elderly patients were not prescribed with VKAs owing to the perceived bleeding risk, in particular related to ICH.[48] Given the lower risk for ICH reported for NOACs,[49] these new drugs could be a relevant alternative for elderly patients,[48] with an appropriate reduction in dose when necessary.[50]

Given the strict relation between age and renal function, careful consideration of renal impairment is required. The impact of age on NOAC use for stroke prevention in AF patients is summarized in **Table 3**. In the RE-LY trial, for example, patient age significantly influenced the risk of bleeding, and a 'treatment-by-age interaction' was

Table 3		
NOAC efficacy according to age strata		
NOAC	**Age <75 NOACs vs Warfarin HR (95% CI)**	**Age ≥75 NOACs vs Warfarin HR (95% CI)**
Dabigatran 110 mg	0.93 (0.70–1.22)	0.88 (0.66–1.17)
Dabigatran 150 mg	0.63 (0.46–0.86)	0.67 (0.49–0.90)
Rivaroxaban	0.95 (0.76–1.19)	0.80 (0.63–1.02)
Apixaban	Age <65, 1.16 (0.77–1.73) Age 65–74, 0.72 (0.54–0.96)	0.71 (0.53–0.95)
Edoxaban 30 mg Edoxaban 60 mg	NA	NA

Abbreviations: HR, hazard ratio; NA, not applicable; NOACs, non-vitamin K antagonist oral anticoagulants.

observed.[51] Indeed, dabigatran 150 mg bd compared with adjusted-dose warfarin was associated with a lower risk of major bleeding in those aged less than 75 years, but there was a trend toward higher risk of major bleeding in those 75 years or older. This interaction was evident for extracranial hemorrhagic events but, importantly, both dabigatran doses were associated with a lower risk of ICH, irrespective of age. In contrast, dabigatran 110 mg bid compared with warfarin was associated with a lower risk of major bleeds in patients less than 75 years but a similar risk in those aged 75 years or older.

For rivaroxaban, age had no impact on the ROCKET AF trial findings[52] In the ARISTOTLE study, apixaban 2.5 mg was administered twice daily in patients with 2 or more of the following criteria: 80 years of age or older, body weight 60 kg or less, or a serum creatinine level of 1.5 mg/dL or greater (133 μmol/L)[8]; however, only approximately 400 trial participants received this lower dose. Advanced age was considered a risk factor for major bleeds with apixaban.

Chronic Kidney Disease

Chronic kidney disease (CKD) represents a major health problem, with an increasing prevalence among the general population.[53] Moreover, several cardiovascular risk factors such as hypertension, dyslipidemia, smoking, and a previous history of cardiovascular disease have been identified as factors influencing both CKD onset and progression.[54] The presence of CKD strongly influences the patients' clinical course, both in the general population[54,55] and in AF.[56,57]

The 2-way relationship between CKD and AF is well-known. CKD patient have a higher risk for developing AF[58,59]; conversely, a considerable proportion of CKD patients is reported in AF patients cohorts.[60,61] The coexistence of CKD in AF patients is a risk factor for increased thromboembolic events, but does not improve thromboembolic risk prediction tools.[57] Furthermore, renal impairment has been also identified as a possible risk factor for bleeding in AF patients[62] and renal impairment is part of the HAS-BLED bleeding score.[29]

CKD also influences heavily the prescription of OAC in AF patients. In fact, Bonde and colleagues[63] show how in a high-risk group of AF patients with CKD, the rate of VKA prescription was low, probably related to the fear of bleeding in these clinical setting, despite the effective role of VKA in reducing stroke.[63]

Since the introduction of NOACs into daily clinical practice, the evaluation of renal function has become a pivotal issue in the management of NVAF patients. All NOACs have a renal dependency for excretion, although to different degrees.[12,64] Of note, patients with severe renal impairment were excluded in all NOAC studies.[64] Currently, a dose reduction related to the presence of moderate to severe renal impairment is recommended by guidelines for dabigatran, rivaroxaban, and edoxaban; only VKA therapy is recommended in patients with end-stage renal disease.[2]

Beyond these considerations, a review of CKD patients treated with NOACs demonstrated that they are as effective and safe as VKA in this population.[65,66] Even if burdened by doubts on its risk–benefit balance,[64] monitoring of renal function is recommended.[2,12,64–66]

Coronary and Peripheral Vascular Disease

AF has always been associated with thromboembolism.[67] Emerging evidence reinforces the idea that AF should be also considered as predisposing to cardiovascular events, such as myocardial infarction and sudden death.

In patients with AF, the risk of myocardial infarction is increased, as well as that of stroke.[68–70] Similarly, peripheral arterial disease (PAD) is associated with AF, and the prevalence of both symptomatic and asymptomatic PAD is high in AF patients.[71,72] AF patients also seem to have a greater risk of developing PAD.[73,74] Importantly,

AF patients with PAD seems also to carry a much greater stroke risk.[73]

The presence of AF and coronary artery disease increases the difficulty of having to decide on the appropriate antithrombotic therapy regime, especially where the AF patient presents with acute coronary syndrome and/or undergoes percutaneous coronary intervention.[75,76] Decision making requires a consideration of 4 aspects, as follows: stroke prevention (needing anticoagulation), prevention of recurrent cardiac ischemia (requiring antiplatelet therapy), preventing stent thrombosis (requiring antiplatelet therapy), and serious bleeding (by combining OAC with antiplatelet therapy).

Current guidelines recommend the use of triple therapy in AF patients for the initial period, however limiting the use to periods as short as possible depending on the risk of bleeding.[18–20] After a period of triple therapy, dual therapy with OAC plus a single antiplatelet (preferably clopidogrel) then with stable vascular disease (arbitrarily defined as 1 year), OAC alone. If VKA is used a target INR of 2.0 to 2.5 is desirable, but a time in therapeutic range of greater than 70% is recommended. If a NOAC is used, the lower tested dose for stroke prevention in AF is recommended. In the joint European consensus document, the decision about triple therapy duration should be taken according to various clinical factors (ie, bleeding and thromboembolic risk, type of stent, type of procedure used).[76]

In patients with PAD, antiplatelet therapy with aspirin has been recommended.[77] Taking into account the contemporary presence of PAD in AF patients, this issue is scarcely addressed by clinical trials in the AF setting.[78] Recent data from the ROCKET AF trial provided some evidence that rivaroxaban seem to be as effective as warfarin in reducing ischemic stroke or systemic thromboembolism in AF patients with PAD, even if with a higher rate of bleeding episodes.[79] Only the ESC guidelines explicitly considering PAD as part of the vascular disease criterion of CHA_2DS_2-VASc,[19] recommend the use of VKA therapy in AF patients with PAD.[19]

Perioperative Management

If needed, NOACs can be interrupted before invasive or surgical procedures and restarted promptly afterward. This is related to the risk of bleeding if the drugs are not discontinued especially for major procedures such as thoracic, abdominal or major orthopedic surgery.[50]

Temporary discontinuation should be strictly tailored according to patient's characteristics (kidney function, age, history of bleeding complications, and concomitant medication) and surgical factors.[50]

Bridging procedures are not recommended in patients treated with OACs, but this remains commonly (and inappropriately) used.[80] Indeed, the "Bridging Anticoagulation in Patients who Require Temporary Interruption of Warfarin Therapy for an Elective Invasive Procedure or Surgery" (BRIDGE) trial[81] demonstrated that bridging procedures with low-molecular-weight heparin have no benefit in preventing thromboembolic events, but increased the risk of major bleeding events.[81] In general, NOACs can be interrupted between 24 and 48 hours before the scheduled procedure, according to the bleeding risk related to the procedure and patient's renal function. NOACs could be restarted after 6 to 12 hours for procedures where there is hemostasis.[50]

FROM TRIALS TO REAL-WORLD CLINICAL PRACTICE

A growing body of evidence is increasing on the safety and efficacy of NOACs in the real-life management of thromboembolic risk in AF.[82] For example, Larsen and colleagues[83] first reported safety data from the Danish nationwide cohort study, showing that both doses of dabigatran were associated with less bleeding and mortality, with no excess of myocardial infarction compared with warfarin. In a large US study (>134,000 patients) investigating a cohort of propensity matched new-starters prescribed with dabigatran (largely 150 mg, and some with 75 mg because the 110 mg dose is not licensed in the United States) and warfarin, dabigatran was as effective as warfarin (hazard ratio for stroke, 0.77; 95% CI, 0.54–1.09), with a better safety profile (hazard ratio for major hemorrhages, 0.75: 95% CI, 0.65–0.87),[84] thus confirming data coming from the RE-LY trial.[6]

Furthermore, 2 large retrospective studies from US cohorts demonstrated that dabigatran is even more effective than warfarin in reducing stroke occurrence and greatly safer in terms of ICH occurrence, even if burdened with higher rates of gastrointestinal bleeding episodes.[84,85] Similar data were also confirmed in other US real-world datasets,[86,87] as well as a large cohort of Canadian elderly patients.[88] The Dresden NOAC Registry reported a composite outcome of stroke/systemic thromboembolism event/transient ischemic attack rate of 2.93 per 100 patient-years with a major bleeding rate of 2.3 per 100 patient-years.[89]

A large observational, prospective, multinational study on rivaroxaban use in 6784 real-life patients, the XANTUS (Xarelto for Prevention of Stroke in Patients With Atrial Fibrillation) study,[90] reported that rivaroxaban was associated with lower rates of both major bleeding and thromboembolic adverse events. Conversely, an International Classification of Diseases-base propensity matched study comparing patients treated with rivaroxaban and warfarin, found no difference both in terms of major bleeding and thromboembolic events.[91] Other large registry studies are going on[92] would increase the data supporting use of NOACs in clinical daily practice.

SUMMARY

OAC is essential for stroke prevention in AF patients. OAC therapy is commonly given as well-controlled VKA and can reduce the risk of stroke in AF patients by almost two-thirds, as well as reducing all-cause mortality. NOACs have now provided therapeutic options with predictable pharmacodynamic and pharmacokinetic properties that are at least as efficacious as warfarin in the prevention of stroke and thromboembolism but are more convenient to use. Indeed, given their intrinsic characteristics NOACs address several limitations of VKA in day-to-day clinical practice.[93] Nonetheless, gaps in translation remain,[64] and further areas of research are evident.[94] An exciting advance is the availability of specific antidotes to NOACs, the first being idarucizumab, an antibody fragment developed to reverse the anticoagulant effects of dabigatran.[95,96]

There is increasing evidence demonstrating that for some specific patients' subgroups (ie, the elderly or those with renal impairment), the NOACs would be superior to warfarin in terms of efficacy and/or safety.[12] Our approach to OAC therapy in AF patients should be addressed in relation to an overall and comprehensive evaluation of patient's characteristics, aiming to a more and more tailored prescription, that is, fit the drug to the patient profile (and vice versa).[93] Decision making between a NOAC and VKA can be facilitated using the SAMe-TT_2R_2 score to guide clinicians,[97] because this simple score helps us identify patients who are likely to do well on VKA with a good time in therapeutic range (SAMe-TT_2R_2 score 0–2), or those less likely to do well on a VKA (with SAMe-TT_2R_2 score >2), where more regular review, education and follow-up monitoring is needed, or – better still – start a NOAC, instead of a trial of warfarin.[98–102] Finally, to obtain best adherence and persistence in treating AF patients in the longer term, patients' values and preferences should be taken into consideration.[103]

REFERENCES

1. Mozaffarian D, Benjamin EJ, Go AS, et al. Heart disease and stroke statistics–2015 update: a report from the American Heart Association. Circulation 2014;131(4):e29–322.

2. January CT, Wann LS, Alpert JS, et al. 2014 AHA/ACC/HRS Guideline for the management of patients with atrial fibrillation: a report of the American College of Cardiology/American Heart Association Task Force on Practice Guidelines and the Heart Rhythm Society. Circulation 2014;130(23): e199–267.

3. Lakshminarayan K, Solid CA, Collins AJ, et al. Atrial fibrillation and stroke in the general Medicare population: a 10-year perspective (1992 to 2002). Stroke 2006;37(8):1969–74.

4. De Caterina R, Husted S, Wallentin L, et al. Vitamin K antagonists in heart disease: current status and perspectives (Section III). Thromb Haemost 2013; 110(6):1087–107.

5. Husted S, de Caterina R, Andreotti F, et al. Non-vitamin K antagonist oral anticoagulants (NOACs): no longer new or novel. Thromb Haemost 2014; 111(5):781–2.

6. Connolly SJ, Ezekowitz MD, Yusuf S, et al. Dabigatran versus warfarin in patients with atrial fibrillation. N Engl J Med 2009;361(12):1139–51.

7. Patel MR, Mahaffey KW, Garg J, et al. Rivaroxaban versus warfarin in nonvalvular atrial fibrillation. N Engl J Med 2011;365(10):883–91.

8. Granger CB, Alexander JH, McMurray JJV, et al. Apixaban versus warfarin in patients with atrial fibrillation. N Engl J Med 2011;365(11):981–92.

9. Giugliano RP, Ruff CT, Braunwald E, et al. Edoxaban versus warfarin in patients with atrial fibrillation. N Engl J Med 2013;369(22):2093–104.

10. Providência R, Grove EL, Husted S, et al. A meta-analysis of phase III randomized controlled trials with novel oral anticoagulants in atrial fibrillation: comparisons between direct thrombin inhibitors vs. factor Xa inhibitors and different dosing regimens. Thromb Res 2014;134(6):1253–64.

11. Chan NC, Paikin JS, Hirsh J, et al. New oral anticoagulants for stroke prevention in atrial fibrillation: impact of study design, double counting and unexpected findings on interpretation of study results and conclusions. Thromb Haemost 2014;111(5): 798–807.

12. Schulman S. New oral anticoagulant agents - general features and outcomes in subsets of patients. Thromb Haemost 2014;111(4):575–82.

13. Fuster V, Rydén LE, Cannom DS, et al. ACC/AHA/ESC 2006 guidelines for the management of patients with atrial fibrillation: full text: a report of the American College of Cardiology/American Heart Association Task Force on practice guidelines and the European Society of Cardiology Committee for Practice Guidelines (Writing Committee to Revise the 2001 guidelines for the management of patients with atrial fibrillation) developed in collaboration with the European Heart Rhythm Association and the Heart Rhythm Society. Europace 2006;8(9):651–745.

14. Singer DE, Albers GW, Dalen JE, et al. Antithrombotic therapy in atrial fibrillation: American College of Chest Physicians Evidence-based clinical practice guidelines (8th Edition). Chest 2008; 133(6 Suppl):546S–92S.

15. Fuster V, Rydén LE, Cannom DS, et al. ACC/AHA/ESC 2006 guidelines for the management of patients with atrial fibrillation-executive summary: a report of the American College of Cardiology/American Heart Association Task Force on Practice Guidelines and the European Society of Cardiology Committee for Practice Guidelines (Writing Committee to Revise the 2001 Guidelines for the Management of Patients with Atrial Fibrillation). Eur Heart J 2006;27(16):1979–2030.

16. Camm AJ, Kirchhof P, Lip GYH, et al. Guidelines for the management of atrial fibrillation: the Task Force for the Management of Atrial Fibrillation of the European Society of Cardiology (ESC). Eur Heart J 2010;31(19):2369–429.

17. Lip GYH, Nieuwlaat R, Pisters R, et al. Refining clinical risk stratification for predicting stroke and thromboembolism in atrial fibrillation using a novel risk factor-based approach: the Euro Heart Survey on Atrial Fibrillation. Chest 2010;137(2): 263–72.

18. You JJ, Singer DE, Howard PA, et al. Antithrombotic therapy for atrial fibrillation: antithrombotic therapy and prevention of thrombosis, 9th ed: American College of Chest Physicians Evidence-Based Clinical Practice Guidelines. Chest 2012;141(2 Suppl): e531S–75S.

19. Camm AJ, Lip GYH, De Caterina R, et al. 2012 focused update of the ESC Guidelines for the management of atrial fibrillation: an update of the 2010 ESC Guidelines for the management of atrial fibrillation. Developed with the special contribution of the European Heart Rhythm Association. Eur Heart J 2012;33(21):2719–47.

20. Verma A, Cairns JA, Mitchell LB, et al. 2014 focused update of the Canadian Cardiovascular Society Guidelines for the management of atrial fibrillation. Can J Cardiol 2014;30(10):1114–30.

21. National Clinical Guideline Centre (UK). Atrial Fibrillation: The management of atrial fibrillation. London: National Institute for Health and Care Excellence (UK); 2014.

22. Senoo K, Lau YC, Lip GY. Updated NICE guideline: management of atrial fibrillation (2014). Expert Rev Cardiovasc Ther 2014;12(9):1037–40.

23. Bushnell C, McCullough LD, Awad IA, et al. Guidelines for the prevention of stroke in women: a statement for healthcare professionals from the American Heart Association/American Stroke Association. Stroke 2014;45(5):1545–88.

24. Pancholy SB, Sharma PS, Pancholy DS, et al. Meta-analysis of gender differences in residual stroke risk and major bleeding in patients with nonvalvular atrial fibrillation treated with oral anticoagulants. Am J Cardiol 2014;113(3):485–90.

25. Cove CL, Albert CM, Andreotti F, et al. Female sex as an independent risk factor for stroke in atrial fibrillation: possible mechanisms. Thromb Haemost 2014;111(3):385–91.

26. Avgil Tsadok M, Jackevicius CA, Rahme E, et al. Sex differences in stroke risk among older patients with recently diagnosed atrial fibrillation. JAMA 2012;307(18):1952–8.

27. Gomberg-Maitland M, Wenger NK, Feyzi J, et al. Anticoagulation in women with non-valvular atrial fibrillation in the stroke prevention using an oral thrombin inhibitor (SPORTIF) trials. Eur Heart J 2006;27(16):1947–53.

28. Lip GYH, Rushton-Smith SK, Goldhaber SZ, et al. Does sex affect anticoagulant use for stroke prevention in nonvalvular atrial fibrillation? The prospective global anticoagulant registry in the FIELD-Atrial Fibrillation. Circ Cardiovasc Qual Outcomes 2015;8(2 Suppl 1):S12–20.

29. Pisters R, Lane DA, Nieuwlaat R, et al. A novel user-friendly score (HAS-BLED) to assess 1-year risk of major bleeding in patients with atrial fibrillation: the Euro Heart Survey. Chest 2010;138(5): 1093–100.

30. Chao T-F, Liu C-J, Wang K-L, et al. Should atrial fibrillation patients with 1 additional risk factor of the CHA2DS2-VASc score (beyond sex) receive oral anticoagulation? J Am Coll Cardiol 2015; 65(7):635–42.

31. Gokhale S, Caplan LR, James ML. Sex differences in incidence, pathophysiology, and outcome of primary intracerebral hemorrhage. Stroke 2015;46:886–92.

32. Lip GYH, Laroche C, Boriani G, et al. Sex-related differences in presentation, treatment, and outcome of patients with atrial fibrillation in Europe: a report from the Euro Observational Research Programme Pilot survey on Atrial Fibrillation. Europace 2015;17(1):24–31.

33. Jackson LR, Peterson ED, Okeagu E, et al. Review of race/ethnicity in non vitamin K antagonist oral anticoagulants clinical trials. J Thromb Thrombolysis 2015;39(2):222–7.

34. Chiang C-E, Wang K-L, Lip GYH. Stroke prevention in atrial fibrillation: an Asian perspective. Thromb Haemost 2014;111(5):789–97.

35. Shen AY-J, Yao JF, Brar SS, et al. Racial/ethnic differences in ischemic stroke rates and the efficacy of warfarin among patients with atrial fibrillation. Stroke 2008;39(10):2736–43.

36. Kabra R, Cram P, Girotra S, et al. Effect of race on outcomes (stroke and death) in patients >65 years with atrial fibrillation. Am J Cardiol 2015;116(2): 230–5.

37. Ogawa S, Aonuma K, Tse H-F, et al. The APHRS's 2013 statement on antithrombotic therapy of patients with nonvalvular atrial fibrillation. J Arrhythmia 2013;29(3):190–200.

38. Chao T-F, Wang K-L, Liu C-J, et al. Age threshold for increased stroke risk among patients with atrial fibrillation. J Am Coll Cardiol 2015;66(12):1339–47.

39. Eckman MH, Wise RE, Speer B, et al. Integrating real-time clinical information to provide estimates of net clinical benefit of antithrombotic therapy for patients with atrial fibrillation. Circ Cardiovasc Qual Outcomes 2014;7(5):680–6.

40. Wang K-L, Lip GYH, Lin S-J, et al. Non-vitamin K antagonist oral anticoagulants for stroke prevention in Asian patients with nonvalvular atrial fibrillation: meta-analysis. Stroke 2015;46(9):2555–61.

41. Hori M, Connolly SJ, Zhu J, et al. Dabigatran versus warfarin: effects on ischemic and hemorrhagic strokes and bleeding in Asians and non-Asians with atrial fibrillation. Stroke 2013;44(7):1891–6.

42. Goto S, Zhu J, Liu L, et al. Efficacy and safety of apixaban compared with warfarin for stroke prevention in patients with atrial fibrillation from East Asia: a subanalysis of the Apixaban for Reduction in Stroke and Other Thromboembolic Events in Atrial Fibrillation (ARISTOTLE) Trial. Am Heart J 2014;168(3):303–9.

43. Wong KSL, Hu DY, Oomman A, et al. Rivaroxaban for stroke prevention in East Asian patients from the ROCKET AF trial. Stroke 2014;45(6):1739–47.

44. Chang JT. Interventions for the prevention of falls in older adults: systematic review and meta-analysis of randomised clinical trials. BMJ 2004; 328(7441):680.

45. O'Brien EC, Simon DN, Allen LA, et al. Reasons for warfarin discontinuation in the outcomes registry for better Informed treatment of atrial fibrillation (ORBIT-AF). Am Heart J 2014;168(4):487–94.

46. Bahri O, Roca F, Lechani T, et al. Underuse of oral anticoagulation for individuals with atrial fibrillation in a nursing home setting in France: comparisons of resident characteristics and physician attitude. J Am Geriatr Soc 2015;63(1):71–6.

47. Donzé J, Clair C, Hug B, et al. Risk of falls and major bleeds in patients on oral anticoagulation therapy. Am J Med 2012;125(8):773–8.

48. Turagam MK, Velagapudi P, Flaker GC. Stroke prevention in the elderly atrial fibrillation patient with comorbid conditions: focus on non-vitamin K antagonist oral anticoagulants. Clin Interv Aging 2015;10:1431–44.

49. Chatterjee S, Sardar P, Biondi-Zoccai G, et al. New oral anticoagulants and the risk of intracranial hemorrhage: traditional and Bayesian meta-analysis and mixed treatment comparison of randomized trials of new oral anticoagulants in atrial fibrillation. JAMA Neurol 2013;70(12):1486–90.

50. Heidbuchel H, Verhamme P, Alings M, et al. Updated European Heart Rhythm Association Practical Guide on the use of non-vitamin K antagonist anticoagulants in patients with non-valvular atrial fibrillation. Europace 2015;17(10):1467–507.

51. Eikelboom JW, Wallentin L, Connolly SJ, et al. Risk of bleeding with 2 doses of dabigatran compared with warfarin in older and younger patients with atrial fibrillation: an analysis of the randomized evaluation of long-term anticoagulant therapy (RE-LY) trial. Circulation 2011;123(21):2363–72.

52. Halperin JL, Hankey GJ, Wojdyla DM, et al. Efficacy and safety of rivaroxaban compared with warfarin among elderly patients with nonvalvular atrial fibrillation in the rivaroxaban once daily, oral, direct factor Xa inhibition compared with vitamin k antagonism for prevention of stroke and embolism. Circulation 2014;130(2):138–46.

53. Qaseem A, Hopkins RH, Sweet DE, et al. Screening, monitoring, and treatment of stage 1 to 3 chronic kidney disease: a clinical practice guideline from the American College of Physicians. Ann Intern Med 2013;159(12):835–47.

54. Levin A, Stevens PE. Summary of KDIGO 2012 CKD Guideline: behind the scenes, need for guidance, and a framework for moving forward. Kidney Int 2014;85:49–61.

55. Gansevoort RT, Correa-Rotter R, Hemmelgarn BR, et al. Chronic kidney disease and cardiovascular risk: epidemiology, mechanisms, and prevention. Lancet 2013;382(9889):339–52.

56. Bansal N, Fan D, Hsu C-Y, et al. Incident atrial fibrillation and risk of death in adults with chronic kidney disease. J Am Heart Assoc 2014;3(5):e001303.

57. Zeng W-T, Sun X-T, Tang K, et al. Risk of thromboembolic events in atrial fibrillation with chronic kidney disease. Stroke 2015;46(1):157–63.

58. Alonso A, Lopez FL, Matsushita K, et al. Chronic kidney disease is associated with the incidence of atrial fibrillation: the Atherosclerosis Risk in Communities (ARIC) study. Circulation 2011;123(25):2946–53.

59. Baber U, Howard VJ, Halperin JL, et al. Association of chronic kidney disease with atrial fibrillation among adults in the United States: REasons for Geographic and Racial Differences in Stroke (REGARDS) Study. Circ Arrhythm Electrophysiol 2011;4(1):26–32.

60. Hart RG, Eikelboom JW, Brimble KS, et al. Stroke prevention in atrial fibrillation patients with chronic kidney disease. Can J Cardiol 2013;29(7 Suppl):S71–8.

61. Roldán V, Marín F, Fernández H, et al. Renal impairment in a "real-life" cohort of anticoagulated patients with atrial fibrillation (implications for thromboembolism and bleeding). Am J Cardiol 2013;111(8):1159–64.

62. Jun M, James MT, Manns BJ, et al. The association between kidney function and major bleeding in older adults with atrial fibrillation starting warfarin treatment: population based observational study. BMJ 2015;350:h246.

63. Bonde AN, Lip GYHH, Kamper A-L, et al. Net clinical benefit of antithrombotic therapy in patients with atrial fibrillation and chronic kidney disease. J Am Coll Cardiol 2014;64(23):2471–82.

64. Hylek EM, Ko D, Cove CL. Gaps in translation from trials to practice: non-vitamin K antagonist oral anticoagulants (NOACs) for stroke prevention in atrial fibrillation. Thromb Haemost 2014;111(5):783–8.

65. Harel Z, Sood MM, Perl J. Comparison of novel oral anticoagulants versus vitamin K antagonists in patients with chronic kidney disease. Curr Opin Nephrol Hypertens 2015;24(2):183–92.

66. Harel Z, Sholzberg M, Shah PS, et al. Comparisons between novel oral anticoagulants and vitamin K antagonists in patients with CKD. J Am Soc Nephrol 2014;25(3):431–42.

67. Go AS, Hylek EM, Phillips KA, et al. Prevalence of diagnosed atrial fibrillation in adults: national implications for rhythm management and stroke prevention: the AnTicoagulation and Risk Factors in Atrial Fibrillation (ATRIA) Study. JAMA 2001;285(18):2370–5.

68. Soliman EZ, Safford MM, Muntner P, et al. Atrial fibrillation and the risk of myocardial infarction. JAMA Intern Med 2014;174(1):107–14.

69. Soliman EZ, Lopez F, O'Neal WT, et al. Atrial fibrillation and risk of ST-segment-elevation versus non-ST-segment-elevation myocardial infarction: the Atherosclerosis Risk in Communities (ARIC) Study. Circulation 2015;131(21):1843–50.

70. Chao T-F, Huang Y-C, Liu C-J, et al. Acute myocardial infarction in patients with atrial fibrillation with a CHA2DS2-VASc score of 0 or 1: a nationwide cohort study. Heart Rhythm 2014;11(11):1941–7.

71. Violi F, Daví G, Hiatt W, et al. Prevalence of peripheral artery disease by abnormal ankle-brachial index in atrial fibrillation: implications for risk and therapy. J Am Coll Cardiol 2013;62(23):2255–6.

72. Raparelli V, Proietti M, Napoleone L, et al. Asymptomatic peripheral artery disease and antiplatelet management. Vasa 2014;43(5):309–25.

73. O'Neal WT, Efird JT, Nazarian S, et al. Peripheral arterial disease and risk of atrial fibrillation and stroke: the multi-ethnic study of atherosclerosis. J Am Heart Assoc 2014;3(6):e001270.

74. Proietti M, Calvieri C, Malatino L, et al. Relationship between carotid intima-media thickness and non valvular atrial fibrillation type. Atherosclerosis 2015;238(2):350–5.

75. Rubboli A, Faxon DP, Juhani Airaksinen KE, et al. The optimal management of patients on oral anticoagulation undergoing coronary artery stenting. The 10th Anniversary Overview. Thromb Haemost 2014;112(6):1080–7.

76. Lip GYH, Windecker S, Huber K, et al. Management of antithrombotic therapy in atrial fibrillation patients presenting with acute coronary syndrome and/or undergoing percutaneous coronary or valve interventions: a joint consensus document of the European Society of Cardiology Working Group on. Eur Heart J 2014;35(45):3155–79.

77. Tendera M, Aboyans V, Bartelink M-L, et al. ESC Guidelines on the diagnosis and treatment of peripheral artery diseases: document covering atherosclerotic disease of extracranial carotid and vertebral, mesenteric, renal, upper and lower extremity arteries: the Task Force on the Diagnosis and Treatment of Peripheral Artery Diseases of the European Society of Cardiology (ESC). Eur Heart J 2011;32(22):2851–906.

78. Subherwal S, Patel MR, Chiswell K, et al. Clinical trials in peripheral vascular disease: pipeline and trial designs: an evaluation of the ClinicalTrials.gov database. Circulation 2014;130(20):1812–9.

79. Jones WS, Hellkamp AS, Halperin J, et al. Efficacy and safety of rivaroxaban compared with warfarin in patients with peripheral artery disease and non-valvular atrial fibrillation: insights from ROCKET AF. Eur Heart J 2014;35(4):242–9.

80. Beyer-Westendorf J, Gelbricht V, Förster K, et al. Peri-interventional management of novel oral anticoagulants in daily care: results from the prospective Dresden NOAC registry. Eur Heart J 2014; 35(28):1888–96.

81. Douketis JD, Spyropoulos AC, Kaatz S, et al. Perioperative bridging anticoagulation in patients with atrial fibrillation. N Engl J Med 2015;373(9): 823–33.

82. Eikelboom JW, Weitz JI. "Realworld" use of non-vitamin K antagonist oral anticoagulants (NOACs): Lessons from the Dresden NOAC Registry. Thromb Haemost 2015;113(6):1159–61.

83. Larsen TB, Rasmussen LH, Skjøth F, et al. Efficacy and safety of dabigatran etexilate and warfarin in "real-world" patients with atrial fibrillation: a prospective nationwide cohort study. J Am Coll Cardiol 2013;61(22):2264–73.

84. Graham DJ, Reichman ME, Wernecke M, et al. Cardiovascular, bleeding, and mortality risks in elderly Medicare patients treated with dabigatran or warfarin for nonvalvular atrial fibrillation. Circulation 2015;131(2):157–64.

85. Lauffenburger JC, Farley JF, Gehi AK, et al. Effectiveness and safety of dabigatran and warfarin in real-World US Patients with non-valvular atrial fibrillation: a retrospective cohort study. J Am Heart Assoc 2015;4(4). http://dx.doi.org/10.1161/JAHA. 115.001798.

86. Seeger JD, Bykov K, Bartels DB, et al. Safety and effectiveness of dabigatran and warfarin in routine care of patients with atrial fibrillation. Thromb Haemost 2015;114(6):1277–89.

87. Villines TC, Schnee J, Fraeman K, et al. A comparison of the safety and effectiveness of dabigatran and warfarin in non-valvular atrial fibrillation patients in a large healthcare system. Thromb Haemost 2015;114(6):1290–8.

88. Avgil-Tsadok M, Jackevicius CA, Essebag V, et al. Dabigatran use in elderly patients with atrial fibrillation. Thromb Haemost 2015;115(1):152–60.

89. Beyer-Westendorf J, Ebertz F, Förster K, et al. Effectiveness and safety of dabigatran therapy in daily-care patients with atrial fibrillation. Results from the Dresden NOAC Registry. Thromb Haemost 2015;113(6):1247–57.

90. Camm AJ, Amarenco P, Haas S, et al. XANTUS: a real-world, prospective, observational study of patients treated with rivaroxaban for stroke prevention in atrial fibrillation. Eur Heart J 2015. http://dx.doi.org/10.1093/eurheartj/ehv466.

91. Laliberté F, Cloutier M, Nelson WW, et al. Real-world comparative effectiveness and safety of rivaroxaban and warfarin in nonvalvular atrial fibrillation patients. Curr Med Res Opin 2014;30(7): 1317–25.

92. Huisman MV, Rothman KJ, Paquette M, et al. Antithrombotic treatment patterns in 10 871 patients with newly diagnosed non-valvular atrial fibrillation: the GLORIA-AF Registry Program, Phase II. Am J Med 2015;128(12):1306–13.e1.

93. Shields AM, Lip GYH. Choosing the right drug to fit the patient when selecting oral anticoagulation for stroke prevention in atrial fibrillation. J Intern Med 2015;278(1):1–18.

94. Hankey GJ. Unanswered questions and research priorities to optimise stroke prevention in atrial fibrillation with the new oral anticoagulants. Thromb Haemost 2014;111(5):808–16.

95. Pollack CVJ, Reilly PA, Eikelboom J, et al. Idarucizumab for dabigatran reversal. N Engl J Med 2015;373(6):511–20.

96. Pollack CVJ, Reilly PA, Bernstein R, et al. Design and rationale for RE-VERSE AD: a phase 3 study of idarucizumab, a specific reversal agent for dabigatran. Thromb Haemost 2015; 114(1):198–205.

97. Apostolakis S, Sullivan RM, Olshansky B, et al. Factors affecting quality of anticoagulation control among patients with atrial fibrillation on warfarin:

the SAMe-TT(2)R(2) score. Chest 2013;144(5): 1555–63.

98. Ruiz-Ortiz M, Bertomeu V, Cequier Á, et al. Validation of the SAMe-TT2R2 score in a nationwide population of nonvalvular atrial fibrillation patients on vitamin K antagonists. Thromb Haemost 2015; 114(4):695–701.

99. Roldan V, Cancio S, Galvez J, et al. The same-TT2R2 score Predicts poor anticoagulation control in AF patients: a prospective "Real-world" Inception cohort study. Am J Med 2015;128(11): 1237–43.

100. Lip GY, Haguenoer K, Saint-Etienne C, et al. Relationship of the SAMe-TT2R2 score to poor-quality anticoagulation, stroke, clinically relevant bleeding, and mortality in patients with atrial fibrillation. Chest 2014;146(3):719–26.

101. Proietti M, Lip GYH. Simple decision making between a vitamin K antagonist and non-vitamin K antagonist oral anticoagulant (NOACs): using the same-TT2R2 score. Eur Heart J: Cardiovasc Pharmacotherapy 2015;1:150–2.

102. Fauchier L, Poli D, Olshansky B. The SAMe-TT2R2 score and quality of anticoagulation in AF: can we predict which patient benefits from anticoagulation? Thromb Haemost 2015;114(4):657–9.

103. Lane DA, Aguinaga L, Blomström-Lundqvist C, et al. Cardiac tachyarrhythmias and patient values and preferences for their management: the European Heart Rhythm Association (EHRA) consensus document endorsed by the Heart Rhythm Society (HRS), Asia Pacific Heart Rhythm Society (APHRS), and Sociedad Latinoame. Europace 2015. http://dx.doi.org/10.1093/europace/euv233.

Left Atrial Appendage Closure for Stroke Prevention
Devices, Techniques, and Efficacy

Sandia Iskandar, MD[a], James Vacek, MD, MS[a],
Madhav Lavu, MD[a], Dhanunjaya Lakkireddy, MD, FHRS[b],*

KEYWORDS

- Left atrial appendage closure devices • Atrial fibrillation • Percutaneous approach
- Surgical approach • Endocardial left atrial appendage closure devices
- Hybrid endocardial-epicardial left atrial closure devices

KEY POINTS

- Left atrial appendage closure can be performed either surgically or percutaneously.
- Surgical approaches include direct suture, excision and suture, stapling, and clipping.
- Percutaneous approaches include endocardial, epicardial, and hybrid endocardial-epicardial techniques.
- Left atrial appendage anatomy is highly variable and complex; therefore, preprocedural imaging is crucial to determine device selection and sizing, which contribute to procedural success and reduction of complications.
- Currently the WATCHMAN is the only device that is approved for left atrial appendage closure in the United States. It has been shown to be noninferior to warfarin.

INTRODUCTION

Stroke prevention is the most important aspect of atrial fibrillation (AF) treatment. Currently, 2.3 million individuals in the United States suffer from AF, and this number is expected to double by 2050.[1–4] Fifteen percent of all strokes are due to cardioembolic stroke, and up to 30% of all strokes in patients older than 80 years of age are due to AF.[5,6] As the aging population increases, the use of oral anticoagulation becomes more challenging.

Warfarin has been the mainstay effective treatment for stroke prevention; however, it is only used in 50% of patients who qualify,[7] and only 50% to 60% of these subjects maintain INR (international normalized ratio) in the therapeutic range (2–3). Recently, the novel oral anticoagulants (NOACs) have gained popularity because of their ease of use and predictable anticoagulant effects, but the discontinuation rate over 20 months of follow-up is as high as 37%.[8–10] Concomitant coronary artery disease with AF also creates new

Disclosures: D. Lakkireddy has served on the Advisory Panelsl/Boards of Lifetech and SentreHEART.
Conflict of Interest: None of the authors have any conflict of interest.
[a] Division of Cardiovascular Diseases, Cardiovascular Research Institute, Mid America Cardiology, University of Kansas Medical Center and Hospital, 3901 Rainbow Blvd, Kansas City, KS 66196, USA; [b] Division of Cardiovascular Diseases, Center for Excellence in Atrial Fibrillation & EP Research, Bloch Heart Rhythm Center, Cardiovascular Research Institute, University of Kansas Medical Center, Mid America Cardiology, University of Kansas Hospitals, 3901 Rainbow Boulevard, Kansas City, KS 66196, USA
* Corresponding author.
E-mail address: dlakkireddy@kumc.edu

Cardiol Clin 34 (2016) 329–351
http://dx.doi.org/10.1016/j.ccl.2015.12.009
0733-8651/16/$ – see front matter © 2016 Elsevier Inc. All rights reserved.

cardiology.theclinics.com

challenges in those who are on dual antiplatelet therapy for coronary artery stents; the addition of oral anticoagulation will further increase the risk of bleeding.[11]

Because of these problems, new strategies are continuously being developed to improve outcomes for AF subjects, especially for those who are at high risk of stroke and bleeding. The left atrial appendage (LAA) is the major source of thrombus in most patients with AF. Blood stasis associated with AF, and the extensive trabeculation of the LAA contribute to thrombus formation.[12] According to an echocardiographic study, 90% of AF-related stroke originates from thrombi in the LAA.[13] This finding led to the development of LAA closure (LAAC) methods and devices to prevent thrombi from entering the systemic circulation.

LAAC can be performed by either surgical or percutaneous approaches. The percutaneous approach has been developed for the past 20 years and can be divided into endocardial, epicardial, and hybrid procedures. Although these devices have been used widely with high procedural success, especially in Europe and Asia, most of these devices have not been tested in randomized clinical trial, except for the WATCHMAN device.

This article begins with a review of the basic anatomy and physiology of the LAA; then the various LAAC approaches and devices currently available, procedural techniques, efficacy, and potential complications are discussed.

LEFT ATRIAL APPENDAGE ANATOMY AND PHYSIOLOGY

The LAA is an embryologic remnant of the left atrium (LA). It is an outpouching cavity arising from the LA located between the left superior pulmonary vein (LSPV) and the mitral valve annulus. The anatomy of the LAA is highly variable in terms of its volume, neck, depth, and number of lobes.[14,15] The orifice of the LAA cavity is oval and has a diameter of 10 to 40 mm. The inside of the LAA is formed by a smooth endocardial surface and pectinate muscles that form impressive ridges (trabeculations) and cavities where blood clots usually form (**Fig. 1**).[15]

Variation in Left Atrial Appendage Anatomy

The size, shape, and the number of lobes of LAAs vary markedly between individuals. Although most individuals have single lobe, some can

have up to 4 lobes.[16–18] The ostium is usually oval, but some individuals have ovaloid (18%), triangular (8%), or round (6%) ostium (**Fig. 2**).[18,19] The LAA ostium typically lies horizontal to the LSPV but can also be superior or inferior to it.[20] The LAA morphologic variations are classified by its complexity and microstructure. These variations include the chicken-wing, windsock, cactus, and cauliflower designations (**Fig. 3**), which are associated with differing stroke risks independent of the CHADS2 score.[21] One study has shown that the chicken-wing type has the least stroke risk in comparison to other types.[21] In addition, an increased number of lobes are associated with an increased risk of LAA thrombus.[22]

FUNCTION
Contractility

In the normal heart, the LAA plays a role in atrial contractility, and therefore, contributes to the "atrial kick"(the active phase of atrial filling); however, because of remodeling, which usually occurs in long-term persistent AF, the LAA eventually loses its contractility, and therefore, no longer contributes to ventricular filling.

Fluid Hemostasis

Like the right atrium (RA), the LAA plays a role in fluid hemostasis via secretion of atrial natriuretic peptide (ANP), although its secretion is lower in comparison to the RA.[15] ANP is excreted in response to volume overload and promotes diuresis, which reduces circulating blood volume. Interestingly, patients who undergo ligation of the LAA have a marked reduction in renin, aldosterone, and noradrenaline levels.[23]

LEFT ATRIAL APPENDAGE EXCLUSION: SURGICAL APPROACH

Surgical LAAC has long been performed along with mitral valve surgery[13]; however, this surgical approach is limited by a high incidence of incomplete closure with a potential for thrombus formation and future thromboembolic events and the potential of morbidity with prolongation of the open-heart procedure.[3,24] Up to a 36% incidence of incomplete exclusion with surgical ligation has been observed.[3,25] The flaccid state of the LAA on cardiac bypass and proximity of the circumflex artery to the base of the LAA have been proposed as causes of suboptimal success with surgical approaches. Excision of the LAA provides more consistent results and the 2014 American Heart Association/American College

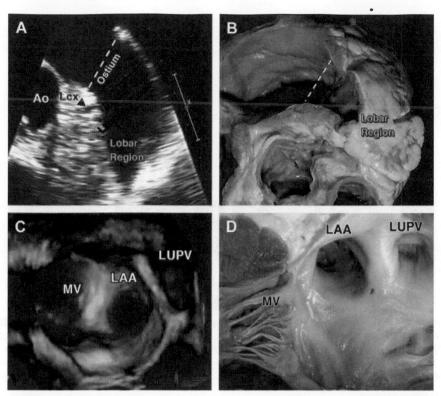

Fig. 1. Echo-anatomy of the LAA. The LAA regions are illustrated in a 2-dimensional (2D) TEE view (45°) (*A*) and in a corresponding anatomic image (*B*). The black arrowhead in (*A*) marks the left circumflex coronary artery (Lcx). The relationship between the LAA, the left upper pulmonary vein (LUPV), and the mitral valve (MV) is shown in a 3D TEE aspect (*C*) and in an anatomic picture (*D*). Ao, aorta. (*From* Wunderlich NC, Beigel R, Swaans MJ, et al. Percutaneous interventions for left atrial appendage exclusion: options, assessment, and imaging using 2D and 3D echocardiography. JACC Cardiovasc Imaging 2015;8(4):477; with permission.)

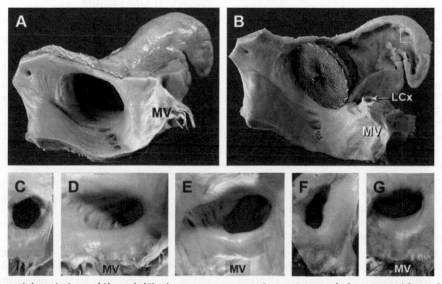

Fig. 2. LAA ostial variations. (*A*) and (*B*) show gross anatomic specimen of the LAA with a chicken-wing morphology without (*A*) and with (*B*) ACP. (*C–G*) Various ostial morphologies that can be seen associated with LAAs: round (*C*), elliptical (*D*), triangular (*E*), and ovaloid (*F*, water drop–like; *G*, footlike). (*From* Cabrera JA, Saremi F, Sánchez-Quintana D. Left atrial appendage: anatomy and imaging landmarks pertinent to percutaneous transcatheter occlusion. Heart 2014;100:1643; with permission.)

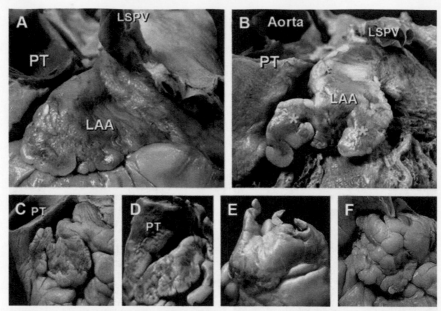

Fig. 3. LAA morphology and spatial relationships. (*A*) Relation to pulmonary trunk and LSPV. (*B*) Multilobed LAA (*asterisk*) in relation to LSPV, pulmonary trunk, and aorta. (*C–F*) Variations of LAA morphology: chicken-wing (*C*), windsock (*D*), cactus (*E*), and cauliflower (*F*) shapes. PT, pulmonary trunk. (*From* Cabrera JA, Saremi F, Sánchez-Quintana D. Left atrial appendage: anatomy and imaging landmarks pertinent to percutaneous transcatheter occlusion. Heart 2014;100:1641; with permission.)

of Cardiology/Heart Rhythm Society guidelines for the management of AF provide a class IIB/level of evidence C recommendation for surgical excision of the LAA in patients undergoing cardiac surgery.[24] In the meantime, the LAAOS (Left Atrial Appendage Occlusion Study) III, the largest study to explore the efficacy of LAA exclusion for stroke patients in patients undergoing on - pump surgical cardiac procedures, is in progress.[26]

Endocardial Suture Closure

This technique is typically performed concomitant to other cardiac procedures. Today, mitral valve surgery can be done with a minimally invasive technique via video-assisted minithoracotomy. During this procedure, once on bypass, after valve repair and left atrial ablation, the LAA is sutured directly using a 4-0 running suture in 2 layers. It is crucial to make deep bites to ensure tight tissue approximation for durable occlusion.[15] Transesophageal echocardiogram (TEE) must be performed to ensure LA closure because even a slight remaining perfusion of LAA can pose lethal problems.[27] Initial observational studies of surgical LAAC at the time of mitral valve surgery have demonstrated uneven results with incomplete closure rates of 36% as demonstrated by TEE.[25]

Stapler Occlusion

Abdominal staplers (autosuture) can be used to excise the LAA in both open and minimally invasive procedures (total thoracoscopic procedure).

Epicardial Clip Closure

Atriclip (AtriCure Inc, West Chester, OH, USA) is approved by the US Food and Drug Administration (FDA) for surgical exclusion of the LAA. The Atriclip can be placed either via a minimally invasive approach using a long handle or via an open approach using a short handle. Robot-assisted clip deployment is under development. The Atriclip is composed of 2 titanium rods with nitinol hinges covered by braided polyester lining. The Atriclip comes in 4 sizes (from 35 mm to 50 mm). The nitinol hinges apply constant force, leading to LAA occlusion. Short-term stability is obtained by the force of the clip, whereas long-term durability is obtained by tissue ingrowth (**Fig. 4**).[15]

Procedure

During this procedure, the LAA is gently grasped with a forceps and manipulated into the open jaws of the clip. Once the clip is in place, the jaws can be closed, and closure can be assessed on TEE. If the clip position is not satisfactory, the clip can be replaced by opening the jaw and repositioning it. In the first-generation LAA clip, secondary

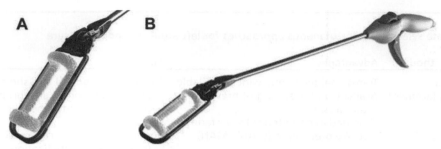

Fig. 4. (*A*) AtriClip deployment loop. It is used to occlude the left atrial appendage from its base to prevent blood from entering the pouch. (*B*) AtriClip deployment system. The full system consists of deployment loop, shaft, handle, activation lever, and deployment tab. (*Courtesy of* Atricure, Mason, OH; with permission.)

positioning is not possible due to possible tissue injury by the metal jaw; however, with the Atriclip, multiple repositioning is possible to achieve perfect closure. Once the final position has been reached, the sutures are cut and the clip is fixed in place, after which the single-use deployment tool is removed.[15]

Efficacy

The initial series demonstrated a successful closure in 60 of 61 patients at 90 days follow-up with imaging either by computed tomography (CT) or TEE. A larger multicenter trial is currently underway to evaluate the safety of the AtriClip in patients thought to be too high risk for anticoagulation.[28]

PERCUTANEOUS APPROACH

This section begins with the basic concept of a percutaneous LAAC procedure followed by a discussion of different endocardial LAA occlusion devices, which include the WATCHMAN, Amplatzer Cardiac Plug (ACP), and other endocardial closure devices not currently available in the United States. All of them are made of a nitinol cage, polytetrafluoroethylene (PTFE) or polyethylene terephthalate (PET) that is positioned on the endocardial surface of the LAA ostium, preventing a thrombus originating in the LAA from entering the systemic circulation. Next, the hybrid endocardial-epicardial approach (LARIAT) and the epicardial approach (Aegis; Aegis Medical, Vancouver, Canada) are discussed. The WATCHMAN is the only device that has FDA approval as an alternative to warfarin for stroke prevention (**Table 1**).

Basic Concept of Percutaneous Left Atrial Appendage Closure Procedure

The procedure is typically performed in the hybrid operating room to allow rapid response to potential complications necessitating surgery. For all devices, imaging is extremely important in guiding the physician to select the ideal patients and evaluate anatomy, and in deciding the type of device that best fits the patient's anatomy.

Preprocedural Imaging

Before starting the procedure, TEE must be performed. TEE is the gold standard for thrombus detection within the LAA. Understanding the anatomy of the LAA is critical for procedural safety. To facilitate successful implantation, width and depth of the LAA as well as number and position of different lobes are important to know. Studies have shown that the width of the LAA orifice can vary from 15 to 35 mm and length from 20 to 45 mm[17] with various anatomic configurations, as discussed above.[29]

Transseptal Access

Generally, the process is similar for all endocardial and hybrid approaches; however, orientation of TEE and fluoroscopy are slightly different to optimally visualize the device anatomy in the LAA. Transseptal puncture is guided by TEE and fluoroscopy with pressure control. To avoid undersizing the LAA, the mean filling pressure of the LA should be in the high normal range (>10 mm Hg). The puncture typically should be at the posterior-inferior atrial septum. The more anterior or inferior the LAA is located, the higher the transseptal puncture should be performed, whereas the more cranial the LAA, the more inferior the puncture should be. Anterior puncture going through a patent foramen ovale (PFO) should be avoided due to difficulty to turn the guide catheter adequately to the anterior located axis of the LAA. Heparin is administered before or immediately after transseptal puncture to achieve an activated clotting time of 200 to 300 seconds (**Fig. 5**).[29]

WATCHMAN (BOSTON SCIENTIFIC, NATICK, MA, USA)

The WATCHMAN device is a self-expanding nitinol structure with fixation barbs and a membrane made of PET covering the nitinol structure (**Fig. 6**). It is

Table 1
Appropriate selection of percutaneous approaches for left atrial appendage closure

Device/Method	Advantages	Limitations
Transseptal device placement	Transseptal technique widely available Available in the setting of previous cardiac surgery Validated as noninferior to warfarin for stroke prevention (WATCHMAN)	Need for procedural and short-term anticoagulation or antithrombotic regimen until endothelialization occurs Foreign body left in central circulation (small risk of embolization, erosion, dislodgement) Device must be sized to match LAA Previous atrial septal defect closure may preclude transseptal delivery
Epicardial	No foreign body left behind No need for procedural anticoagulation because no contact with central circulation and no transseptal puncture (which exposes blood to tissue factor) Adjustable size loop to accommodate variable LAA shape/morphology without need for sizing Pericardial control facilitates management of effusion should one develop	Human experience not yet reported Previous cardiac surgery limits pericardial access and maneuverability Epicardial access techniques less widely available than transseptal puncture
Hybrid	No foreign body left behind Pericardial control facilitates management of effusion should one develop	Need for both transseptal and epicardial access with risks of both, and delivery failure if cannot achieve both Superiorly directed LAA, multiple lobes, and pectus excavatum may preclude use

From Friedman PA, Holmes DR. Non-surgical left atrial appendage closure for stroke prevention in atrial fibrillation. J Cardiovasc Electrophysiol 2011;22(10):1190; with permission.

implanted via transseptal puncture and occludes the LAA at the level of LAA ostium.[30]

Device

WATCHMAN devices come in 5 sizes and are delivered through dedicated 14-French sheaths with 12-French inner diameter and 75-cm working length. There are 3 dedicated access sheaths: double curve, single curve, and anterior curve. There are 3 radiopaque marker bands (33, 27, and 21 mm) on the distal sheath, which should be aligned to the LAA ostium according to the selected device. The standard is the double-curve sheath (>90% cases), which allows easier access into superiorly directed distal lobes **(Fig. 7)**.[31]

Data

The WATCHMAN device has been evaluated in 2 randomized clinical trials: the PROTECT-AF (WATCHMAN Left Atrial Appendage System for

Embolic Protection in Patients with Atrial Fibrillation) and PREVAIL (Prospective Randomized Evaluation of the WATCHMAN Left Atrial Appendage Closure Device in Patients with Atrial Fibrillation vs long-term Warfarin therapy) trial. The first study showed noninferiority of the WATCHMAN device to warfarin; however, there were 12% procedural complications, including pericardial effusion requiring drainage, embolic stroke, device migration, and device sepsis. The second study was designed to confirm the results of the PROTECT-AF study and validated the safety of the implant procedure. This study met early safety endpoints with more than 50% reduction in complication rates, although noninferiority was not achieved.[32]

Anticoagulation

The PROTECT-AF and PREVAIL both used anticoagulation therapy for 45 days. The ASAP study (Aspirin Plavix Feasibility Study), which used aspirin and Plavix for 6 months instead of oral

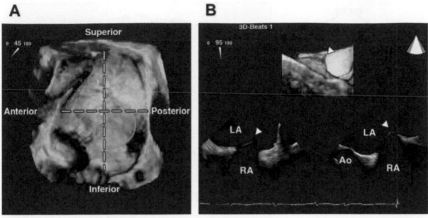

Fig. 5. Transseptal puncture anatomy. (*A*) Viewed from a position in the middle of the interatrial septum (*crossing of the white dashed lines*), the preferred TS puncture site is located usually slightly posterior and inferior as demonstrated in (*A*) (*green area*) in a left atrial 3D TEE aspect. (*B*) Simultaneous 3D TEE (*top*) and X-plane imaging (*bottom*) demonstrate the tentlike indentation of the interatrial septum (*white arrowheads*). This imaging approach facilitates the determination of the preferred puncture site. Factors that can impact the TS puncture, such as the size and location of the fossa ovalis, the thickness of the interatrial septum, the presence of a persistent foramen ovale, an atrial septum defect, an atrial septum aneurysm, or an eustachian valve, should be assessed in addition (not shown). TS, transseptal. (*From* Wunderlich NC, Beigel R, Swaans MJ, et al. Percutaneous interventions for left atrial appendage exclusion: options, assessment, and imaging using 2D and 3D echocardiography. JACC Cardiovasc Imaging 2015;8(4):481; with permission.)

anticoagulants (OAC) for 45 days, revealed that the ischemic stroke rate was less than expected based on the CHADS2 and CHA2DS2-Vasc score (7.3% per year),[33,34] which supports the approach that the WATCHMAN may be safely used without oral anticoagulation.[34]

Procedure
Preprocedural imaging and transseptal puncture as previously described
Implantation of the WATCHMAN device The WATCHMAN device should be advanced in the sheath until the marker of the device catheter matches the most distal marker on the access sheath. The next step is to pull back the access sheath over the device until the device catheter and access sheath are connected (**Fig. 8**). At this point, the device should remain in position because forward pushing of the device increases the risk of LAA injury. The device is deployed by retracting the sheath and the device catheter simultaneously while the device is held in place (**Fig. 9**). Once the device is deployed within the LAA, correct positioning of the WATCHMAN device at the LAA ostium must be demonstrated by echocardiography and angiography.

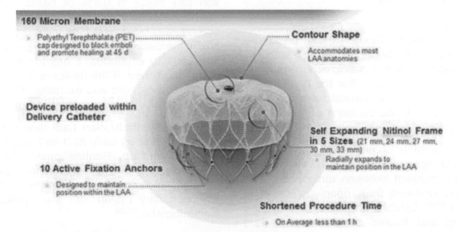

Fig. 6. WATCHMAN device. (Image provided courtesy of Boston Scientific. © 2016 Boston Scientific Corporation or its affiliates. All rights reserved.)

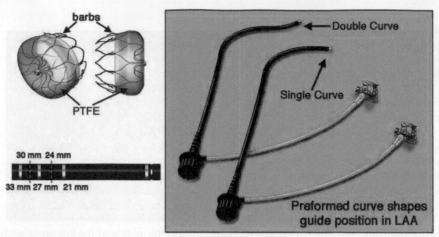

Fig. 7. WATCHMAN and 14-French access sheaths (*double and single curve*). There are 3 radiopaque marker bands (33, 27, and 21 mm) on the distal sheath, which should be aligned to the LAA "ostium" according to the selected device. (*From* Saw J, Lempereur M. Percutaneous left atrial appendage closure: procedural techniques and outcomes. JACC Cardiovasc Interv 2014;7(11):1208; with permission.)

Device release To avoid device embolization, there are 4 release criteria that should be evaluated[29]: (1) Position: the plane of maximum diameter of the device should be at or just distal to the orifice of the LAA; (2) Anchor: to confirm proper anchoring, withdraw the access sheath 1 to 2 cm from the face of the device and, after injecting small contrast, gently retract and push the deployment knob to see the combined movement of the device and the LAA tissue; (3) Size: confirm the correct device by measuring the plane of the maximum diameter using TEE in the 4 standard views: 0°, 45°, 90°, and 135° and ensure the thread is visible. The device size should be 80% to 92% of the nominal diameter; (4) Seal: confirm with color Doppler to ensure that all lobes are distal to the device and are sealed. The device should be repositioned if there is less than a 3-mm gap between the LAA wall and the device.[29]

Complications

Pericardial effusion Although most pericardial effusions occur early, subacute and late effusions are also possible. A transthoracic echocardiogram (TTE) performed 48 hours after the procedure is recommended to rule out pericardial effusion and to confirm stable device positioning.[29]

Air embolism Air emboli may enter LA due to accidental injection of air, due to trapped air despite flushing the catheter, or by air intrusion driven by a gradient between atmospheric and intracardiac pressure from deep inspiration of the patient.[29,35] Cerebral air embolism is usually self-limiting and treated supportively. In rare cases, air embolism to the coronary circulation can occur and most commonly affects the right

coronary artery due to the anterior position of the ostium. This air embolism often resolves on its own; however, if the patients become hemodynamically unstable, aspiration of the air or rigorous contrast dye injection into coronary artery may be helpful.[29]

Thrombus formation during device implantation LAA thrombus can form during device implantation. In this case, if the delivery sheath is in a satisfactory position, implantation is still possible because the device can catch the thrombus in the LAA. If the sheath has not been maneuvered into the LAA, aspiration of the blood and thrombus through the side port should be attempted, followed by removal of the sheath.[29]

Early device embolization Early device embolization can occur in 0.2% of cases. Ideally, the WATCHMAN device must be fully expanded and compressed by at least 10% to 30% of its original size. If the device is too deep in the LAA and therefore not fully expanded, it has to be recaptured and repositioned. If the device is too proximal, a complete recapture and exchange of the device are necessary.[29]

Late device embolization Late device embolization can occur as early as 1 to 2 days after device implantation. Routine postprocedure TTE to exclude new or expanding pericardial effusion and screen for device embolization is necessary even if the patients are asymptomatic.[29,36]

Leak A leak can be seen after WATCHMAN implantation. A leak that is less than 5 mm is not

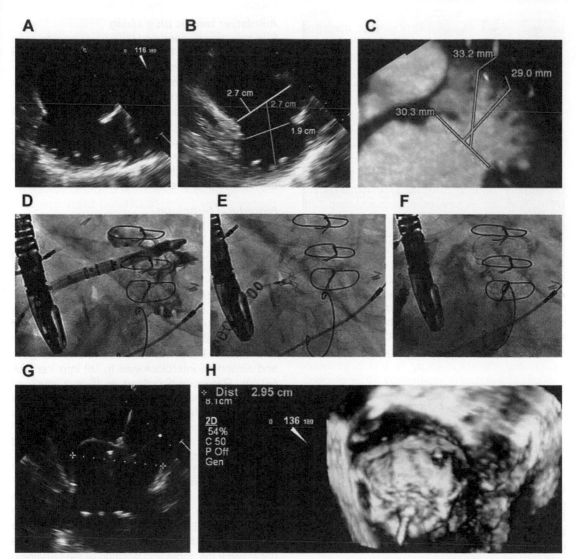

Fig. 8. Example of WATCHMAN implantation. (*A*) TEE image at 116° showing LAA with trabeculations in a fan shape. (*B*) TEE at 97° with measurements. (*C*) Preprocedure cardiac CT angiography showing complex LAA with protruding proximal pectinate ridge, widest dimension of 30.3 mm, and usable depth of 29 to 33.2 mm. (*D*) The 14-French double-curve sheath advanced deep over the marker pigtail. (*E*) The 33-mm WATCHMAN deployed. (*F*) Device released after ensuring PASS (position, anchor, size, seal) criteria were achieved. (*G*) TEE widest shoulder measurement of 29.5 mm representing 10.6% compression and no significant residual leak. (*H*) 3D TEE showing acceptable slight protrusion of the shoulder of the WATCHMAN into the LA, with PET fabric covering the device. (*From* Saw J, Lempereur M. Percutaneous left atrial appendage closure: procedural techniques and outcomes. JACC Cardiovasc Interv 2014;7(11):1210; with permission.)

likely to cause stroke in comparison to those with no leak (PROTECT-AF trial).[37] If the TEE in 45 days shows a greater than 5-mm leak, warfarin must be continued, and follow-up TEE in another 3 months should be performed. If the leak remains greater than 5 mm, the implant is considered a failure and the patient needs to remain on OAC. However, if the leak decreases to less than 5 mm, therapy can be changed to aspirin and clopidogrel.[29]

AMPLATZER CARDIAC PLUG (ST. JUDE MEDICAL, ST. PAUL, MN, USA)

The Amplatzer cardiac plug is a self-expandable nitinol platform with a distal lobe and proximal disc connected with a central waist (**Fig. 10**). It is a modification of the Amplatzer septal occluder originally designed for atrial septal defect closure.[30] The ACP has been marketed for use with antiplatelet therapy only, albeit with little

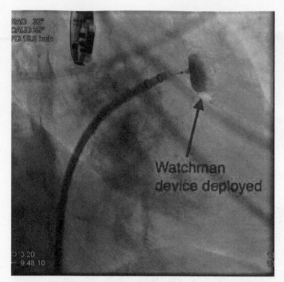

Fig. 9. WATCHMAN device deployment. Contrast injection filling the LAA before WATCHMAN device delivery. (*From* Lin AC, Knight BP. Left atrial appendage closure. Prog Cardiovasc Dis 2015;58(2):198; with permission.)

supportive evidence. Many implantations in Europe have been performed without oral anticoagulation.[38]

Amulet (St. Jude Medical)

The Amulet is a second-generation ACP with a wider lobe, longer waist, recessed proximal end screw, and more stabilizing wires. These features improve device stability and theoretically may reduce thrombus formation on the atrial side of the device. The Amulet also comes in 8 sizes and can accommodate larger LAAs (up to 32 mm).[39]

Preprocedural imaging

As with any other LAAC device, preprocedural imaging is extremely important for sizing and device selections. TEE is useful to evaluate LAA anatomy for accurate measurements. Cardiac CT angiography may be a noninvasive alternative to TEE, because it is good for ruling out LAA thrombi, especially when delayed imaging is acquired.[31,40]

Size selection

Appropriate size selection is crucial for the success of the implantation. There are basic principles for optimal sizing. First, the left atrial disc of the ACP has to fit within the LAA and serve as an anchor to prevent embolization of the device from the LAA. Second, the right atrial disc has to sit within or near the ostium of the LAA.[41]

Amplatzer cardiac plug sizing

Size selection depends on the widest landing zone on fluoroscopy or TEE. The measurement of the landing zone and orifice is important at both short- and long-axis views on TEE. The landing zone is measured at 10 mm within the orifice perpendicular to the neck axis. The LAA depth is measured from the orifice to the back wall along the neck axis.[31] It is recommended to upsize the device by 3 to 5 mm from the widest measured landing zone. The oversizing improves stability of the device and proper anchoring of the lobe.[31]

Procedural technique

After the transseptal puncture (previously described), a 5-French pigtail catheter is advanced into the LAA, and fluoroscopy is performed in multiple projections (**Fig. 11**).

Access sheath advancement

A 260-cm J-tipped stiff 0.035-inch wire is advanced into the LSPV for sheath access, and the appropriate-sized access sheath is advanced to the LSPV. The sheath is then withdrawn slightly and turned counterclockwise to fall into the LAA ostium. Gafoor and colleagues,[42] in a study of 10 patients receiving ACP, demonstrated the "shaping the sheath" technique to better access the LAA and ensure stable positioning. This technique led to decreased fluoroscopic time and device recaptures.

Device deployment and release

The ACP lobe is deployed by withdrawing the delivery sheath, and after confirming the optimal position by TEE and fluoroscopy, the remainder of the lobe is deployed. Finally, the disc can be deployed if the angle and position of the remaining lobe at the landing zone are optimal. If the device positioning is inadequate and the platinum marker enters beyond the radiopaque band, the device needs to be entirely removed and the sheath replaced. If there is uncertainty about device stability, a gentle pull of the disc may be performed, but vigorous wiggle testing is contraindicated. Once a satisfactory position is achieved, the device is released with counterclockwise rotation of the delivery cable within the LAA ostium.[31]

Data

A pilot study of 52 patients with an absolute contraindication to warfarin demonstrated a 98.1% ACP implant success rate.[43] Following implantation, patients were maintained on either single- or dual-antiplatelet therapy at the investigator's discretion.[43] Nonrandomized trials with the first-generation LAA plug demonstrated feasibility, effectiveness in reducing thromboembolic

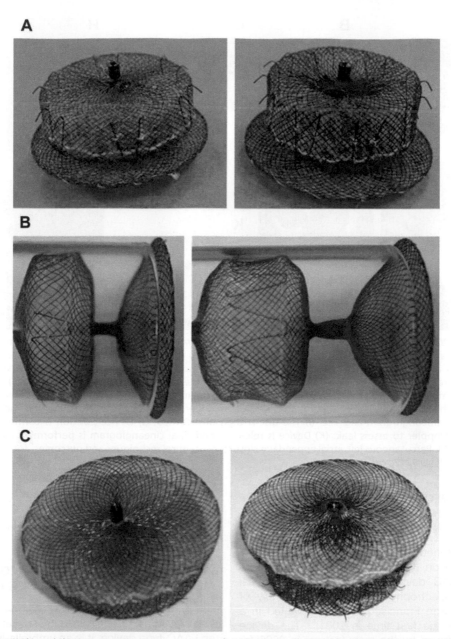

Fig. 10. ACP (*left*) and the newer AMPLATZER Amulet Left Atrial Appendage Occluder (*right*) indicating the greater distal lobe length of the Amulet (ie, thickness reaching into LAA) (*A*), waist (*B*), and inversion of the disc and screw (*C*). (*From* Freixa X, Chan JL, Tzikas A, et al. The Amplatzer Cardiac Plug 2 for left atrial appendage occlusion: novel features and first-in-man experience. EuroIntervention 2013;8(9):1095; with permission from Europa Digital & Publishing.)

cerebral events, and a high rate of technical success.[44–48]

Complications

Device embolization

Delayed device embolization can occur despite proper positioning at implant. Aminian and colleagues[49] reported a case of device entrapment at the superior mitral apparatus causing severe mitral regurgitation due to chordae rupture.

Perforation

Because of the close proximity between the pulmonary artery and LAA, perforation of the artery, tamponade, and death after appendage closure using cardiac plug device have been reported.[50]

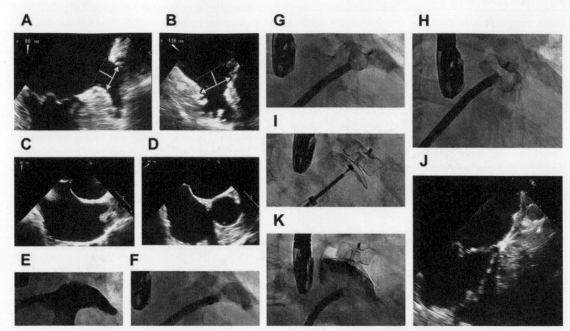

Fig. 11. ACP/Amulet implantation. (*A*) Short- and (*B*) long-axis baseline TEE views showing measurements of the orifice (*red arrows*) and the landing zone (*yellow arrows*) at 10 mm (*yellow line*) within the orifice. Transseptal puncture in an inferior position on bicaval TEE view (*C*) and posterior position on short-axis TEE view (*D*). (*E*) Cineangiogram with marker pigtail in the LAA, and same measurements taken as with TEE. (*F*) TorqueVue 45 × 45 sheath is advanced with the distal tip aligned with the landing zone. (*G*) First step of ACP/Amulet deployment is unsheathing to a ball configuration. (*H*) The remainder of the lobe is unsheathed, and the position is checked on cineangiogram and TEE. (*I*) The disc is then unsheathed. (*J*) Device position is confirmed on TEE with color Doppler to assess leak. (*K*) Device is released, and final cineangiogram is performed. (*From* Saw J, Lempereur M. Percutaneous left atrial appendage closure: procedural techniques and outcomes. JACC Cardiovasc Interv 2014;7(11):1212; with permission.)

PERCUTANEOUS LEFT ATRIAL APPENDAGE TRANSCATHETER OCCLUSION (APPRIVA MEDICAL INC, SUNNYVALE, CA, USA)

The percutaneous left atrial appendage transcatheter occlusion (PLAATO) was the first percutaneous LAAC device developed by Dr Michael Lesh, an electrophysiologist from University of California San Francisco. It was implanted in a human for the first time in 2001.[51] The device was withdrawn by the manufacturer in 2006 for commercial reasons.

Device

PLAATO is a self-expanding nitinol cage measuring 15 to 32 mm in diameter with 3 anchors on each strut for stabilization. It is covered with PTFE membrane to occlude blood flow into the LAA (**Fig. 12**).[31]

Data

PLAATO's safety and feasibility were demonstrated in several nonrandomized studies.[29] In the PLAATO feasibility study of 64 patients with AF and contraindication to OAC, the stroke risk was lower in the

PLAATO group (3.8% vs 6.6% in 5-year follow-up).[52] Complications such as device embolization and cardiac tamponade had been reported.[52–54]

WAVECREST OCCLUDER DEVICE (COHEREX MEDICAL INC, SALT LAKE CITY, UT, USA)
Device

The Wavecrest device is the latest development of an LAAC-type device. It is an umbrella-like device made of expanded PTFE[30] with 20 anchoring points (**Fig. 13**). The device is designed to simplify implant procedure and to reduce complications associated with other LAAC devices.[55] The material facing the LA has a unique ability to minimize thrombus formation and allow rapid endothelialization.[35] It also has a unique distal injection port to assess device stability during implant. This device can be a good alternative for patients with a very short appendage not suitable for WATCHMAN or ACP.[50] The device was approved in Europe in 2013. Plans are underway to conduct clinical trials leading to regulatory approval in the United States and Japan.

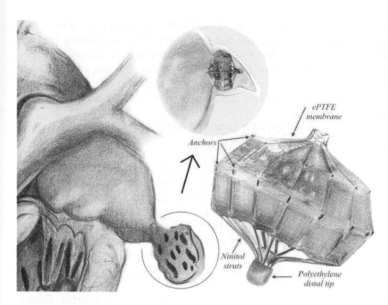

Fig. 12. PLAATO system. The device is constructed of a nitinol frame and an implant occlusion membrane consisting of a laminated expanded PTFE. Note the small anchors along the frame passing through the occlusive membrane, which assist with device anchoring and stability. (*From* Romero J, Natale A, Engstrom K, et al. Left atrial appendage isolation using percutaneous (endocardial/epicardial) devices: pre-clinical and clinical experience. Trends Cardiovasc Med 2015;26 [pii:S1050-1738(15)00154-1]; with permission.)

Technique

This device is deployed similarly to other endovascular devices. However, the delivery sheath is not intended for deep access and manipulation inside the appendage, because the device is designed for proximal placement.[56] The projected landing zone on TEE includes the distance from the left circumflex coronary artery to 10 mm distal to the apex of the lateral ridge. Its position proximal to all lobes guarantees the best occlusion and reduces the risk of pericardial effusion.[56]

Data

The Wavecrest I trial of 73 patients showed a 93% acute procedural success. Complete LAAC was achieved at 45 days in 92% of patients. There were 2 pericardial effusions, but no procedural stroke, device embolization, or device-associated thrombus reported[34] (https://clinicaltrials.gov/ct2/show/NCT02239887).

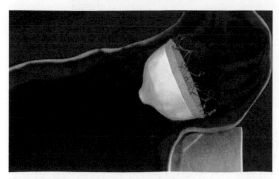

Fig. 13. Wavecrest closure device. (*From* Lin AC, Knight BP. Left atrial appendage closure. Prog Cardiovasc Dis 2015;58(2):195–201; with permission.)

THE TRANSCATHETER PATCH (CUSTOM MEDICAL DEVICES, ATHENS, GREECE)

The trans-catheter patch is a soft, bioabsorbable, frameless balloon deliverable device used for the occlusion of heart defects (**Fig. 14**). This device can be adjusted for the shape and size of the LAA. The patches are made from polyurethane foam (Foamex, Media, PA, USA), and the balloon is made from latex (NuMED, Hopkinton, NY, USA). It is attached to the LAA with surgical adhesives, thereby reducing the risk of perforation.[2,34]

Technique

The surgical adhesive is made of polyethylene glycol and is applied to the distal half of the device

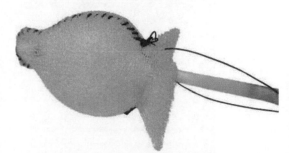

Fig. 14. Transcatheter patch device for occlusion of heart defects is tailored from polyurethane foam. Diluted contrast inflates the supporting balloon to diameters of 15 to 25 mm. A 2-mm nylon loop is sutured at the bottom of the patch, and a double nylon thread is connected for retrieval purposes. (*From* Toumanides S, Sideris EB, Agricola T, et al. Transcatheter patch occlusion of the left atrial appendage using surgical adhesives in high-risk patients with atrial fibrillation. J Am Coll Cardiol 2011;58(21):2236–40; with permission.)

activated by direct alkaline solution injection. Transseptal access is performed using standard technique, and the patch is delivered by balloon. The balloon is inflated to 15- to 25-mm diameter by diluted contrast. A 2-mm nylon loop is then sutured at the bottom of the patch to which the double nylon thread is connected for retrieval purposes. The supportive balloon catheter is removed 45 minutes after surgical adhesive activation. Next, the balloon is deflated and the catheter is retracted. Position and stability of the patch are confirmed by pulling lightly on the retrieval thread under the echocardiogram. After confirming satisfactory positioning, the patch can be released by removing the double nylon thread.[2]

Data

This device was studied in 20 high-risk patients with AF with 17 successful placements. In 3 patients, the patch failed to attach and was retrieved.

In these 3 patients, angiography was used, whereas the rest used TEE, suggesting that the contrast may affect the patch adhesion. There was one intraprocedural complication due to thrombus formation requiring treatment. There was no periprocedural stroke reported.[2]

OTHER DEVICES NOT YET TESTED IN HUMAN

LAmbre (Lifetech Scientific Corp, Shenzhen, China) is another kind of self-expanding nitinol-based device that shows promising results in the canine model. The device is composed of an umbrella and a cover connected by a short central waist (Fig. 15).[44] The main feature of this device is the small delivery system (8–10-French sheath) and the ability for full recapturing and repositioning. Human trials are underway to further evaluate its safety and efficacy.[44]

Cardia Ultrasept LAA Occluder (Cardia, Eagan, MN, USA) consists of a distal cylindrical bulb

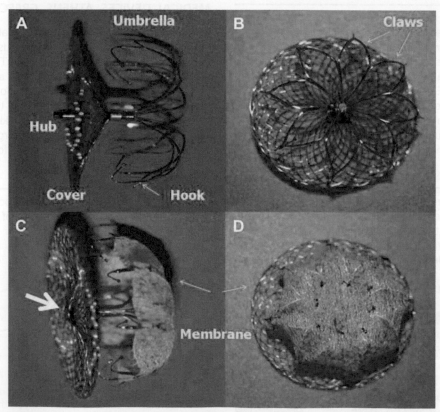

Fig. 15. The LAmbre is a nitinol-based, self-expanding device consisting of a fabric-enriched cover and an umbrella connected with a short central waist, and 1 attachment hub (A). The umbrella comprises 8 claws with individual stabilizing hooks attaching to them (B). The hub is recessed to the surface of the cover (*white arrow*) and an additional membrane was introduced to the umbrella in the newer version of LAmbre (C, D). (*From* Lam YY, Yan BP, Doshi SK, et al. Preclinical evaluation of a new left atrial appendage occluder (Lifetech LAmbre device) in a canine model. Int J Cardiol 2013;168(4):3996–4001; with permission; and *Data from* Patel MR, Mahaffey KW, Garg J, et al. Rivaroxaban versus warfarin in nonvalvular atrial fibrillation. N Engl J Med 2011;365(10):883–91.)

anchoring into the LAA and a separate articulated sail unfolding the ostium.[57]

Occlutech LAA Occluder (Occlutech International, Helsingborg, Sweden) is a conical-shaped device designed to improve expansile force and wire loops at the side to anchor the LAA trabeculae.[58]

HYBRID EPICARDIAL-ENDOCARDIAL APPROACH
LARIAT (SentreHeart, Redwood City, CA, USA)

In the United States, the LARIAT suture delivery system has not been approved for LAAC and stroke prevention in AF. The device was approved by the FDA for soft tissue approximation, although it has been used off-label for LAAC worldwide.[59] It is a hybrid endocardial-epicardial approach to ligate the LAA from the outside of the pericardium, thereby leaving no foreign material inside the endocardium (**Fig. 16**).

Patient selection
Before the procedure, it is important to evaluate the LAA anatomy to exclude LAA characteristics that preclude successful device advancement.[3]

Role of imaging
Computed tomographic scan Preprocedural cardiac CT scan with 3-dimensional (3D) reconstruction is able to evaluate some anatomic variants precluding use of this device. These variants include an LAA diameter greater than 40 mm, superiorly oriented LAA with apex directed behind the pulmonary artery, multilobed LAA with different orientation in different planes exceeding 40 mm, and posteriorly rotated heart.[3]

Transesophageal echocardiogram Preprocedurally, TEE is performed to exclude LAA thrombus and intraprocedurally to verify the anatomic position of

the balloon catheter (EndoCATH, SentreHEART, Redwood City, CA).[31]

Other exclusion criteria
Based on the initial clinical experience by Bartus and colleagues,[59] there were some relative contraindications for the LARIAT procedure. These contraindications include a history of pericarditis, open heart surgery, pectus excavatum, myocardial infarction within 3 months, prior embolic event within the last 30 days, New York Heart Association class IV, ejection fraction less than 30%, and history of thoracic radiation.

LARIAT device
This device has 3 components: a 15-mm compliant occlusion balloon catheter (EndoCATH), 0.025- to 0.035-inch magnet-tipped guidewires (FindrWIRZ), and a 12-French LARIAT suture delivery device (**Fig. 17**).[31,59]

Technique
Pericardial access and transseptal access When performing pericardial access, an anterior approach is used through the subxiphoid process using an 17-gauge epidural needle with fluoroscopic guidance in the anteroposterior and lateral views. Next, a 0.035-inch guidewire is advanced and left in the pericardial space. The transseptal access is then performed as previously described. Subsequently, the EndoCATH along with the 0.025-inch endocardial guidewire are advanced into the LAA apex through the transseptal catheter.[31]

Connection of the epicardial-endocardial magnet-tipped guidewire Before connecting the epicardial-endocardial magnet-tipped guidewire, dilation of epicardial access is performed to insert the 14-French guide cannula (**Fig. 18**). The epicardial 0.035 magnet-tipped guidewire is then placed through the epicardial sheath and directed toward

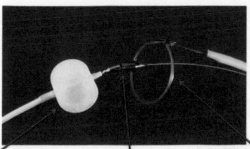

Endovascular balloon catheter   Magnet-tipped guidewires   Epicardial snare mounted with a pretied suture loop

Fig. 16. LARIAT suture delivery system. (*From* Lin AC, Knight BP. Left atrial appendage closure. Prog Cardiovasc Dis 2015;58(2):195–201; with permission; and *Courtesy of* SentreHeart, Redwood City, CA; with permission.)

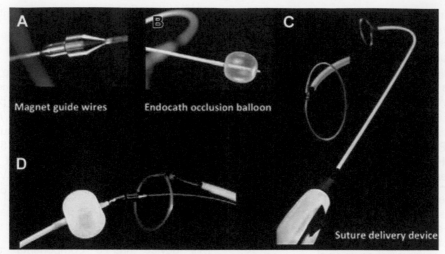

Fig. 17. Components for the percutaneous LAA ligation procedure. The components of the percutaneous LAA ligation procedure include (*A*) a 0.025-inch endocardial magnet-tipped and 0.035-inch epicardial magnet-tipped guidewire, each with a magnet of opposite polarity enabling an end-to-end alignment; (*B*) a 15-mm compliant occlusion balloon catheter to identify the LAA os with TEE; (*C*) the LARIAT suture delivery device. The higher-power inset demonstrates the pretied size 0 Teflon-coated, braided polyester suture (*blue*) mounted within a radiopaque adjustable snare. (*D*) Use of the components as a system to ligate the LAA. (*From* Romero J, Natale A, Engstrom K, et al. Left atrial appendage isolation using percutaneous (endocardial/epicardial) devices: pre-clinical and clinical experience. Trends Cardiovasc Med 2015;26 [pii:S1050-1738(15)00154-1]; with permission; and *Courtesy of* SentreHeart, Redwood City, CA; with permission.)

the LAA to connect with the endocardial magnet.[31]

Snare capture of the left atrial appendage with closure confirmation and release of the pre-tied suture for left atrial appendage ligation After

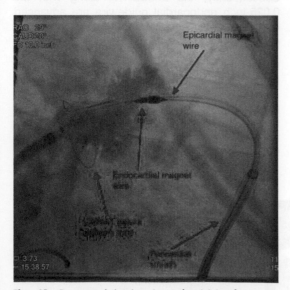

Fig. 18. Contrast injection into the LAA after positioning the LARIAT at the level of the LAA os and before suture delivery. (*From* Lin AC, Knight BP. Left atrial appendage closure. Prog Cardiovasc Dis 2015;58(2):195–201; with permission; and *Courtesy of* SentreHeart, Redwood City, CA; with permission.)

the EndoCATH balloon is inflated at the LAA ostium, the LARIAT suture is guided to the LAA along the epicardial magnet and looped over the LAA to snare it. The snare is closed after confirmation on the LA angiogram and Doppler TEE to ensure complete closure of the LAA (<1 mm flow on cross-section). The suture is finally released and seals off the LAA from the rest of the heart, causing the LAA to shrink over time.[4,60]

Pericardial drain placement After the procedure, the pericardial drain is left in place and removed the following day if output is minimal. Patients can usually be discharged 24 to 48 hours after the procedure.[3]

When to Consider the LARIAT Procedure

- The LARIAT procedure may be considered in AF patients with high risk of stroke and bleeding, or when even a short-term anticoagulation is contraindicated or not tolerated. In this procedure, theoretically, OAC is not required because, unlike other endocardial devices, the LARIAT left no foreign body in the endocardial surface of the LA. Nevertheless, patients need to be educated that they are still at risk for thromboembolism. Patients who can tolerate OAC should continue taking this medication until follow-up imaging to assess leak is performed.[3,59]

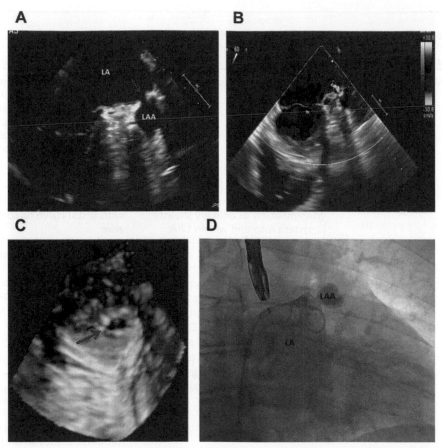

Fig. 19. Residual communication between the LA and LAA by TEE (*A–C*) images of residual communication. (*D*) Angiographic image of residual communication. Red arrows show the site of residual leak. (*From* Soni K, Kesarwani M, Badhwar N, et al. Percutaneous closure of a residual left atrial appendage leak after lariat procedure. JACC Cardiovasc Interv 2015;8(7):998–1000; with permission; and Hansen ML, Sorensen R, Clausen MT, et al. Risk of bleeding with single, dual, or triple therapy with warfarin, aspirin, and clopidogrel in patients with atrial fibrillation. Arch Intern Med 2010;170(16):1433–41.)

- The LARIAT procedure may be considered in patients with nonparoxysmal AF and possible AF triggers in the LAA. The LARIAT procedure can potentially eliminate AF triggers in LAA and increase the success rate of AF ablation. In a study of 69 patients with persistent AF undergoing LARIAT LAA ligation followed by AF catheter ablation at least 30 days after the procedure, there was a substantially higher rate of freedom from AF without antiarrhythmic drug treatment in the LARIAT plus AF ablation group versus the AF ablation only control group (65% vs 39%, *P* = .002).[30,61] The combination of catheter ablation and percutaneous LAAC in a single procedure is technically feasible, although it is associated with significant risk of major complications.[62]

- The LARIAT procedure may be considered when the LAA is too large for either the WATCHMAN or the ACP devices, as long as the maximal ostial diameter is less than 40 mm.[56]

Complications

Thrombus on left atrial appendage orifice

Cumulative published experience[63–68] showed a 2.2% incidence of LAA orifice thrombus during follow-up surveillance. The thrombus formation may result from an inflammatory reaction at the ligation site, epithelial denuding at the LAA orifice during balloon catheter retrieval, and suboptimal suture deployment.[3,59] The knot loosening and tissue necrosis at the suture site are potential mechanisms of thromboembolic complications.[3,59]

Table 2
Major procedural compilations of percutaneous left atrial appendage closure devices

Complication	Cause	Preventative Strategy
Pericardial effusion	Initial transseptal puncture	TEE guidance (eg, X-plane) Avoid severe tenting of the interatrial septum (increases the risk of free-wall puncture): alternative strategies (eg, application of radiofrequency energy) Puncturing at the fossa ovalis
	Guidewire or catheter into LAA after initial transseptal puncture Manipulation of delivery sheath/system into and within LAA	Advance dilator into LAA under fluoroscopy over 0.32-inch wire with distal curve or coronary wire Advance delivery sheath into LAA over pigtail catheter rather than guidewire Posterior-inferior puncture to optimize coaxial approach to LAA; avoid using PFO, which guides entry superiorly and suboptimally to work within LAA
	LARIAT endocardial wire pulls epicardial wire into the LAA Device deployment and retrieval	Recognize tension on LARIAT endocardial wire when connected to epicardial wire including when balloon being placed at ostium Maintain delivery sheath position; minimize retrievals and reimplantations if possible
Procedural stroke	Pre-existing thrombus in LAA Insufficient anticoagulation Air embolus from delivery sheath/system	Careful baseline TEE Monitor anticoagulation, if possible; consider anticoagulation before transseptal puncture Flush sheath only after entering LAA, and after device exchange, if performed
Device embolization	Inappropriate size, inappropriate position	Tug test; confirm device compression (WATCHMAN should be 8%–20% compressed) or appropriate fluoroscopic appearance Confirm device position and seal by TEE and fluoroscopy
Vascular (hematoma, arteriovenous fistula, pseudoaneurysm, bleeding)	Venous access	Careful technique; consider ultrasound guidance as needed
Pericardial pain	Common after LARIAT closure? Pericardial inflammation/LAA necrosis	Anecdotal: prophylactic NSAIDs, oral colchicine course, intrapericardial therapy (eg, local anesthetic flushes)

Adapted from Price MP. Prevention and management of complications of left atrial appendage closure devices. Intervent Cardiol Clin 2014;3:303; with permission.

Leaks

Leaks are frequently seen after LARIAT procedures. If the leak is greater than 5 mm, a repeat LARIAT procedure is not usually performed due to potential adhesions after the initial procedure.[21,69–71] In this case, alternate endocardial devices can be used depending on the size of the leak.[3] The implications of a small leak are unknown. Studies have shown that a small leak less than 5 mm does not increase thromboembolic events[72] (**Fig. 19**).

Pericarditis

Profound inflammatory response contributes to pericarditis and Dressler syndrome. Prophylaxis with colchicine or nonsteroidal anti-inflammatory drugs (NSAIDs) is often used to prevent Dressler syndrome.[64]

Pericardial effusion/Tamponade

Simultaneous epicardial and transseptal access increase the risk of pericardial effusion and bleeding.[4] Late pericardial effusion can be transudative or exudative and may represent volume retention from reduced ANP release after LAA ligation.[73]

Technical approach to avoid complications

The technical approach to prevent complications is summarized in **Tables 2** and **3**. Using a micropuncture needle for pericardial access may decrease the risk of right ventricle (RV) laceration.[3] When adhesions are encountered during the procedure, one needs to consider aborting the procedure, because procedural success is low with high complication rates.[3]

Data

The safety and efficacy of the LARIAT procedure were reported in several observational studies. Single-center studies by Massumi and colleagues[60] and Stone and colleagues,[74] and a multicenter study by Bartus and colleagues,[64] demonstrated greater than 95% procedural success rates with relatively low complications. In contrast, a single-center study by Price and colleagues[68] reported significantly higher complications with low success rates. However, the inclusion and exclusion criteria were not defined; therefore, it is difficult to analyze the safety and efficacy of the LARIAT procedure based on this study.

Table 3
Potential prevention strategies for procedural complications of LARIAT left atrial appendage occlusion devices

Complication	Cause	Preventative Strategy
Pericardial effusion	Initial TSP Guidewire or catheter trauma to LAA after TSP Manipulation of delivery system in pericardium Pericardial access	TEE guidance Avoidance of severe IAS tenting Advancement of transsepta 1 sheath dilator into LAA under fluoroscopy over 0.32-inch wire with distal curve on coronary wire TEE surveillance for RV compression with sheath advancement to avoid RV abrasion Micropuncture access needle Placement of a "bail out" wire in the pericardium for quick pericardial drain placement
LAA laceration or perforation	LARIAT advancement and deployment	Cognizance of endocardial and epicardial wire forces on LAA Minimization of LARIAT delivery system prolapse onto LA Careful suture tightening
Procedural stroke	LAA thrombus Insufficient anticoagulation Air embolus	Careful baseline TEE Close AC monitoring Careful flushing of transseptal sheath
Vascular complications	Hematoma, arteriovenous fistula, pseudoaneurysm, bleeding, hematoma	Careful technique with ultrasound guidance as needed

Abbreviations: IAS, interatrial septum; TSP, transseptal puncture.
From Srivastava MC, See VY, Dawood MY, et al. A review of the LARIAT device: insights from the cumulative clinical experience. Springerplus 2015;4:522; with permission.

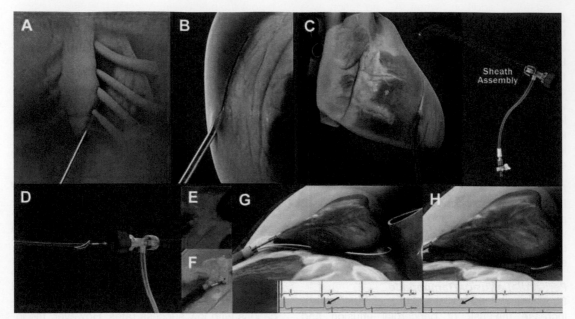

Fig. 20. Epicardial system for percutaneous LAAC. (*A, B*) Percutaneous puncture to gain access to the pericardial space. (*C*) Placement of sheath in pericardial space using Seldinger technique. (*D*) Introduction of multielectrode LAA grabber with a preloaded looped suture into sheath. (*E, F*) Positioning of grabber toward LAA using electrograms from the electrodes embedded in and immediately proximal to the grabber jaws. (*G*) The grabber is used to identify the appendage and record its electrograms, whereas the hollow suture loop delivery tool is used to place the loop around the base of the LAA. (*H*) On tightening of the suture, the LAA ostium is closed. The arrows show the LAA electrogram obtained from electrodes embedded in the grabber jaws. Within seconds of closure, the LAA electrical activity is eliminated (note absence of electrogram at *arrow*) and the surface P wave becomes shorter because the LAA no longer contributes to the P wave (not shown). Simultaneous TEE is used to confirm placement at the LAA ostium and its complete closure. (*Courtesy of* Mayo Clinic Foundation, Rochester, MN; with permission.)

Postprocedure imaging

Surveillance TEE is performed 4 to 6 weeks after implant to assess thrombus and leaks.

EPICARDIAL APPROACH
The Aegis System

The Aegis system is a novel epicardial occlusion device that does not require transseptal access (**Fig. 20**). This epicardial grabber is introduced via percutaneous subxiphoid pericardial access and avoids the need for procedural and short-term postprocedural anticoagulation. The grabber has an electrode that can allow the operator to distinguish between epicardial adipose tissue and the LAA.[19,75]

SUMMARY

LAAC devices are promising tools for stroke prevention in selected patients who are not candidates for oral anticoagulation. It is important to select an appropriate device based on the LAA anatomy and patient characteristics. New devices with improved design are continuously being developed to improve outcomes. More studies

need to be done to compare these devices with the NOACs and between different devices.

REFERENCES

1. Go AS, Hylek EM, Phillips KA, et al. Prevalence of diagnosed atrial fibrillation in adults: national implications for rhythm management and stroke prevention: the AnTicoagulation and Risk Factors in Atrial Fibrillation (ATRIA) Study. JAMA 2001;285(18): 2370–5.
2. Toumanides S, Sideris EB, Agricola T, et al. Transcatheter patch occlusion of the left atrial appendage using surgical adhesives in high-risk patients with atrial fibrillation. J Am Coll Cardiol 2011;58(21): 2236–40.
3. Srivastava MC, See VY, Dawood MY, et al. A review of the LARIAT device: insights from the cumulative clinical experience. Springerplus 2015;4:522.
4. Safavi-Naeini P, Razavi M, Saeed M, et al. A review of the LARIAT suture delivery device for left atrial appendage closure. J Tehran Heart Cent 2015; 10(2):69–73.
5. Wolf PA, Abbott RD, Kannel WB. Atrial fibrillation: a major contributor to stroke in the elderly.

The Framingham Study. Arch Intern Med 1987; 147(9):1561–4.

6. Wolf PA, Abbott RD, Kannel WB. Atrial fibrillation as an independent risk factor for stroke: the Framingham Study. Stroke 1991;22(8):983–8.

7. Fuster V, Ryden LE, Cannom DS, et al. ACC/AHA/ ESC 2006 guidelines for the management of patients with atrial fibrillation-executive summary: a report of the American College of Cardiology/ American Heart Association Task Force on Practice Guidelines and the European Society of Cardiology Committee for Practice Guidelines (Writing Committee to Revise the 2001 Guidelines for the Management of Patients with Atrial Fibrillation). Eur Heart J 2006;27(16):1979–2030.

8. Connolly SJ, Ezekowitz MD, Yusuf S, et al. Dabigatran versus warfarin in patients with atrial fibrillation. N Engl J Med 2009;361(12):1139–51.

9. Granger CB, Alexander JH, McMurray JJ, et al. Apixaban versus warfarin in patients with atrial fibrillation. N Engl J Med 2011;365(11):981–92.

10. Patel MR, Mahaffey KW, Garg J, et al. Rivaroxaban versus warfarin in nonvalvular atrial fibrillation. N Engl J Med 2011;365(10):883–91.

11. Hansen ML, Sorensen R, Clausen MT, et al. Risk of bleeding with single, dual, or triple therapy with warfarin, aspirin, and clopidogrel in patients with atrial fibrillation. Arch Intern Med 2010;170(16): 1433–41.

12. Al-Saady NM, Obel OA, Camm AJ. Left atrial appendage: structure, function, and role in thromboembolism. Heart 1999;82(5):547–54.

13. Blackshear JL, Odell JA. Appendage obliteration to reduce stroke in cardiac surgical patients with atrial fibrillation. Ann Thorac Surg 1996;61(2):755–9.

14. Mansour M, Refaat M, Heist EK, et al. Three-dimensional anatomy of the left atrium by magnetic resonance angiography: implications for catheter ablation for atrial fibrillation. J Cardiovasc Electrophysiol 2006;17(7):719–23.

15. Salzberg SP, Tolboom H. Management of the left atrial appendage. Multimed Man Cardiothorac Surg 2011;2011(1118). mmcts.2010.004432.

16. Heist EK, Refaat M, Danik SB, et al. Analysis of the left atrial appendage by magnetic resonance angiography in patients with atrial fibrillation. Heart Rhythm 2006;3(11):1313–8.

17. Veinot JP, Harrity PJ, Gentile F, et al. Anatomy of the normal left atrial appendage: a quantitative study of age-related changes in 500 autopsy hearts: implications for echocardiographic examination. Circulation 1997;96(9):3112–5.

18. Wang Y, Di Biase L, Horton RP, et al. Left atrial appendage studied by computed tomography to help planning for appendage closure device placement. J Cardiovasc Electrophysiol 2010; 21(9):973–82.

19. Syed FF, DeSimone CV, Friedman PA, et al. Left atrial appendage exclusion for atrial fibrillation. Cardiol Clin 2014;32(4):601–25.

20. Wongcharoen W, Tsao HM, Wu MH, et al. Morphologic characteristics of the left atrial appendage, roof, and septum: implications for the ablation of atrial fibrillation. J Cardiovasc Electrophysiol 2006; 17(9):951–6.

21. Di Biase L, Burkhardt JD, Gibson DN, et al. 2D and 3D TEE evaluation of an early reopening of the LARIAT epicardial left atrial appendage closure device. Heart Rhythm 2014;11(6):1087–8.

22. Yamamoto M, Seo Y, Kawamatsu N, et al. Complex left atrial appendage morphology and left atrial appendage thrombus formation in patients with atrial fibrillation. Circ Cardiovasc Imaging 2014; 7(2):337–43.

23. Lakkireddy D. Left atrial appendage exclusion as adjunct strategy for AF ablation. San Francisco (CA): Heart Rhythm Society Annual Sessions; 2014.

24. January CT, Wann LS, Alpert JS, et al. 2014 AHA/ACC/ HRS guideline for the management of patients with atrial fibrillation: executive summary: a report of the American College of Cardiology/American Heart Association Task Force on practice guidelines and the Heart Rhythm Society. Circulation 2014;130(23): 2071–104.

25. Katz ES, Tsiamtsiouris T, Applebaum RM, et al. Surgical left atrial appendage ligation is frequently incomplete: a transesophageal echocardiographic study. J Am Coll Cardiol 2000;36(2):468–71.

26. Whitlock R, Healey J, Vincent J, et al. Rationale and design of the left atrial appendage occlusion study (LAAOS) III. Ann Cardiothorac Surg 2014; 3(1):45–54.

27. Kanderian AS, Gillinov AM, Pettersson GB, et al. Success of surgical left atrial appendage closure: assessment by transesophageal echocardiography. J Am Coll Cardiol 2008;52(11):924–9.

28. Ailawadi G, Gerdisch MW, Harvey RL, et al. Exclusion of the left atrial appendage with a novel device: early results of a multicenter trial. J Thorac Cardiovasc Surg 2011;142(5):1002–9, 1009.e1.

29. Mobius-Winkler S, Majunke N, Sandri M, et al. Percutaneous left atrial appendage closure: technical aspects and prevention of periprocedural complications with the watchman device. World J Cardiol 2015;7(2):65–75.

30. Lin AC, Knight BP. Left atrial appendage closure. Prog Cardiovasc Dis 2015;58(2):195–201.

31. Saw J. Percutaneous left atrial appendage closure for stroke prevention. Trends Cardiovasc Med 2015;26:200–1.

32. Holmes DR Jr, Kar S, Price MJ, et al. Prospective randomized evaluation of the Watchman Left Atrial Appendage Closure device in patients with atrial

fibrillation versus long-term warfarin therapy: the PREVAIL trial. J Am Coll Cardiol 2014;64(1):1–12.

33. Reddy VY, Mobius-Winkler S, Miller MA, et al. Left atrial appendage closure with the Watchman device in patients with a contraindication for oral anticoagulation: the ASAP study (ASA Plavix Feasibility Study with Watchman Left Atrial Appendage Closure Technology). J Am Coll Cardiol 2013;61(25):2551–6.

34. Romero J, Natale A, Engstrom K, et al. Left atrial appendage isolation using percutaneous (endocardial/epicardial) devices: pre-clinical and clinical experience. Trends Cardiovasc Med 2015;26 [pii:S1050-1738(15)00154-1].

35. Franzen OW, Klemm H, Hamann F, et al. Mechanisms underlying air aspiration in patients undergoing left atrial catheterization. Catheter Cardiovasc Interv 2008;71(4):553–8.

36. Holmes DR, Reddy VY, Turi ZG, et al. Percutaneous closure of the left atrial appendage versus warfarin therapy for prevention of stroke in patients with atrial fibrillation: a randomised non-inferiority trial. Lancet 2009;374(9689):534–42.

37. Viles-Gonzalez JF, Kar S, Douglas P, et al. The clinical impact of incomplete left atrial appendage closure with the Watchman Device in patients with atrial fibrillation: a PROTECT AF (Percutaneous Closure of the Left Atrial Appendage versus Warfarin Therapy for Prevention of Stroke in Patients with Atrial Fibrillation) substudy. J Am Coll Cardiol 2012; 59(10):923–9.

38. Masoudi FA, Calkins H, Kavinsky CJ, et al. 2015 ACC/HRS/SCAI left atrial appendage occlusion device Societal Overview: a professional societal overview from the American College of Cardiology, Heart Rhythm Society, and Society for Cardiovascular Angiography and Interventions. Catheter Cardiovasc Interv 2015;86(5):791–807.

39. Saw J, Lempereur M. Percutaneous left atrial appendage closure: procedural techniques and outcomes. JACC Cardiovasc Interv 2014;7(11): 1205–20.

40. Romero J, Husain SA, Kelesidis I, et al. Detection of left atrial appendage thrombus by cardiac computed tomography in patients with atrial fibrillation: a meta-analysis. Circ Cardiovasc Imaging 2013;6(2):185–94.

41. Vaitkus PT, Wang DD, Guerrero M, et al. Left atrial appendage closure with Amplatzer septal occluder in patients with atrial fibrillation: CT-based morphologic considerations. J Invasive Cardiol 2015;27(5): 258–62.

42. Gafoor S, Heuer L, Schulz P, et al. "A bend in time": shaping the sheath facilitates left atrial appendage closure. Catheter Cardiovasc Interv 2015;86(5): E224–8.

43. Urena M, Rodes-Cabau J, Freixa X, et al. Percutaneous left atrial appendage closure with the AMPLATZER cardiac plug device in patients with nonvalvular atrial fibrillation and contraindications to anticoagulation therapy. J Am Coll Cardiol 2013; 62(2):96–102.

44. Lam YY, Yip GW, Yu CM, et al. Left atrial appendage closure with AMPLATZER cardiac plug for stroke prevention in atrial fibrillation: initial Asia-Pacific experience. Catheter Cardiovasc Interv 2012;79(5): 794–800.

45. Lopez-Minguez JR, Eldoayen-Gragera J, Gonzalez-Fernandez R, et al. Immediate and one-year results in 35 consecutive patients after closure of left atrial appendage with the Amplatzer cardiac plug. Rev Esp Cardiol 2013;66(2):90–7.

46. Park JW, Bethencourt A, Sievert H, et al. Left atrial appendage closure with Amplatzer cardiac plug in atrial fibrillation: initial European experience. Catheter Cardiovasc Interv 2011;77(5):700–6.

47. Tzikas A, Shakir S, Gafoor S, et al. Left atrial appendage occlusion for stroke prevention in atrial fibrillation: multicentre experience with the AMPLATZER Cardiac Plug. EuroIntervention 2015;10(10).

48. Wunderlich NC, Beigel R, Swaans MJ, et al. Percutaneous interventions for left atrial appendage exclusion: options, assessment, and imaging using 2D and 3D echocardiography. JACC Cardiovasc Imaging 2015;8(4):472–88.

49. Aminian A, Chouchane I, Compagnie M, et al. Delayed and fatal embolization of a left atrial appendage closure device. Circ Cardiovasc Interv 2014;7(4):628–30.

50. Hanazawa K, Brunelli M, Saenger J, et al. Close proximity between pulmonary artery and left atrial appendage leading to perforation of the artery, tamponade and death after appendage closure using cardiac plug device. Int J Cardiol 2014; 175(2):e35–6.

51. Sievert H, Lesh MD, Trepels T, et al. Percutaneous left atrial appendage transcatheter occlusion to prevent stroke in high-risk patients with atrial fibrillation: early clinical experience. Circulation 2002;105(16): 1887–9.

52. Block PC, Burstein S, Casale PN, et al. Percutaneous left atrial appendage occlusion for patients in atrial fibrillation suboptimal for warfarin therapy: 5-year results of the PLAATO (Percutaneous Left Atrial Appendage Transcatheter Occlusion) Study. JACC Cardiovasc Interv 2009; 2(7):594–600.

53. Ostermayer SH, Reisman M, Kramer PH, et al. Percutaneous left atrial appendage transcatheter occlusion (PLAATO system) to prevent stroke in high-risk patients with non-rheumatic atrial fibrillation: results from the international multi-center feasibility trials. J Am Coll Cardiol 2005;46(1):9–14.

54. Ussia GP, Mule M, Cammalleri V, et al. Percutaneous closure of left atrial appendage to prevent embolic

events in high-risk patients with chronic atrial fibrillation. Catheter Cardiovasc Interv 2009;74(2):217–22.

55. Coherex WAVECREST I Left Atrial Appendage Occlusion Study. 2015. Available at: https://clinicaltrials.gov/ct2/show/NCT02239887.

56. Meier B, Blaauw Y, Khattab AA, et al. EHRA/EAPCI expert consensus statement on catheter-based left atrial appendage occlusion. Europace 2014; 16(10):1397–416.

57. Cheng Y, Conditt G, Yi G, et al. First in vivo evaluation of a flexible self-apposing left atrial appendage closure device in the canine model. Catheter Cardiovasc Interv 2015;86(1):173–81.

58. Whisenant B, Weiss P. Left atrial appendage closure with transcatheter-delivered devices. Intervent Cardiol Clin 2015;3(2):209–18.

59. Bartus K, Morelli RL, Szczepanski W, et al. Anatomic analysis of the left atrial appendage after closure with the LARIAT device. Circ Arrhythm Electrophysiol 2014;7(4):764–7.

60. Massumi A, Chelu MG, Nazeri A, et al. Initial experience with a novel percutaneous left atrial appendage exclusion device in patients with atrial fibrillation, increased stroke risk, and contraindications to anticoagulation. Am J Cardiol 2013;111(6): 869–73.

61. Lakkireddy D, Kanmanthareddy A, et al. Left atrial appendage ligation and ablation for persistent atrial fibrillation (LAALA-AF registry). JACC Clin Electrophysiol 2015;(1):153–60.

62. Calvo N, Salterain N, Arguedas H, et al. Combined catheter ablation and left atrial appendage closure as a hybrid procedure for the treatment of atrial fibrillation. Europace 2015;17(10):1533–40.

63. Baker MS, Paul Mounsey J, Gehi AK, et al. Left atrial thrombus after appendage ligation with LARIAT. Heart Rhythm 2014;11(8):1489.

64. Bartus K, Han FT, Bednarek J, et al. Percutaneous left atrial appendage suture ligation using the LARIAT device in patients with atrial fibrillation: initial clinical experience. J Am Coll Cardiol 2013;62(2): 108–18.

65. Briceno DF, Fernando RR, Laing ST. Left atrial appendage thrombus post LARIAT closure device. Heart Rhythm 2014;11(9):1600–1.

66. Giedrimas E, Lin AC, Knight BP. Left atrial thrombus after appendage closure using LARIAT. Circ Arrhythm Electrophysiol 2013;6(4):e52–3.

67. Koranne KP, Fernando RR, Laing ST. Left atrial thrombus after complete left atrial appendage exclusion with LARIAT device. Catheter Cardiovasc Interv 2015;85(2):E54–7.

68. Price MJ, Gibson DN, Yakubov SJ, et al. Early safety and efficacy of percutaneous left atrial appendage suture ligation: results from the U.S. transcatheter LAA ligation consortium. J Am Coll Cardiol 2014; 64(6):565–72.

69. Mosley WJ 2nd, Smith MR, Price MJ. Percutaneous management of late leak after lariat transcatheter ligation of the left atrial appendage in patients with atrial fibrillation at high risk for stroke. Catheter Cardiovasc Interv 2014;83(4):664–9.

70. Pillai AM, Kanmanthareddy A, Earnest M, et al. Initial experience with post Lariat left atrial appendage leak closure with Amplatzer septal occluder device and repeat Lariat application. Heart Rhythm 2014; 11(11):1877–83.

71. Yeow WL, Matsumoto T, Kar S. Successful closure of residual leak following LARIAT procedure in a patient with high risk of stroke and hemorrhage. Catheter Cardiovasc Interv 2014;83(4):661–3.

72. Pillarisetti J, Reddy YM, Gunda S, et al. Endocardial (Watchman) vs epicardial (Lariat) left atrial appendage exclusion devices: understanding the differences in the location and type of leaks and their clinical implications. Heart Rhythm 2015;12(7):1501–7.

73. Gunda S, Kanmanthareddy A, Vallakati A, et al. Characterization of pleural effusion after left atrial appendage exclusion using the lariat procedure. J Cardiovasc Electrophysiol 2015;26(5):515–9.

74. Stone D, Byrne T, Pershad A. Early results with the LARIAT device for left atrial appendage exclusion in patients with atrial fibrillation at high risk for stroke and anticoagulation. Catheter Cardiovasc Interv 2015;86(1):121–7.

75. Hu TY, Yogeswaran V, Deshmukh, et al. Device-based approach to prevention of stroke in atrial fibrillation. The Journal of Innovations in Cardiac Rhythm Management, JICRM 2015;6: 2038–50.

Index

Note: Page numbers of article titles are in **boldface** type.

A

Acute ischemic stroke
  subtypes of
    TOAST classification of, 270
Acute myocardial infarction (AMI)
  cardioembolic stroke following, 207–208
  noncardioembolic strokes following, 208
Aegis system
  in stroke prevention, 348
AF. *See* Atrial fibrillation (AF)
Age
  as factor in OAC therapy in AF–related stroke
    prevention, 321
AHREs. *See* Atrial high-rate events (AHREs)
AMI. *See* Acute myocardial infarction (AMI)
Amplatzer cardiac plug
  in stroke prevention, 337–339
Anticoagulation
  AF and stroke related to
    recent observations on, **317–328** (*See also*
      Atrial fibrillation (AF), stroke and; Oral
      anticoagulation (OAC) therapy)
  in patients with heart failure
    AF, 220–221
    guidelines for, 221–222
    novel oral methods, 221
    in sinus rhythm, 218–220
  periprocedural
    AF–related catheter ablation and, 310–311
Arteriovenous malformations (AVMs)
  pulmonary, **241–246** (*See also* Pulmonary
    arteriovenous malformations (PAVMs))
ASDs. *See* Atrial septal defects (ASDs)
Atrial fibrillation (AF)
  ablation for
    stroke risk associated with, **307–316** (*See also*
      Catheter ablation, AF–related)
  AHREs and, 300–302
  anticoagulation in patients with heart failure in,
    220–221
  cognitive decline related to, **279–285**
    described, 279–280
    discussion, 283–284
    introduction, 279
    mechanisms underlying, 280–283
      brain morphometric changes, 283
      changes in brain perfusion, 282–283
      hypercoagulable states and brain infarcts,
        280–281

      proinflammatory state, 282
  in cryptogenic stroke
    cardiac monitoring for, **287–297** (*See also*
      Cryptogenic stroke, AF in, cardiac
      monitoring for)
  described, 255, 299–300
  device-detected, **299–306** (*See also* Atrial
    high-rate events (AHREs))
    introduction, 299–300
  epidemiology of, 256–257
  following MI, 209–211
  introduction, 255–256, 299–300, 317
  prevalence of, 299, 317
  stroke and, 300
    anticoagulation observations related to,
      317–328 (*See also* Oral anticoagulation
      (OAC) therapy)
    current clinical guidelines, 318–319
    from trials to real-world clinical practice,
      323
    epidemiology of, **255–268**
      ischemic stroke subtypes, 257–264
    prevention of
      OAC with VKAs in, 317
  treatment of
    stroke prevention in, 329–330
Atrial high-rate events (AHREs)
  AF and, 300–302
  CIEDs with atrial lead in detection of, **299–306**
    unanswered questions related to, 304
  thromboembolism and, 302–304
Atrial septal defects (ASDs)
  background of, 225–226
  cardioembolic strokes related to, **225–230**
    background of, 225–226
    causes of, 226–227
    epidemiology of, 226
    management of, 227–229
      closure in, 227–229
      medical, 229
    presentation of, 225–226
  described, 225
  incidence of, 225
  presentation of, 225–226

B

Biventricular hearts
  paradoxical emboli related to, 250–252

http://dx.doi.org/10.1016/S0733-8651(16)30010-0
0733-8651/16/$ – see front matter © 2016 Elsevier Inc. All rights reserved.

Brain infarctions
  hypercoagulable states and
    AF and cognitive decline related to, 280–281
Brain morphometric changes
  AF and cognitive decline related to, 283
Brain perfusion changes
  AF and cognitive decline related to, 282–283

C

Cardiac implantable electronic devices (CIEDs)
  with atrial lead
    in AHREs detection (See Atrial fibrillation (AF);
      Atrial high-rate events (AHREs))
Cardiac monitoring
  for AF in cryptogenic stroke, 287–297 (See also
    Cryptogenic stroke, AF in, cardiac monitoring
    for)
Cardioembolic stroke(s)
  abnormalities associated with, 270
  ASDs and, 225–230 (See also Atrial septal defects
    (ASDs))
  following MI, 207–214
    AF, 209–211
    introduction, 207–208
    left ventricular thrombus formation, 208–209
  imaging appearance of, 273–277
Cardiomyopathy(ies)
  embolic stroke in, 215–224 (See also Embolic
    stroke(s), in cardiomyopathy)
Catheter ablation
  AF–related
    cerebrovascular complications of, 308–310
      silent cerebral ischemia, 308–310
      stroke, 308
      TIAs, 308
    introduction, 307–308
    periprocedural anticoagulation in, 310–311
    stroke risk associated with, 307–316
      ablation energy source and, 312
      ablation protocol and periprocedural
        cardioversion and, 312–313
      patient characteristics and, 311–312
      sheaths and catheters and, 312
Cerebral ischemia
  silent
    AF–related ablation and, 308–310
    mechanisms of, 309–310
Chronic kidney disease (CKD)
  as factor in OAC therapy in AF–related stroke
    prevention, 321–322
CIEDs. See Cardiac implantable electronic devices
  (CIEDs)
CKD. See Chronic kidney disease (CKD)
Cognitive decline
  AF and, 279–285 (See also Atrial fibrillation (AF),
    cognitive decline related to)

Congenital malformations
  paradoxical emboli related to, 247–254 (See also
    Paradoxical embolism, congenital
    malformations leading to)
Coronary disease
  as factor in OAC therapy in AF–related stroke
    prevention, 322
Cryptogenic stroke
  AF in
    cardiac monitoring for, 287–297
      cost-effectiveness of, 295
      future implications for, 295
      holter monitoring, 288–289
      inpatient monitoring, 288
      MCOT, 290
      meta-analyses of monitoring techniques,
        293–295
      observational studies of external monitors,
        288–290
      observational studies of insertable cardiac
        monitors, 291–292
      outpatient event monitoring, 289–290
      randomized controlled trials comparing
        external monitoring strategies,
        290–291
      randomized controlled trials of insertable
        cardiac monitors vs. external monitors,
        292–293
    causes of, 287–288
    PFO and, 231–232
      management of, 237–238
CRYSTAL AF, 292–293

D

Ductus venosus
  paradoxical emboli related to, 248–249

E

Embolic stroke(s)
  acute
    imaging modalities in, 273
    management of
      emergency, 270–272
  in cardiomyopathy, 215–224
    anticoagulation in patients with heart failure in
      AF, 220–221
    anticoagulation in patients with heart failure in
      sinus rhythm, 218–220
    epidemiology of, 215–217
    introduction, 215
    novel oral anticoagulation in heart failure, 221
    pathogenesis of, 217–218
  clinical presentation of, 270
  radiological portrait of, 269–278
    introduction, 269–270

Embolism(i)
  paradoxical
    congenital malformations leading to, **247–254**
      (*See also* Paradoxical embolism, congenital
      malformations leading to)
Ethnicity
  as factor in OAC therapy in AF–related stroke
    prevention, 320–321

G

Gender
  as factor in OAC therapy in AF–related stroke
    prevention, 320

H

Heart(s)
  biventricular
    paradoxical emboli related to, 250–252
  univentricular
    paradoxical emboli related to, 249–250
Heart failure
  in AF
    anticoagulation in patients with, 220–221
  anticoagulation in
    guidelines for, 221–222
  in sinus rhythm
    anticoagulation in patients with, 218–220
  stroke in
    epidemiology of, 215–217
    pathogenesis of, 217–218
Holter monitoring
  for AF in cryptogenic stroke, 288–289
Hypercoagulable states
  brain infarcts and
    AF and cognitive decline related to, 280–281

I

Inferior vena cava draining to left atrium
  paradoxical emboli related to, 248
Ischemic stroke(s)
  acute
    subtypes of
      TOAST classification of, 270
  prevalence of, 317
  subtypes of
    epidemiology of
      AF related to, 257–264
Isolated systemic venous abnormalities
  paradoxical emboli related to, 248–249

L

LARIAT procedure
  in stroke prevention, 343–348

Left atrial appendage
  anatomy and physiology of, 330
  function of, 330
Left atrial appendage closure
  in stroke prevention, **329–351**
    introduction, 329–330
    surgical approach to, 330–333
      Aegis system in, 348
      Amplatzer cardiac plug in, 337–339
      devices not yet tested in humans,
        342–343
      endocardial suture closure in, 332
      epicardial clip closure in, 332–333
      hybrid epicardial-endocardial approach,
        343–348
      LARIAT procedure in, 343–348
      percutaneous approach, 333
      PLAATO in, 339
      stapler occlusion in, 332
      trans-catheter patch in, 341–342
      WATCHMAN device implantation in,
        333–337
      Wavecrest occluder device in, 340–341
Left ventricular thrombus formation
  following MI, 208–209

M

MCOT. *See* Mobile cardiac outpatient telemetry
  (MCOT)
Mobile cardiac outpatient telemetry (MCOT)
  for AF in cryptogenic stroke, 290
Myocardial infarction (MI)
  acute
    cardioembolic stroke following, 207–208
    noncardioembolic stroke following, 208
  cardioembolic stroke following, **207–214** (*See also*
    Cardioembolic stroke, following MI)

N

Noncardioembolic strokes
  following AMI, 208

O

OAC therapy. *See* Oral anticoagulation (OAC) therapy
Oral anticoagulation (OAC) therapy
  in AF–related stroke prevention
    recent observations on, 320–323
      age, 321
      CKD, 321–322
      coronary and peripheral vascular disease,
        322
      ethnicity, 320–321
      gender, 320
      perioperative management, 322–323

Oral (*continued*)
  VKAs with
    in AF–related stroke prevention, 317
Outpatient event monitoring
  for AF in cryptogenic stroke, 289–290

P

Paradoxical embolism
  congenital malformations leading to, **247–254**
    biventricular hearts, 250–252
    introduction, 247–248
    isolated systemic venous abnormalities,
      248–249
    univentricular hearts, 249–250
Patent foramen ovale (PFO), **231–240**
  cryptogenic stroke and, 231–232
    management of, 237–238
  introduction, 231
  management of, 233–238
    medical therapy in, 233
    ongoing studies in, 238
    percutaneous therapy in, 234
    randomized trials in
      evidence for, 234–236
      limitations of, 236–237
    surgical therapy in, 233–234
  recurrent stroke and, 232–233
PAVMs. *See* Pulmonary arteriovenous malformations
  (PAVMs)
Percutaneous left atrial appendage transcatheter
  occlusion (PLAATO)
  in stroke prevention, 339
Peripheral vascular disease
  as factor in OAC therapy in AF–related stroke
    prevention, 322
Persistent left superior vena cava
  paradoxical emboli related to, 248
PFO. *See* Patent foramen ovale (PFO)
PLAATO. *See* Percutaneous left atrial appendage
  transcatheter occlusion (PLAATO)
Proinflammatory state
  AF and cognitive decline related to, 282
Pulmonary arteriovenous malformations (PAVMs),
  241–246
  clinical findings, 241–243
  described, 241
  diagnosis of, 243–244
  incidence of, 241
  introduction, 241
  stroke risk related to, **241–246**
  treatment of, 244–245

R

Recurrent stroke
  PFO and, 232–233

Right superior vena cava draining to left atrium
  paradoxical emboli related to, 248

S

Silent cerebral ischemia
  AF–related ablation and, 308–310
  mechanisms of, 309–310
Sinus rhythm
  heart failure in
    anticoagulation in patients with, 218–220
Stroke(s)
  acute
    imaging modalities in, 273
  AF and, 300
    anticoagulation observations related to,
      317–328 (*See also* Atrial fibrillation (AF),
      stroke and; Oral anticoagulation (OAC)
      therapy)
    epidemiology of, **255–268** (*See also* Atrial
      fibrillation (AF), stroke and)
  AF–related ablation and, **307–316** (*See also*
    Catheter ablation, AF–related)
  ASDs and
    causes of, 226–227
    epidemiology of, 226
  cardioembolic (*See* Cardioembolic stroke(s))
  causes of, 287–288
  costs related to, 287
  cryptogenic (*See* Cryptogenic stroke)
  disabilities related to, 287
  embolic (*See* Embolic stroke(s))
  epidemiology of, 257
  in heart failure
    epidemiology of, 215–217
    pathogenesis of, 217–218
  ischemic (*See* Ischemic stroke(s))
  noncardioembolic
    following AMI, 208
  PAVMs and, **241–246** (*See also* Pulmonary
    arteriovenous malformations (PAVMs))
  prevalence of, 269, 287
  prevention of
    left atrial appendage closure in, **329–351** (*See
      also* Left atrial appendage closure, in stroke
      prevention)
  recurrent
    PFO and, 232–233
  TOAST classification for, 270, 287
  types of, 269–270

T

Thromboembolism
  AHREs and, 302–304
TIAs. *See* Transient ischemic attacks (TIAs)
TOAST classification, 287

of acute ischemic stroke subtypes, 270
Trans-catheter patch
    in stroke prevention, 341–342
Transcatheter therapy
    in PAVMs management, 244–245
Transient ischemic attacks (TIAs)
    AF–related ablation and, 308

U

Univentricular hearts
    paradoxical emboli related to, 249–250

V

Vitamin K antagonists (VKAs)
    OAC therapy with
        in AF–related stroke prevention, 317
VKAs. *See* Vitamin K antagonists (VKAs)

W

WATCHMAN device
    in stroke prevention, 333–337
Wavecrest occluder device
    in stroke prevention, 340–341

Moving?

Make sure your subscription moves with you!

To notify us of your new address, find your **Clinics Account Number** (located on your mailing label above your name), and contact customer service at:

Email: journalscustomerservice-usa@elsevier.com

800-654-2452 (subscribers in the U.S. & Canada)
314-447-8871 (subscribers outside of the U.S. & Canada)

Fax number: 314-447-8029

Elsevier Health Sciences Division
Subscription Customer Service
3251 Riverport Lane
Maryland Heights, MO 63043

*To ensure uninterrupted delivery of your subscription, please notify us at least 4 weeks in advance of move.

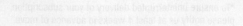

Printed and bound by CPI Group (UK) Ltd, Croydon, CR0 4YY

03/10/2024

01040384-0009